T0202226

# Upper Airway Stimulation Therapy for Obstructive Sleep Apnea

# Upper Airway Stimulation Therapy for Obstructive Sleep Apnea

## *Medical, Surgical and Technical Aspects*

Edited by

## Karl Doghramji, MD
*Professor of Psychiatry, Neurology, and Medicine*
*Medical Director, Jefferson Sleep Disorders Center*
*Program Director, Fellowship in Sleep Medicine*
*Thomas Jefferson University, Philadelphia, PA, USA*

## Maurits S. Boon, MD
*Associate Professor*
*Residency Program Director*
*Co-Director of Jefferson Voice and Swallowing Center*
*Department of Otolaryngology—Head and Neck Surgery*
*Thomas Jefferson University, Philadelphia, PA, USA*

## Colin T. Huntley, MD
*Assistant Professor*
*Associate Residency Program Director*
*Department of Otolaryngology—Head and Neck Surgery*
*Thomas Jefferson University*
*Philadelphia, PA, USA*

## Kingman P. Strohl, MD
*Professor of Medicine and Physiology & Biophysics*
*Case Western Reserve University School of Medicine*
*Center for Sleep Disorders Research*
*Northeast Ohio VA Medical Center, Cleveland, OH, USA*

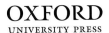

OXFORD
UNIVERSITY PRESS

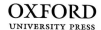

Oxford University Press is a department of the University of Oxford. It furthers the University's objective of excellence in research, scholarship, and education by publishing worldwide. Oxford is a registered trade mark of Oxford University Press in the UK and certain other countries.

Published in the United States of America by Oxford University Press
198 Madison Avenue, New York, NY 10016, United States of America.

© Oxford University Press 2021

All rights reserved. No part of this publication may be reproduced, stored in a retrieval system, or transmitted, in any form or by any means, without the prior permission in writing of Oxford University Press, or as expressly permitted by law, by license, or under terms agreed with the appropriate reproduction rights organization. Inquiries concerning reproduction outside the scope of the above should be sent to the Rights Department, Oxford University Press, at the address above.

You must not circulate this work in any other form
and you must impose this same condition on any acquirer.

Library of Congress Cataloging-in-Publication Data
Names: Doghramji, Karl, editor. | Boon, Maurits S., editor. |
Huntley, Colin T., editor. | Strohl, Kingman P., editor.
Title: Upper airway stimulation therapy for obstructive sleep apnea : medical, surgical and technical aspects /
edited by Karl Doghramji, Maurits S. Boon, Colin T. Huntley, and Kingman P. Strohl.
Description: New York, NY : Oxford University Press, [2021] |
Includes bibliographical references and index.
Identifiers: LCCN 2020031477 (print) | LCCN 2020031478 (ebook) |
ISBN 9780197521625 (paperback) | ISBN 9780197521649 (epub) |
ISBN 9780197521656 (online)
Subjects: MESH: Sleep Apnea, Obstructive—therapy | Electric Stimulation
Therapy—methods | Airway Management—methods
Classification: LCC RC737.5 (print) | LCC RC737.5 (ebook) | NLM WF 143 |
DDC 616.2/09—dc23
LC record available at https://lccn.loc.gov/2020031477
LC ebook record available at https://lccn.loc.gov/2020031478

DOI: 10.1093/med/9780197521625.001.0001

This material is not intended to be, and should not be considered, a substitute for medical or other professional advice. Treatment for the conditions described in this material is highly dependent on the individual circumstances. And, while this material is designed to offer accurate information with respect to the subject matter covered and to be current as of the time it was written, research and knowledge about medical and health issues is constantly evolving and dose schedules for medications are being revised continually, with new side effects recognized and accounted for regularly. Readers must therefore always check the product information and clinical procedures with the most up-to-date published product information and data sheets provided by the manufacturers and the most recent codes of conduct and safety regulation. The publisher and the authors make no representations or warranties to readers, express or implied, as to the accuracy or completeness of this material. Without limiting the foregoing, the publisher and the authors make no representations or warranties as to the accuracy or efficacy of the drug dosages mentioned in the material. The authors and the publisher do not accept, and expressly disclaim, any responsibility for any liability, loss, or risk that may be claimed or incurred as a consequence of the use and/or application of any of the contents of this material.

9 8 7 6 5 4 3 2 1

Printed by Sheridan Books, Inc., United States of America

# Contents

# Contributors

**Safwan Badr, MD**
Professor and Chair
Division of Pulmonary Critical Care and
    Sleep Medicine
Department of Internal Medicine
Wayne State University School of Medicine
Detroit, MI, USA

**Maurits S. Boon, MD**
Associate Professor, Residency Program
    Director
Co-Director of Jefferson Voice and
    Swallowing Center
Department of Otolaryngology—Head and
    Neck Surgery
Thomas Jefferson University
Philadelphia, PA, USA

**Jolie L. Chang, MD**
Associate Professor of Otolaryngology—
    Head and Neck Surgery
Chief of the Division of Sleep Surgery
University of California
San Francisco, CA, USA

**Denise Dewald, MD, MA**
Senior Research Fellow in Sleep Medicine
Case Western Reserve University
Department of Medicine
Division of Pulmonary, Critical Care, and
    Sleep Medicine
University Hospitals Cleveland
    Medical Center
Cleveland, OH, USA

**Karl Doghramji, MD**
Professor of Psychiatry, Neurology, and
    Medicine
Medical Director, Jefferson Sleep
    Disorders Center
Program Director, Fellowship in Sleep
    Medicine
Thomas Jefferson University
Philadelphia, PA, USA

**Katrin Hasselbacher, MD**
ENT Specialist/Head and Neck Surgeon
Department of Otorhinolaryngology
University of Lübeck
Lübeck, Germany

**Clemens Heiser, MD**
Consultant for Otorhinolaryngology, Head
    and Neck Surgeon, Sleep Physician
Department of Otorhinolaryngology, Head
    and Neck Surgery
Technical University of Munich
Munich, Germany

**Winfried Hohenhorst, MD**
Head of Department of Otolaryngology,
    Head and Neck Surgery, and
    Interventional Sleep Medicine
Alfried Krupp Krankenhaus
Essen, Germany

**Colin T. Huntley, MD**
Assistant Professor, Associate Residency
    Program Director
Department of Otolaryngology—Head and
    Neck Surgery
Thomas Jefferson University
Philadelphia, PA, USA

**David T. Kent, MD**
Assistant Professor of Otolaryngology,
    Head and Neck Surgery
Vanderbilt University Medical Center
Nashville, TN, USA

**Eric J. Kezirian, MD, MPH**
Professor and Vice Chair
USC Caruso Department of
    Otolaryngology—Head and Neck
    Surgery
Keck School of Medicine
University of Southern California
Los Angeles, CA, USA

**Alan Kominsky, MD**
Assistant Professor
Head and Neck Institute
Cleveland Clinic
Cleveland, OH, USA

**Ho-sheng Lin, MD**
Professor and Chair
Department of Otolaryngology—Head and
    Neck Surgery
Wayne State University
Detroit, MI, USA

**Sara W. Liu, MD**
Head and Neck Institute
Cleveland Clinic
Cleveland, OH, USA

**Kevin Motz, MD**
Clinical Fellow
Department of Otolaryngology
Johns Hopkins University School of
    Medicine
Baltimore, MD, USA

**Susheel P. Patil, MD, PhD**
Assistant Professor of Medicine
Department of Medicine
Johns Hopkins University School of
    Medicine
Baltimore, MD, USA

**Vaibhav H. Ramprasad, MD**
Resident Physician
Department of Otolaryngology
University of Pittsburgh Medical Center
Pittsburgh, PA, USA

**Madeline J. L. Ravesloot, MD, PhD, MSc**
Department of Otolaryngology—Head and
    Neck Surgery
OLVG
Amsterdam, The Netherlands

**Julianna Rodin, MD**
Resident Physician
Department of Otolaryngology—Head and
    Neck Surgery
Thomas Jefferson University Hospitals
Philadelphia, PA, USA

**Abhay Varun Sharma, MD**
Department of Otolaryngology Head and
    Neck Surgery
University of South Florida Morsani
    College of Medicine
Tampa, FL, USA

**Kerolos Shenouda, MD**
Physician
Department of Otolaryngology—Head and
    Neck Surgery
Wayne State University
Detroit, MI, USA

**J. Ulrich Sommer, MD, PhD**
Physician
ENT
Helios University Hospital Wuppertal
Wuppertal, Germany

**Ryan J. Soose, MD**
Director, Division of Sleep Surgery
Associate Professor, Department of
    Otolaryngology
University of Pittsburgh School of
    Medicine
Pittsburgh, PA, USA

**Armin Steffen, MD**
Head of ENT sleep laboratory
Department for Otorhinolaryngology
University of Lübeck
Ratzeburger, Germany

**Kingman P. Strohl, MD**
Professor of Medicine and Physiology &
    Biophysics
Case Western Reserve University School of
    Medicine
Center for Sleep Disorders Research,
    Northeast Ohio VA Medical System
Case Western Reserve University
Cleveland, OH, USA

**Maria V. Suurna, MD**
Assistant Professor of Otolaryngology—
    Head and Neck Surgery
Director of Sleep Surgery
Weill Cornell Medicine
New York City, NY, USA

**Erica R. Thaler, MD**
Professor of Otorhinolaryngology: Head
    and Neck Surgery
University of Pennsylvania
Philadelphia, PA, USA

**Nico de Vries, MD, PhD**
Professor, ENT, Head and Neck Surgeon
Department of Otorhinolaryngology, Head
    and Neck Surgery
OLVG
Amsterdam, The Netherlands

**Jonathan Waxman, MD, PhD**
Department of Otolaryngology—Head and
    Neck Surgery
Wayne State University
Detroit, MI, USA

**B. Tucker Woodson, MD**
Department of Otolaryngology and
    Human Communication
Medical College of Wisconsin
Milwaukee, WI, USA

# About the Editors

**Karl Doghramji, MD,** is Professor of Psychiatry, Neurology, and Medicine at Thomas Jefferson University. He also serves as Medical Director of the Jefferson Sleep Disorders Center and Program Director of the Fellowship in Sleep Medicine. Dr. Doghramji works as a clinician, researcher, educator, and physician leader, and is actively engaged in interdisciplinary care with academic contributions in the fields of psychiatry, sleep medicine, otolaryngology, neurology, and pulmonary medicine.

**Maurits S. Boon, MD,** is board certified in Otolaryngology—Head and Neck Surgery as well Sleep Medicine. He is the Residency Program Director for the Department of Otolaryngology—Head and Neck Surgery. He has focused his career on both surgical and non-surgical treatments for sleep-disordered breathing. He was one of the first adopters of upper airway stimulation in the United States and has published extensively on the topic.

**Colin T. Huntley, MD,** is board certified in Otolaryngology—Head and Neck Surgery as well Sleep Medicine. He is the Associate Residency Program Director for the Department of Otolaryngology—Head and Neck Surgery. He has focused his clinical and research career on both surgical and non-surgical treatments for sleep disordered breathing. He has published extensively on the management of sleep disordered breathing, including the use of upper airway stimulation.

**Kingman P. Strohl, MD,** is an established clinical investigator in respiratory and sleep medicine, an active clinician, and an author of more than 250 peer-reviewed publications and 150 invited works. His work encompasses the fields of respiratory physiology, consequences of sleep and sleep apnea, genetic architecture of respiratory control, and sleep education at the pre-doctoral and post-doctoral levels.

# Introduction

Karl Doghramji, Maurits S. Boon, Colin T. Huntley, and Kingman P. Strohl

Obstructive sleep apnea (OSA) is a highly prevalent condition that affects 9% to 38% of the general population.[1] Untreated OSA is associated with an increased risk of various other disorders, including myocardial infarction, stroke, renal disease, cardiac arrhythmias, heart failure, and pulmonary/systemic hypertension.[2–4] It also increases the risk of sudden cardiac death,[5] cardiac death during sleeping hours,[6] and death from any cause, independently of other OSA risk factors.[7] The syndrome was first identified as obstructive sleep apnea syndrome in the United States in the late 1970s, and initial therapy was tracheostomy, which was effective in diminishing excessive hypersomnolence and pulmonary hypertension. However, low patient acceptance and challenges in long-term therapy with tracheotomy led to the development of alternative therapies. By the mid-1980s positive pressure therapy and uvulopalatopharyngoplasty (UPPP) were commonly used,[8] and multiple therapies have been introduced since, including various forms of continuous positive airway pressure (CPAP), oral mandibular advancement and nasal expiratory pressure devices, anatomic surgery to the upper airway structures, bariatric surgery, and others.[9]

CPAP is now widely accepted as the first and most effective approach in management. It is the most commonly used treatment modality. It has been shown to improve quality of life; to mitigate disturbed sleep, daytime somnolence, and depressive symptoms; and to lower blood pressure. It may also reduce mortality and the risk of stroke and various cardiovascular disturbances.[10] However, CPAP therapy is complicated by low compliance rates following long-term therapy; 2 years after treatment initiation, up to 60% of patients cannot use or tolerate CPAP.[11] Surgical managements, while effective in some, are not as predictably efficacious or durable.[12] For instance, UPPP reduces a severe apnea–hypopnea index (AHI) by an average of 30% to 50%, but residual AHI remains in the mild to moderate range (<20 per hour) after 2 years.[13]

The Sendai group in Japan began studies in the 1980s into stimulating upper airway muscles to produce functional expansion during sleep as a treatment for OSA. Miki et al.[14] noted that transoral stimulation of the genioglossus muscle in dogs decreased airflow resistance. Their initial report of use in humans was in 1988 involved transcutaneous electrical stimulation of the submental region (genioglossus).[15] Stimulation was shown to reduce apneic episodes using several respiratory metrics. In 1989, the same group reported that transcutaneous electrical stimulation of the submental region (genioglossus muscle) in patients with OSA improved the apnea index and time in deep sleep using a demand-type skin surface stimulator based on tracheal breath sounds.[15] The magnitude of improvement in inspiratory but not expiratory values was shown to depend on the stimulation frequency and voltage.[16] However, negative and inconsistent results led to a diminution of interest in transcutaneous stimulation in favor of direct nerve stimulation.

The main inherent advantages of nerve stimulation over transcutaneous stimulation are that it can be more selective in the muscle groups that are recruited. Since selective stimulation occurs at very low amplitudes below perception, or at least below a certain sensory threshold that might interfere with sleep, fewer adverse effects are likely. Hypoglossal nerve stimulation (HNS) is designed to activate nerve branches innervating the intrinsic and extrinsic muscles of the tongue, positioning the hydrostat in the oral cavity. This treatment addresses the role of inadequate neural activation rather than the anatomy/passive mechanical properties treated by CPAP, site-selected surgery, or oral appliances.[17]

In 1993 studies demonstrated that HNS was capable of keeping the airway open during sleep in OSA patients and permitting sleep.[17] A phase I trial of efficacy was reported in 2001.[18] Over the next 10 to 12 years, HNS was developed commercially as therapy for OSA.[19] Four companies have been involved in the clinical development of upper airway stimulation (Imthera, Inspire, Apnex, and Nyxoah), each with a slightly different approach as to how to trigger stimulation.

Imthera and Inspire technologies have been available in Europe for several years, under postmarketing rules. Inspire therapy completed its pivotal trial in late 2013, met criteria for success, and gained approval from the U.S. Food and Drug Administration in April 2014. Commercial implants began in Europe in 2013 and the United States in 2014. A more detailed review of the history of development of this technology is available in Chapter 14 of this book.

Since its commercial introduction, upper airway stimulation (UAS) therapy has rapidly become a vital component of the multidisciplinary management of OSA. Although the procedure is performed primarily by otolaryngologists, the evaluation and management of the patient also relies on the collaborative work of specialists in sleep medicine, pulmonary medicine, neurology, and psychiatry, among others. Evaluation and implantation programs are now readily available in North America and in Europe. In addition to its obvious clinical benefits, UAS has provided a platform for scientific work and has been the focus of hundreds of publications.

This textbook was written to provide the current state of knowledge regarding UAS for treatment of OSA. It reviews the pathophysiologic basis of OSA and the specific mechanism by which UAS provides airway support in this disorder. Thereafter, it provides more practical insight into this therapy related to patient selection, clinical outcomes, surgical technique, long-term follow-up, adverse events, as well as developing a UAS program. Finally, it provides an overview of unique populations and circumstances that may be encountered, as well as thoughts on the future of this technology.

This textbook is intended for all practitioners who have an interest in or care for sleep disordered breathing, including sleep medicine physicians, pulmonologists, otolaryngologists, primary care practitioners, as well as physician extenders. We hope that you will find it a valuable resource and guide.

# References

1. Kageyama T, Kabuto M, Nitta H, et al. A population study on risk factors for insomnia among adult Japanese women: A possible effect of road traffic volume. *Sleep*. 1997;20(11):963–971.
2. Morgan K, Clarke D. Risk factors for late-life insomnia in a representative general practice sample. *Br J Gen Pract*. 1997;47(416):166–169.
3. Costa e Silva JA, Chase M, Sartorius N, Roth T. Special report from a symposium held by the World Health Organization and the World Federation of Sleep Research Societies: An overview of insomnias and related disorders—recognition, epidemiology, and rational management. *Sleep*. 1996;19(5):412–416.
4. Leger D, Guilleminault C, Bader G, et al. Medical and socio-professional impact of insomnia. *Sleep*. 2002;25(6):625–629.
5. Dodge R, Cline MG, Quan SF. The natural history of insomnia and its relationship to respiratory symptoms. *Arch Intern Med*. 1995;155(16):1797–1800.
6. Katz DA, McHorney CA. Clinical correlates of insomnia in patients with chronic illness. *Arch Intern Med*. 1998;158(10):1099–1107.
7. Pallesen S, Nordhus IH, Nielsen GH, et al. Prevalence of insomnia in the adult Norwegian population. *Sleep*. 2001;24(7):771–779.
8. Strohl KP, Cherniack NS, Gothe B. Physiologic basis of therapy for sleep apnea. *Am Rev Respir Dis*. 1986;134(4):791–802. doi:10.1164/arrd.1986.134.4.791
9. Jordan AS, McSharry DG, Malhotra A. Adult obstructive sleep apnoea. *Lancet*. 2014;383(9918):736–747. doi:10.1016/S0140-6736(13)60734-5
10. Morsy NE, Farrag NS, Zaki NFW, et al. Obstructive sleep apnea: Personal, societal, public health, and legal implications. *Rev Environ Health*. 2019;34(2):153–169. doi:10.1515/reveh-2018-0068
11. Sawyer AM, Gooneratne NS, Marcus CL, et al. A systematic review of CPAP adherence across age groups: Clinical and empiric insights for developing CPAP adherence interventions. *Sleep Med Rev*. 2011;15(6):343–356. doi:10.1016/j.smrv.2011.01.003
12. Sher AE, Schechtman KB, Piccirillo JF. The efficacy of surgical modifications of the upper airway in adults with obstructive sleep apnea syndrome. *Sleep*. 1996;19(2):156–177. doi:10.1093/sleep/19.2.156
13. Sommer UJ, Heiser C, Gahleitner C, et al. Tonsillectomy with uvulopalatopharyngoplasty in obstructive sleep apnea. *Dtsch Arztebl Int*. 2016;113(1–02):1–8. doi:10.3238/arztebl.2016.0001
14. Miki H, Hida W, Inoue H, Takishima T. A new treatment for obstructive sleep apnea syndrome by electrical stimulation of submental region. *Tohoku J Exp Med*. 1988;154(1):91–92. doi:10.1620/tjem.154.91

15. Miki H, Hida W, Chonan T, et al. Effects of submental electrical stimulation during sleep on upper airway patency in patients with obstructive sleep apnea. *Am Rev Respir Dis.* 1989;140(5):1285–1289. doi:10.1164/ajrccm/140.5.1285

16. Hida W, Okabe S, Miki H, et al. Submental stimulation and supraglottic resistance during mouth breathing. *Respir Physiol.* 1995;101(1):79–85. doi:0034568795000112

17. Decker MJ, Haaga J, Arnold JL, et al. Functional electrical stimulation and respiration during sleep. *J Appl Physiol.* 1993;75(3):1053–1061. doi:10.1152/jappl.1993.75.3.1053

18. Schwartz AR, Bennett ML, Smith PL, et al. Therapeutic electrical stimulation of the hypoglossal nerve in obstructive sleep apnea. *Arch Otolaryngol Head Neck Surg.* 2001;127(10):1216–1223. doi:10.1001/archotol.127.10.1216

19. Schwartz AR, Smith PL, Oliven A. Electrical stimulation of the hypoglossal nerve: A potential therapy. *J Appl Physiol.* 2014;116(3):337–344. doi:10.1152/japplphysiol.00423.2013

# The Prevalence and Impact of Obstructive Sleep Apnea and Current Management Landscape

Kevin Motz and Susheel P. Patil

## 2.1. Overview of Obstructive Sleep Apnea

Obstructive sleep apnea (OSA) is a common disorder, affecting roughly 10% of adults.[1] The disorder is characterized by recurrent pharyngeal airway obstruction during sleep leading to complete (apnea) or partial (hypopnea) reduction in airflow despite persistent efforts to breathe. Anatomic, neuroventilatory, and neuromuscular mechanisms contribute to these episodes of pharyngeal obstruction.[2] Apneas and hypopneas are typically associated with increased intrathoracic pressure swings, intermittent hypoxia, and/or brief arousals from sleep. The acute pathophysiologic consequences of these events include hypothalamic-pituitary-adrenal axis activation, oxidative stress, increased sympathetic activity, increased cardiac preload and afterload, and sleep disruption. In the long term, OSA is associated with a range of consequences, including excessive daytime sleepiness, impaired sleep-related quality of life, motor vehicle accidents, neurocognitive dysfunction, cardiovascular disease (e.g., hypertension, myocardial infarction, stroke, and heart failure), and metabolic dysfunction.[3] In this chapter, we review the prevalence, diagnosis, and consequences of OSA as well as currently available treatments.

# 2.2. OSA Prevalence, Presentation, and Diagnosis

## 2.2.1. Prevalence and Factors Associated with OSA

OSA, defined by an apnea–hypopnea index (AHI) of ≥5 events per hour, is highly prevalent, with an estimated worldwide prevalence of 936 million individuals between the ages of 30 and 69 being affected.[4] Expert consensus has defined the severity of OSA as mild (AHI 5 to 15 events per hour), moderate (AHI 15 to 30 events per hour), and severe (AHI ≥30 events per hour).[5] The prevalence of OSA is substantially affected by the different definitions of hypopnea, which include a conservative (associated with a 4% desaturation) and clinical (associated with a 3% desaturation OR arousal) definition.[5] The clinical definition can increase the AHI two- to three-fold depending on OSA severity compared to the conservative definition and can affect prevalence estimates of the distribution of OSA severity.[6,7]

Using polysomnography alone, the Wisconsin Sleep Cohort Study determined the estimated prevalence of OSA in the United States among persons 30 to 70 years of age to be 26%, with 10% having moderate or severe OSA.[1] When OSA is defined by AHI ≥5 events per hour with symptoms of sleepiness, the prevalence of OSA was estimated to be approximately 10%. Depending on the definition of hypopneas used, worldwide studies based on more sensitive measures of breathing (e.g., nasal pressure transducers) suggest that the prevalence of OSA ranges from 27.8% to 71.9%.[8]

Several factors influence the prevalence of OSA; among them, gender, obesity, age, and race appear to be important. U.S. estimates suggest that the prevalence of a polysomnography-based diagnosis of OSA in men is 33.9% compared to 17.4% in women, in a mostly non-Hispanic white population.[1] The stark differences in OSA prevalence between men and women are in part attributed to differences in central adiposity and sex hormone differences, including female menopausal status. For example, when controlling for the waist-to-hip ratio, a measure of central adiposity, a similar prevalence was observed between men and women.[9] Furthermore, postmenopausal women, compared to premenopausal women, have a 2.6 times increased risk of OSA after adjustments for obesity and age, with a prevalence of 29.1% approaching that seen in men.[10]

Increases of age and obesity within gender strata also impact the prevalence of OSA.[1,11,12] For example, in men between the age of 30 and 49 and body mass index (BMI) >40 kg/m$^2$, there is an approximately 11-fold increase in OSA prevalence compared to men with BMI <25 kg/m$^2$ (79.5% vs. 7.0%, respectively). In women between the age of 30 and 49, the OSA prevalence is 1.4% in women with BMI <25 kg/m$^2$ compared to 67.9% in women with BMI ≥40 kg/m$^2$. In men, the OSA prevalence is 26.6% and 43.2% in those 30 to 49 years old and in those 50 to 70 years old, respectively. In women, the OSA prevalence is 8.7% and 27.8% in those 30 to 49 years old and those 50 to 70 years old, respectively.[1] As such, these clinical factors can be used to stratify risk for OSA.

Race may also affect the prevalence of OSA. In the Multi-Ethnic Study of Atherosclerosis (MESA), in participants between 54 and 93 years of age, the prevalence of moderate or severe OSA in participants was 32.4% in African Americans, 38.2% in Hispanics, and 39.4% in those of Chinese descent compared to 30.4% in white participants. After accounting for sex, age, and study site, there was a 1.4, 2.1, and 1.4 increased risk of severe OSA in Chinese, Hispanics, and African Americans, respectively, compared to white participants.[13] Differences in craniofacial features and an increased prevalence of comorbidities associated with OSA (e.g., obesity, hypertension, type 2 diabetes mellitus [T2DM], hyperlipidemia) may account for these differences.[14]

## 2.2.2. OSA Clinical Presentations

People with OSA can experience both daytime and nighttime symptoms (Table 2.1). Common daytime symptoms include excessive daytime sleepiness (EDS), fatigue, and morning headaches. EDS, which affects 15% to 50% of people with OSA in the general population,[1,3,15] refers to the experience of sleepiness during times the patient would expect to be alert. Patients may not always appreciate the extent of their sleepiness, which may require careful assessment by the clinician for more subtle presentations. The most widely used tool to assess EDS is the Epworth Sleepiness Scale score (ESS), in which patients rate the extent of their sleepiness in eight different situations, with a score of >10 defining EDS.[16] The ESS should not be the only method to assess sleepiness, given its limited reliability, with 21% of individuals reported to have an ESS difference of 5 or more on repeat administration.[17] Fatigue, often described as tiredness or a lack of energy, is a separate and distinct symptom from EDS but is more commonly reported in OSA patients than EDS.[2,18] Morning headache is another symptom of OSA. Twelve percent to 18% of patients with OSA report morning headaches compared to 5% to 8% in the general population.[19] However, morning headache does not discriminate well between those who do or do not have OSA.[20]

Nighttime symptoms experienced by people with OSA or more commonly observed by bedpartners include obstructive breathing symptoms characterized by snoring, choking/gasping, and witnessed apneas. Snoring, which affects 50% to 60% of those

**TABLE 2.1 Common Clinical Signs and Symptoms in Adult OSA**

| Signs | Symptoms |
|---|---|
| Loud snoring | Excessive daytime somnolence |
| Gasping during sleep | Morning headache |
| Witnessed apnea | Fatigue |
| Obesity | Poor memory or concentration |
| Increased neck circumference | Mood disturbance or irritability |
| Hypertension | Dry mouth upon awakening |
| Nocturia | Frequent nocturnal awakenings |

with OSA, has a rather limited specificity, at 27% to 46%.[3,20] Nocturnal choking/gasping, however, has been reported to be the most reliable symptom in identifying OSA, with a positive likelihood ratio of 3.3 and a positive predictive value between 17% and 35%.[20] Reported apneas may have more limited utility than initially reported, with a positive likelihood ratio of 1.4 and a positive predictive value between 8% and 19%.[20] Other commonly reported symptoms include nocturnal gastroesophageal reflux disorder, nocturia, unexplained awakenings, and insomnia.[3]

In addition to clinical symptoms, certain signs and physical exam findings are associated with OSA. Obesity, defined by BMI $\geq 30$ kg/m$^2$ (as discussed earlier in the chapter), is a predictor of OSA, though it has a sensitivity of 48.1% and a specificity of 68.6%.[21] Neck circumference, a measure of central adiposity, is also predictive of OSA,[22] with increasing neck circumference independent of BMI being associated with OSA. Neck circumferences >17 inches in men and >16 inches in women are used as clinical cutpoints in determining increased risk for OSA.[23] Certain comorbid conditions have a high prevalence of OSA, including treatment-resistant hypertension (73% to 82%), stroke (71%), atrial fibrillation (76% to 85%), T2DM (65% to 85%), coronary artery disease (38% to 65%), and congestive heart failure (12% to 55%), which can raise the clinician's index of suspicion for OSA.[3,20]

In addition to body habitus, stature, and neck circumference, certain physical exam findings are often found in people with OSA. Lateral narrowing of the pharyngeal walls, enlarged palatine tonsils, enlarged tongue size (macroglossia), and an enlarged or elongated uvula are common features that are predictive of OSA, more so in men than women.[24] For example, narrowing of the lateral pharyngeal walls or a uvula >1.5 cm long or >1 cm wide carried an odds ratio of 2.6 and 1.9, respectively. The modified Mallampati (MM) score and the Friedman tongue position (FTP), which assesses the oropharyngeal airway by examining tongue position and size with regard to visualization of the uvula, are also frequently used tools. The MM assessment is performed with the tongue protruded and graded from I to IV based on ability to visualize the uvula (Figure 2.1). The FTP, another anatomically based assessment tool, is similar to the MM but is performed with the tongue in its natural position in the mouth (Figure 2.2A). Higher MM scores (i.e., scores of III or IV) have been associated with an increased likelihood of moderate to severe OSA but are more predictive in men than women.[25,26] Like the MM, the FTP is also associated with OSA, with higher scores associated with OSA status, independent of age, sex, race, and BMI.[27,28] However, the overall correlation between the MM or FTP and OSA severity is poor to modest. One meta-analysis of eight studies demonstrated a correlation of only 0.18 for the MM and 0.39 for the FTP, suggesting limited reliability as a predictive tool.[27] Furthermore, challenges in reproducibility due to the patient's breathing pattern (nasal vs. oral breathing) and the ability to visualize landmarks have been shown to limit the intrarater and interrater variability of these tools.[29,30] The FTP can also be used in combination with tonsil size (Figure 2.2B) and patient weight to predict an OSA patient's

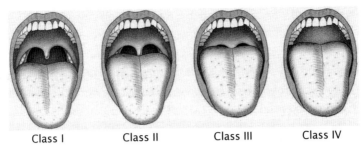

Class I     Class II     Class III     Class IV

**FIGURE 2.1** The Mallampati classification system classifies the oropharyngeal space in regard to visualization of the palate and tonsillar pillars. The original Mallampati is performed with the tongue protruded; modified Mallampati is performed with the tongue in the mouth. Class I: Hard palate, soft palate, uvula, and tonsillar pillars are visualized. Class II: Hard palate, soft palate, and uvula are visualized. Class III: Hard palate and soft palate are visualized. Class IV: Only the hard palate is visualized. Published with permission from Thomas J. Nuckton, MD, MS, David V. Glidden, PhD, Warren S. Browner, MD, MPH, David M. Claman, MD, Physical examination: Mallampati score as an independent predictor of obstructive sleep apnea. *Sleep*, Volume 29, Issue 7, July 2006, Pages 903–908.

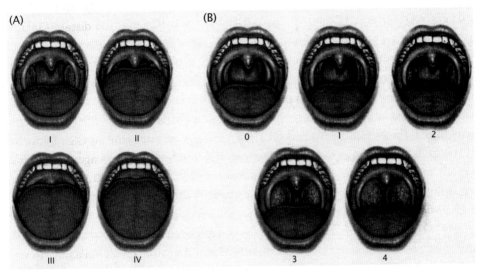

**FIGURE 2.2 (A)** Friedman palate position. This classification is performed with the tongue in its native position inside of the mouth. Grade I: Visualization of the entire uvula and tonsillar pillars. Grade II: Visualization of the uvula but not the tonsils. Grade III: Visualization of the soft palate but not the uvula. Grade IV: Visualization of the hard palate only. **(B)** Friedman tonsil size. Size 1: Tonsils are within the tonsillar pillars. Size 2: Tonsils extend to the pillars. Size 3: Tonsils extend beyond the pillars. Size 4: Tonsils extend to midline. Obtained with permission from Friedman M, Ibrahim H, Bass L. Clinical staging for sleep-disordered breathing. *Otolaryngol Head Neck Surg.* 2002;127:13–21.

response to uvulopalatopharyngoplasty (UPPP); patients who have a low FTP (1,2) and a high tonsil size (3,4) are more favorable candidates.

## 2.2.3. Diagnosis of OSA

The diagnosis of OSA begins with an assessment of common signs and symptoms of OSA. Predictive questionnaires have been developed as a more standardized approach to stratify for the risk of OSA. Questionnaires such as the Berlin and STOP-BANG have been commonly used to identify patients who are at risk for OSA and to guide decision making regarding sleep testing. The STOP-BANG questionnaire, an eight-item validated assessment for OSA originally developed in the presurgery population, assesses signs and symptoms such as snoring, tiredness, observed apneas, hypertension, BMI, age, neck circumference, and gender (Box 2.1a).[31] A score of ≥3 on the STOP-BANG is considered "high risk" and has a sensitivity of 93%, specificity of 36%, and accuracy 80% for an AHI ≥5 per hour, assuming a prevalence of 87% in high-risk patients.[32] The Berlin Questionnaire is a 10-item survey that assesses patient risk for OSA. These 10 questions are grouped into three clusters, which assess obstructive breathing symptoms, sleepiness, and the presence of obesity or hypertension (Box 2.1b). A positive score in two of the three clusters results in a classification of "high risk" for OSA.[33] When used as a screening tool, the Berlin Questionnaire has a sensitivity of 76%, specificity of 45%, and accuracy of 70%, assuming a prevalence of 87% with OSA in high-risk patients.[32] Despite this, clinical screening tools appear to have a similar ability to raise the posttest probability of OSA (STOP-BANG: positive likelihood ratio [LR] 1.4 to 1.8; Berlin: positive LR 1.4 to 1.5) as an overall clinical impression (positive LR 1.7).[20] The primary benefit of screening questionnaires relates to their standardization and ability to be deployed as screening tools in a large population or a busy clinical practice.

Sleep testing should be performed when there is clinical suspicion for OSA in the setting of unexplained sleepiness, unrefreshing sleep, or fatigue and other supporting symptoms.[3] The reference standard for sleep testing is an overnight polysomnography (PSG) study supervised by a sleep technologist. PSG testing involves monitoring of sleep via electroencephalogram, electro-oculogram, and electromyogram activity; breathing via airflow and respiratory effort sensors and oximetry; body position and leg movement; and cardiac status via electrocardiogram. Home sleep apnea testing (HSAT) has become widely used as an alternative to PSG due to patient convenience and lower cost. HSATs have a more limited montage, using primarily monitoring airflow, respiratory effort, oximetry, and movement. HSATs have a reasonable sensitivity of 79% and specificity of 79% but can result in false negatives as high as 25% to 50%, even in patients with a high probability of OSA.[3,34,35] In the setting of a negative or equivocal HSAT and a persistent high probability of OSA, testing with PSG is recommended.[32]

## 2.2.4. Consequences Associated with OSA

The repeated intrathoracic pressure swings, intermittent hypoxia, and brief arousals from sleep observed with obstructive respiratory events create a cascade of events that can result in a broad array of health-related consequences in people with OSA. Approximately 80% of individuals living with OSA remain undiagnosed,[36] resulting in estimated costs of $149.6 billion to the U.S. healthcare system in 2015.[37] The adverse health consequences associated with OSA including neurocognitive impairment (EDS; impaired attention, vigilance, and executive function; depression, cognitive impairment, and reduced quality

## BOX 2.1 OSA Screening Questionnaires

(A) STOP-BANG questionnaire is an 8-item survey that stratifies risk of OSA. 0 to 2 "yes" responses: low risk for OSA; 3 or more "yes" responses: high risk for OSA.

**STOP**

**S**noring?

Do you snore loudly at night (louder than talking or loud enough to be heard through a closed door)?

**T**ired?

Do you often feel tired, fatigued, or sleepy during the daytime hours?

**O**bserved?

Has anyone observed you stop breathing during sleep?

**P**ressure?

Do you have or are you being treated for high blood pressure?

**BANG**

**B**ody mass index >35 kg/m$^2$?

**A**ge older than 50 years?

**N**eck circumference >40 cm?

**G**ender = Male?

(B) Berlin Questionnaire

### Category 1

1. Do you snore?
2. How loud is your snoring?
3. How often do you snore?
4. Does your snoring ever bother other people?
5. Has anyone noticed you quit breathing during your sleep?

### Category 2

1. How often do you feel tired or fatigued after your sleep?
2. During your waking time, do you feel tired, fatigued, or not up to par?
3. Have you ever nodded off or fallen asleep while driving a vehicle?
4. If you do fall asleep or nod off while driving, how often does this occur?

### Category 3

1. Do you have high blood pressure?

Published with permission from Frances Chung, Balaji Yegneswaran, Pu Liao, Sharon A. Chung, Santhira Vairavanathan, Sazzadul Islam, Ali Khajehdehi, Colin M. Shapiro. STOP Questionnaire: A tool to screen patients for obstructive sleep apnea. *Anesthesiology.* 2008;108(5):812–821.

of life), cardiovascular disease (hypertension, coronary artery disease, acute coronary syndromes, transient ischemic attacks or stroke, atrial fibrillation, heart failure), and glucose metabolism (T2DM).

Neurocognitive dysfunction can include a range of consequences. EDS, a result of the repeated fragmentation of sleep from disordered breathing events, is reported in up to 90% of patients with OSA presenting to sleep clinics.[38] EDS has significant consequences, limiting both home and workplace productivity and increasing the risk of motor vehicle accidents, perhaps due to impaired attention and vigilance.[39] Patients with untreated OSA have a 1.2- to 4.9-fold increased risk of motor vehicle accidents.[40] Specific neurocognitive domains such as attention, verbal memory, executive function, and learning have been associated with untreated OSA, though without a clear dose–response relationship.[41] OSA and depression symptoms often overlap, which has raised the possibility of an association. The incidence of depression has been suggested to be increased at 1 year after the diagnosis of OSA at 18.1/1,000 person-years in those with OSA compared to 8.2/1,000 person-years in those without OSA, with women more commonly affected.[42] OSA may also be associated with cognitive impairment.[43] Analyses of brain magnetic resonance imaging scans have suggested that patients with moderate or severe OSA have a twofold increase in cerebral white matter changes and fourfold higher odds of microinfarcts.[44,45] Persons with OSA, in one study, were found to have developed mild cognitive impairment or signs of Alzheimer's disease earlier than those who did not have OSA.[46] Neurocognitive dysfunction can ultimately impair both sleep-related and overall quality of life as shown by lower quality-of-life measures in untreated OSA patients compared to the general population.[47]

OSA also appears to be associated with several cardiovascular-related disorders, likely mediated by intermittent hypoxemia-associated increases in systemic inflammation, oxidative stress, and sympathetic activity. Hypertension is perhaps the most strongly associated. Both the Sleep Heart Health Study and the Wisconsin Cohort Study have demonstrated that OSA is associated with incident hypertension.[48,49] A more recent study from Spain demonstrated that over a 12-year period, the risk of incident hypertension was 1.8- to 2-fold higher in those who declined to use continuous positive airway pressure (CPAP) or were nonadherent to CPAP compared to controls without OSA.[50] Furthermore, the prevalence of OSA may be as high as 83% in patients with treatment-resistant hypertension.[51] Atrial fibrillation has been demonstrated to be more prevalent in those with OSA compared to controls (5% vs. 1%, respectively).[52] In particular, the risk of atrial fibrillation recurrence after ablation is increased by 25% in those with untreated OSA.[53] An association between OSA and incident CAD, as well as OSA and incident heart failure, has been demonstrated in prospective studies, but only in men less than 70 years of age.[54] Subsequently, a longer-term study following controls and participants with OSA demonstrated that those with untreated, severe OSA had 2.9-fold increased odds of a fatal cardiovascular event and 3.20-fold increased odds of a nonfatal cardiac event compared to controls after adjustments for confounders.[55] Subsequent randomized controlled trials of positive airway pressure (PAP) therapy have yet to confirm that treatment of OSA mitigates this increased risk.

OSA also appears to be associated with disorders of glucose metabolism, such as T2DM. An initial epidemiologic study demonstrated that snoring was associated with a twofold higher risk of T2DM after accounting for diabetes risk factors and sleeping-related covariates.[56] Subsequent studies more fully characterizing cohorts using PSG have shown that there is an increased prevalence of T2DM in those with OSA and that sleep disordered breathing is associated with glucose intolerance.[57–59] However, prospective studies have yet to clearly establish that OSA is causal in the development of T2DM.[58,60]

Given the associated comorbidities and economic burden of OSA, the high encumbrance of disease underscores the need for effective therapeutic management of OSA.

# 2.3. Current Treatment Landscape for OSA

Current treatment strategies for OSA focus on preventing the upper airway obstruction that occurs during sleep. OSA management can be divided into nonsurgical and surgical approaches. Among nonsurgical approaches, PAP is the most commonly prescribed treatment for OSA. PAP applied via a mask interface over the nose and/or mouth relieves upper airway obstruction by functioning as a pneumatic splint to maintain airway patency during sleep. Other nonsurgical options for OSA treatment include behavioral treatments (e.g., weight loss, exercise, and positional therapy) and mandibular advancement devices (MADs), also known as oral appliance therapy (OAT).

Surgical management of OSA focuses on relieving upper airway obstruction through ablative, reconstructive, or neurostimulatory approaches. Ablative surgeries such as midline glossectomy, lingual or palatine tonsillectomy, and UPPP aim to reduce pharyngeal collapsibility by increasing pharyngeal volume or stiffness. Reconstructive procedures such as maxillomandibular advancement (MMA), hyoid suspension, and expansion pharyngoplasty aim to reduce obstruction by increasing airway patency through reconstructing, repositioning, or reorienting existing structures. Hypoglossal nerve stimulation seeks to overcome airway obstruction by augmenting pharyngeal neuromuscular tone. Bariatric surgery, when associated with successful weight loss, can also improve OSA severity.[61] Finally, tracheostomy can be performed to bypass the upper airway, though this is usually reserved for refractory patients with significant OSA.

## 2.3.1. Medical Therapies for OSA

### 2.3.1.1. PAP

CPAP, first described in 1981, is the most commonly used treatment modality for patients with OSA.[62] CPAP is postulated to relieve upper airway obstruction by pneumatically splinting the airway open and through increases in lung volumes, which result in tracheal traction and decrease pharyngeal collapsibility.[62,63] CPAP traditionally requires a titration during an overnight sleep study. However, in the last decade the advent of auto-adjustable PAP (APAP), with internal algorithms that can detect respiratory events and automatically adjust pressure settings to prevent subsequent events, has reduced the need for in-laboratory CPAP titrations.

In meta-analyses, PAP, whether CPAP or APAP, reduces the AHI by 86% and effectively reduces the AHI to <5 events per hour.[64] PAP, when consistently used, can improve snoring, EDS, and sleep-related quality of life; reduce motor vehicle crashes; and reduce blood pressure.[64] More controversial is whether CPAP improves cardiovascular outcomes such as myocardial infarction; acute coronary syndrome; hospitalization for heart failure, stroke, or transient ischemic attack; or cardiovascular disease–related death.[64]

Adherence to PAP is important to derive clinical benefits, particularly for noncardiovascular outcomes such as EDS.[65,66] Adherence, as defined by the Center for Medicare and Medicaid Services (CMS), occurs when an individual uses PAP for at least 4 hours per night for at least 5 days a week.[67] Greater use of PAP results in more improvement in symptoms.[65,67] In post-hoc analyses of studies with cardiovascular endpoints, participants using CPAP for more than 4 hours per night may have better outcomes.[68,69] However, these analyses may be confounded by participant adherence to healthier lifestyles and adherence to their medical regimen. CPAP usage is reported to be variable, with adherence rates ranging from 29% to 83%.[70,71] However, a real-world study examining a PAP database of approximately 2.6 million persons demonstrated that 90-day adherence based on the CMS definition was 75%. with an average use of 6.2 hours on days used.[72] Over time, adherence typically declines. with 65% to 80% of patients continuing to use it for more than 4 years.[3,73,74]

Primary reasons for PAP nonadherence are broad and include discomfort, claustrophobia, nasal congestion, skin irritation, and social sigma.[71] Moreover, PAP nonadherence has been associated with younger age, female sex, depression, mild OSA, gastroesophageal reflux disorder, and depression.[75] Multiple innovations in mask comfort, heated humidification, strategies to lower the applied pressure, and behavioral interventions with and without PAP adherence metrics have helped to improve adherence. The availability of multiple mask interfaces with inventive headgear allows patients to sleep more comfortably in their natural position and minimize air leak. In-line heated humidification systems help minimize sinonasal dryness, congestion, and rhinorrhea. Additionally, strategies to lower the delivered pressure and improve tolerance of PAP, using bilevel (BPAP), APAP, and modified pressure profiles, can be used.[64] Due to the frequency of nonadherence to PAP, educational and behavioral interventions for increasing CPAP utilization have been proposed to an attempt to improve compliance. Educational interventions can increase adherence to PAP by 0.6 hours a night.[64] Behavioral interventions, which require more resources and are time intensive, include cognitive-behavioral therapy and motivation enhancement therapy. These can potentially have greater benefit and increase adherence by 1.2 hours a night.[64] Cognitive-behavioral therapy for PAP use focuses on understanding the consequences of untreated OSA, managing expectations from CPAP therapy, and mitigating anxiety around CPAP use.[76] Motivation enhancement therapy helps patients identify and overcome barriers that limit their use of CPAP therapy.[77] Patients who undergo behavioral interventions are 3.1 times more likely to be adherent to PAP than those who do not receive behavioral interventions.[64] Collectively, these patient-centered strategies empower patients to understand and take control of their disease process by building patient-specific strategies that increase individual CPAP use. Nevertheless, since PAP therapy is not optimal for many patients, non-PAP therapy options, whether nonsurgical or surgical, represent important alternatives to mitigate the consequences of OSA.

## 2.3.1.2. Non-PAP Medical Therapies

Non-PAP medical therapies for the treatment of sleep apnea should be used in select patients and trialed in patients who do not tolerate PAP therapy. The most common behavioral therapies include weight loss, exercise, and positional therapy. Weight loss should be the cornerstone of treatment for all obesity-related OSA and should complement ongoing treatment of OSA. Several randomized controlled studies have demonstrated that weight loss can improve OSA severity.[78–80] In aggregate these studies have demonstrated that a 10- to 20-kg weight reduction can result in OSA resolution in 17% to 61% of OSA patients, with the greatest improvements in OSA severity seen in men and those with a higher baseline OSA severity before weight loss.[78,79] However, most individuals experienced weight regain of approximately 30% 1 year after the intervention ceased, though surprisingly changes in OSA severity persisted despite the weight gain.[78,79] In the Sleep AHEAD study, improvements in OSA severity persisted at 4 years despite a 50% weight regain.[78] Exercise, which is often a component of lifestyle regimens that aim for weight loss, have been suggested to improve OSA severity independent of weight loss.[81,82] In a meta-analysis, five randomized controlled trials that examined exercise regimens were included and demonstrated a mean reduction in AHI of 17 events per hour compared to control conditions.[82] The mechanisms by which exercise may improve OSA are unclear; however, reduction in visceral adiposity, increased pharyngeal muscle tone, reduced rostral movement of leg fluid when supine, and improved sleep quality have been postulated.

For patients who have the majority of their obstructive events in the supine position, positional therapy can be an effective strategy for mitigating OSA. Positional OSA can be defined as supine-predominant (supine AHI >2 times nonsupine AHI) or supine-isolated (additionally requires a nonsupine AHI of <5 events per hour).[83] Positional therapy aims to prevent patients from sleeping in a supine position, where they are most vulnerable to airway collapse and obstruction. Positional therapy devices, such as positional alarms that wake the patient when in the supine position, or mechanical devices such as pillows or vests that physically prevent the patient from sleeping in a supine position, have demonstrated moderate short-term efficacy in managing mild to moderate OSA.[84] Unfortunately, long-term compliance with this type of therapy has been shown to be poor.[85] More recently, novel devices worn around the neck or waist have been developed that deliver a vibration when sleeping supine to remind the patient to shift to a nonsupine position.[86,87] For the appropriate and motivated patient, positional therapy can be an effective approach for managing positional OSA.[88]

MADs are the most common form of OAT and are intended to expand the pharyngeal airway by holding the mandible in a protruded position. These devices can be self-molded as a boil-and-bite device or can be custom-made by a dentist or oral surgeon to fit a patient's dental occlusion. Custom-fitted devices appear to be more durable and more effective in treating OSA.[89] MADs are most effective in treating mild to moderate OSA.[90,91] Although OAT may not be as effective as PAP in reducing the AHI, as reviewed in a 2015 clinical practice guideline, improvements in patient-oriented outcomes are reported to be similar, demonstrating improvements in EDS, sleep-related quality of life, and blood pressure.[92] Just like PAP devices, MADs must be worn on a consistent basis throughout the sleeping period to obtain benefits. Compared to PAP, patients prescribed MADs use these devices roughly 0.7 hours more.[92] Although effective, MADs can be difficult for some to tolerate due to patient discomfort, with adherence rates as low as 32%.[93] The most common side effects observed with MADs include temporomandibular joint pain, oral discomfort, drooling, and changes in dental occlusion.[93] For patients who use a MAD, on-treatment sleep testing is recommended to confirm appropriate treatment of OSA and to allow for OAT calibration. Additionally, patients using MADs should have routine dental follow-up to evaluate and track potential changes in dental occlusion related to use.

## 2.3.2. Surgical Therapies for OSA

While PAP and other nonsurgical therapies are usually first implemented in treating OSA, many patients remain intolerant or nonadherent, reinforcing the need for alternative approaches for the management of OSA. PAP-intolerant patients may benefit from single or multiple surgical interventions aimed at either improving PAP adherence or primarily treating their OSA. Nasal obstruction secondary to septal deviation or turbinate hypertrophy is a common reason for PAP intolerance. Surgical interventions (septoplasty and inferior turbinate reduction) that address nasal obstruction can improve PAP adherence and are cost-effective.[94] Surgery for curative management of OSA, using ablative or reconstructive surgery, is generally targeted at identified sites of airway obstruction during different physiologic maneuvers or drug-induced sleep. Successful surgeries for OSA are commonly multilevel and address obstruction at the level of the nasal cavity, nasopharynx, retropalatal, retroglossal, and/or hypopharyngeal airway. Postoperative outcomes for OSA surgery should be assessed objectively 3 to 4 months after surgery by sleep testing, and then again 1 year later. Surgical success is traditionally accepted if a 50% reduction in AHI and an AHI reduction to <20 events per hour is achieved. A surgical cure is defined when AHI <5 events per hour is achieved.

## 2.3.2.1. Drug-Induced Sleep Endoscopy

Drug-induced sleep endoscopy (DISE) uses flexible nasopharyngoscopy to visualize upper airway collapse in sedated patients. The goal of DISE is to identify the specific anatomic areas of collapse in patients with OSA so that surgical therapies can be tailored to the site of obstruction. Commonly identified areas of airway collapse identified on DISE are the soft palate, oropharynx, tongue base, and epiglottis and are the basis for the VOTE classification system (Table 2.2).[95] The specific pattern of collapse (anteroposterior, lateral, or concentric) is also identified; this has implications in guiding surgical therapy.[96] Furthermore, the presence of single or multilevel collapse can be identified to further tailor the surgical approach. However, the DISE findings can be subjective and the interrater reliability is modest, with greater disagreement for the degree of airway obstruction than the presence of obstruction.[97] Whether sedation administered during DISE accurately reflects the obstruction that occurs during natural sleep remains controversial. When DISE is performed, intravenous propofol is traditionally used given its quick onset, short half-life, and induction of upper airway obstruction. The use of alternative pharmacologic agents, such as dexmedetomidine, has been explored in DISE because it demonstrates fewer cardiopulmonary side effects than propofol.[98] Further studies are needed to demonstrate how DISE-related patterns of upper airway obstruction and specific patterns of airway collapse can predict surgical success to improve OSA surgery outcomes.

## 2.3.2.2. Nasal Surgery in OSA

For patients with OSA, nasal surgery can be a useful tool for correcting underlying nasal obstruction and enhancing PAP adherence postoperatively. Approaches for correcting nasal obstruction focus on increasing patency of the internal nasal valve, which comprises the septum (medial), the floor of the nose (inferiorly), the inferior turbinate (laterally), and the upper lateral cartilage (superiorly). Surgical interventions to correct a deviated nasal septum (septoplasty), reduce and lateralize the inferior turbinate (inferior turbinate reduction), and increase the nasal valve angle (nasal valve repair/functional

**TABLE 2.2 VOTE Classification for Staging Findings During DISE**

| Structure | Configuration | | |
| --- | --- | --- | --- |
| | Anterior-Posterior | Lateral | Concentric |
| **V**elum | | | |
| **O**ropharynx and lateral walls | | | |
| **T**ongue base | | | |
| **E**piglottis | | | |

The evaluation of upper airway collapse during DISE can be divided into four anatomic regions for which specific patterns of airway collapse (anterior-posterior, lateral, and concentric) can be determined.
With permission from Kezirian E, Hohenhorst W, de Vries N. Drug-induced sleep endoscopy: The VOTE classification. *Eur Arch Otorhinolaryngol.* 2011;268:1233–1236.

rhinoplasty) can improve nasal obstruction. In patients with OSA, nasal surgery can help to improve symptoms by reducing daytime sleepiness. Nasal surgery also improves PAP tolerance and increases use in noncompliant patients. Moreover, a reduction in the PAP pressure setting to adequately treat OSA has been noted after nasal surgery.[99] Despite improvements in daytime somnolence symptoms, there is no clear evidence to suggest that nasal surgery improves the AHI in OSA patients.[100] Therefore, nasal surgery should not be regarded as corrective surgery for OSA, and patients should be counseled that the goal of nasal surgery is to improve PAP adherence.

### 2.3.2.3. Palatal Surgery for OSA

Surgery of the palate is a common strategy to improve OSA. Velopharyngeal and oropharyngeal obstruction is the most common site of collapse in patients with OSA.[101,102] UPPP, the most commonly performed surgery for OSA, targets oropharyngeal and velopharyngeal obstruction and was introduced in 1981 by Fujita et al.[103] Conventionally, UPPP aims to improve OSA through volumetric tissue reduction secondary to excision of the palatine tonsils and redundant mucosa of the uvula and palate. In addition, the development of postsurgical scar tissue has a stiffening effect that also likely contributes to reduced pharyngeal collapse. Since its development, many different techniques for UPPP have evolved, shifting the strategy from tissue reduction toward reconstructive-type surgery. In an effort to address collapse of the lateral pharyngeal walls, expansion pharyngoplasty was developed. In this procedure the palatopharyngeus muscles is reoriented or pexyed to the hamulus to tighten the lateral pharyngeal walls and prevent them from collapsing. Collectively, the effectiveness of palatal surgery for the treatment of OSA is variable, with the average AHI reduction of approximately 50%; this includes a subset of patients who are not responsive and have persistent disease.[104] Due to this, careful patient selection and counseling are critically important. In general, OSA patients with lower FTP (I and II) and larger tonsils (3 and 4) are better candidates for UPPP, and patients with higher FTP (III and IV), as well as a low hyoid position, are less likely to respond to UPPP.[105]

Another approach to correcting velopharyngeal or palatal obstruction is transpalatal advancement pharyngoplasty. Originally described by Woodson et al.,[106] this approach is reserved for patients with an elongated and vertically oriented soft palate, which characteristically is not well corrected by traditional UPPP. In patients with severe OSA undergoing this procedure alone, a 65% relative reduction in AHI has been reported.[107] Collectively, surgery of the palate should be tailored to a patient's specific pattern of airway collapse, and strategic and thoughtful counseling should be offered to the patient on the expected benefits.

### 2.3.2.4. Oral Tongue and Tongue Base Surgery for OSA

Volumetric reduction of the oral tongue and tongue base is used to reduce obstruction in patients with OSA, targeting hypopharyngeal collapse. Midline glossectomy and lingual tonsillectomy can be performed to reduce the size of the tongue in patients with macroglossia or lingual tonsil hypertrophy, respectively. Midline glossectomy, which openly excises or ablates the tongue in a submucosal, minimally invasive fashion, is an effective method to reduce the AHI in patients with OSA. However, this procedure has been most commonly used and studied as part of multilevel surgery, usually in conjunction with palatal surgery. In patients undergoing multilevel surgery, which included midline glossectomy, surgical success was achieved in 60% of patients.[108] In patients who only had a midline glossectomy as treatment for their OSA, an average AHI reduction of 16.5 events per hour was observed.[108] For patients with OSA, lingual tonsil hypertrophy is commonly missed on routine physical examination and can exacerbate hypopharyngeal obstruction. Therefore, indirect or flexible laryngopharyngoscopy is warranted in patients being considered for surgical therapy for OSA. Lingual tonsillectomy can remove excessive lymphoid tissue at the base of the tongue and has been demonstrated to be effective at reducing the AHI when part of a multilevel surgery.[109] However, this intervention should be reserved for patients with clear evidence of lingual tonsil hypertrophy. Tongue base collapse can also be addressed indirectly through genioglossus advancement. Finally, hyoid suspension procedures can be effective at reducing hypopharyngeal collapse and have been shown to effect modest reductions in AHI.[110]

## 2.3.2.5. Craniofacial Surgery for OSA

Craniofacial surgery for the treatment of OSA focuses on reconstructing the facial skeleton to expand the upper airway. MMA is an effective reconstructive surgery that opens the upper airway and prevents upper airway collapse through advancement of the maxilla and mandible. In patients undergoing MMA for OSA, a surgical success rate of 86% has been reported, with a mean reduction in AHI of approximately 80%. This high rate of success occurs in the setting of many patients having an AHI >60 events per hour and failing previous surgical attempts.[111]

## 2.3.2.6. Tracheostomy for OSA

The use of a tracheostomy to bypass upper airway collapse is the only curative therapy for OSA. Tracheostomy bypasses upper airway collapse and eliminates the potential for airflow limitation secondary to upper airway soft tissue obstruction.[112] Before the advent of PAP therapy it was the only available therapy for OSA. Although tracheostomy can alleviate upper airway obstruction and OSA, it is not uncommon for a pattern of periodic breathing to become unmasked after the procedure, which can subside in some patients after several weeks.[113] Furthermore, despite tracheostomy some patients continue to experience oxyhemoglobin desaturation during sleep related to their obesity or obesity hypoventilation syndrome. Due to advancements in PAP and other therapies, tracheostomy is rarely needed today and is reserved for the most severe and refractory cases of OSA.

### 2.3.2.7. Hypoglossal Nerve Stimulation for OSA

Hypoglossal nerve stimulation to improve airway patency and prevent upper airway obstruction during sleep has evolved as a neurostimulatory therapy for OSA. Reduced pharyngeal dilator muscle tone during sleep contributes to the developed upper airway obstruction; therefore, neuromuscular stimulation has been hypothesized as a viable treatment strategy. Preclinical and clinical investigation of hypoglossal nerve stimulation has demonstrated that increasing neuromuscular tone to the protrusor muscles of the tongue can reduce OSA severity.[114,115] There have been four commercially trialed hypoglossal nerve stimulation devices worldwide. The Inspire hypoglossal nerve stimulation system is currently the only commercially available device in the United States and has shown promise in treating OSA in selected patients.[116]

## 2.4. Conclusions

OSA is a common disease with adverse consequences on overall health and well-being. PAP therapy, the most common initial treatment strategy for OSA, can treat the full severity range but can be limited by patient adherence. Alternative nonsurgical and surgical therapies for OSA are available, but their effectiveness must be considered in the context of the pathophysiologic features that contribute to OSA for that specific patient. Tracheostomy is the only definitive surgical treatment for OSA but is associated with significant morbidity. Emerging treatment strategies for OSA, such as hypoglossal nerve stimulation, represent an exciting and innovative approach to the management of OSA.

## References

1. Peppard PE, Young T, Barnet JH, et al. Increased prevalence of sleep-disordered breathing in adults. *Am J Epidemiol*. 2013;177(9):1006–1014. doi:10.1093/aje/kws342
2. Patil SP, Schneider H, Schwartz AR, Smith PL. Adult obstructive sleep apnea: Pathophysiology and diagnosis. *Chest*. 2007;132(1):325–337. doi:10.1378/chest.07-0040
3. Gottlieb DJ, Punjabi NM. Diagnosis and management of obstructive sleep apnea: A review. *JAMA*. 2020;323(14):1389–1400. doi:10.1001/jama.2020.3514
4. Benjafield AV, Ayas NT, Eastwood PR, et al. Estimation of the global prevalence and burden of obstructive sleep apnoea: A literature-based analysis. *Lancet Respir Med*. 2019;7(8):687–698. doi:10.1016/S2213-2600(19)30198-5
5. Berry R, Brooks R, Gamaldo C, Harding S. *The AASM Manual for the Scoring of Sleep and Associated Events*. Published online 2015.
6. Ruehland WR, Rochford PD, O'Donoghue FJ, et al. The new AASM criteria for scoring hypopneas: Impact on the apnea hypopnea index. *Sleep*. 2009;32(2):150–157. doi:10.1093/sleep/32.2.150
7. Ho V, Crainiceanu CM, Punjabi NM, et al. Calibration model for apnea-hypopnea indices: Impact of alternative criteria for hypopneas. *Sleep*. 2015;38(12):1887–1892. doi:10.5665/sleep.5234
8. Senaratna CV, Perret JL, Lodge CJ, et al. Prevalence of obstructive sleep apnea in the general population: A systematic review. *Sleep Med Rev*. 2017;34:70–81. doi:10.1016/j.smrv.2016.07.002
9. Young T. Analytic epidemiology studies of sleep disordered breathing: What explains the gender difference in sleep disordered breathing? *Sleep*. 1993;16(8 Suppl):S1–S2. doi:10.1093/sleep/16.suppl_8.s1

10. Young T, Finn L, Austin D, Peterson A. Menopausal status and sleep-disordered breathing in the Wisconsin Sleep Cohort Study. *Am J Respir Crit Care Med.* 2003;167(9):1181–1185. doi:10.1164/rccm.200209-1055OC

11. Bixler EO, Vgontzas AN, Ten Have T, et al. Effects of age on sleep apnea in men: I. Prevalence and severity. *Am J Respir Crit Care Med.* 1998;157(1):144–148. doi:10.1164/ajrccm.157.1.9706079

12. Ayalon L, Ancoli-Israel S, Drummond SPA. Obstructive sleep apnea and age: A double insult to brain function? *Am J Respir Crit Care Med.* 2010;182(3):413–419. doi:10.1164/rccm.200912-1805OC

13. Lutsey PL, McClelland RL, Duprez D, et al. Objectively measured sleep characteristics and prevalence of coronary artery calcification: The Multi-Ethnic Study of Atherosclerosis Sleep study. *Thorax.* 2015;70(9):880–887. doi:10.1136/thoraxjnl-2015-206871

14. Sutherland K, Lee RWW, Cistulli PA. Obesity and craniofacial structure as risk factors for obstructive sleep apnoea: Impact of ethnicity: OSA anatomic risk factors and ethnicity. *Respirology.* 2012;17(2):213–222. doi:10.1111/j.1440-1843.2011.02082.x

15. Kapur VK, Baldwin CM, Resnick HE, et al. Sleepiness in patients with moderate to severe sleep-disordered breathing. *Sleep.* 2005;28(4):472–478. doi:10.1093/sleep/28.4.472

16. Johns MW. A new method for measuring daytime sleepiness: The Epworth Sleepiness Scale. *Sleep.* 1991;14(6):540–545. doi:10.1093/sleep/14.6.540

17. Campbell AJ, Neill AM, Scott DAR. Clinical reproducibility of the Epworth Sleepiness Scale for patients with suspected sleep apnea. *J Clin Sleep Med.* 2018;14(05):791–795. doi:10.5664/jcsm.7108

18. Chervin RD. Sleepiness, fatigue, tiredness, and lack of energy in obstructive sleep apnea. *Chest.* 2000;118(2):372–379. doi:10.1378/chest.118.2.372

19. Russell MB, Kristiansen HA, Kværner KJ. Headache in sleep apnea syndrome: Epidemiology and pathophysiology. *Cephalalgia.* 2014;34(10):752–755. doi:10.1177/0333102414538551

20. Myers KA, Mrkobrada M, Simel DL. Does this patient have obstructive sleep apnea?: The rational clinical examination systematic review. *JAMA.* 2013;310(7):731. doi:10.1001/jama.2013.276185

21. Romero E, Krakow B, Haynes P, Ulibarri V. Nocturia and snoring: Predictive symptoms for obstructive sleep apnea. *Sleep Breath Schlaf Atm.* 2010;14(4):337–343. doi:10.1007/s11325-009-0310-2

22. Hoffstein V, Mateika S. Differences in abdominal and neck circumferences in patients with and without obstructive sleep apnoea. *Eur Respir J.* 1992;5(4):377–381.

23. Hartenbaum N, Collop N, Rosen IM, et al. Sleep apnea and commercial motor vehicle operators: Statement from the joint Task Force of the American College of Chest Physicians, American College of Occupational and Environmental Medicine, and the National Sleep Foundation. *J Occup Environ Med.* 2006;48(9 Suppl):S4–37. doi:10.1097/01.jom.0000236404.96857.a2

24. Schellenberg JB, Maislin G, Schwab RJ. Physical findings and the risk for obstructive sleep apnea: The importance of oropharyngeal structures. *Am J Respir Crit Care Med.* 2000;162(2 Pt 1):740–748. doi:10.1164/ajrccm.162.2.9908123

25. Nuckton TJ, Glidden DV, Browner WS, Claman DM. Physical examination: Mallampati score as an independent predictor of obstructive sleep apnea. *Sleep.* 2006;29(7):903–908. doi:10.1093/sleep/29.7.903

26. Dahlqvist J, Dahlqvist Å, Dahlqvist J, et al. Physical findings in the upper airways related to obstructive sleep apnea in men and women. *Acta Otolaryngol (Stockh).* 2007;127(6):623–630. doi:10.1080/00016480600987842

27. Friedman M, Hamilton C, Samuelson CG, et al. Diagnostic value of the Friedman tongue position and Mallampati classification for obstructive sleep apnea: a meta-analysis. *Otolaryngol Head Neck Surg.* 2013;148(4):540–547. doi:10.1177/0194599812473413

28. Schwab RJ, Leinwand SE, Bearn CB, et al. Digital morphometrics. *Chest.* 2017;152(2):330–342. doi:10.1016/j.chest.2017.05.005

29. Sundman J, Bring J, Friberg D. Poor interexaminer agreement on Friedman tongue position. *Acta Otolaryngol (Stockh).* 2017;137(5):554–556. doi:10.1080/00016489.2016.1255776

30. Yu JL, Rosen I. Utility of the modified Mallampati grade and Friedman tongue position in the assessment of obstructive sleep apnea. *J Clin Sleep Med.* 2020;16(2):303–308. doi:10.5664/jcsm.8188

31. Chung F, Yegneswaran B, Liao P, et al. STOP questionnaire: A tool to screen patients for obstructive sleep apnea. *Anesthesiology.* 2008;108(5):812–821. doi:10.1097/ALN.0b013e31816d83e4

32. Kapur VK, Auckley DH, Chowdhuri S, et al. Clinical practice guideline for diagnostic testing for adult obstructive sleep apnea: An American Academy of Sleep Medicine clinical practice guideline. *J Clin Sleep Med.* 2017;13(3):479–504. doi:10.5664/jcsm.6506

33. Netzer NC, Stoohs RA, Netzer CM, et al. Using the Berlin Questionnaire to identify patients at risk for the sleep apnea syndrome. *Ann Intern Med.* 1999;131(7):485–491. doi:10.7326/0003-4819-131-7-199910050-00002

34. Pereira EJ, Driver HS, Stewart SC, Fitzpatrick MF. Comparing a combination of validated questionnaires and level III portable monitor with polysomnography to diagnose and exclude sleep apnea. *J Clin Sleep Med.* 2013;09(12):1259–1266. doi:10.5664/jcsm.3264

35. Zeidler MR, Santiago V, Dzierzewski JM, et al. Predictors of obstructive sleep apnea on polysomnography after a technically inadequate or normal home sleep test. *J Clin Sleep Med.* 2015;11(11):1313–1318. doi:10.5664/jcsm.5194

36. Kapur V, Strohl KP, Redline S, et al. Underdiagnosis of sleep apnea syndrome in U.S. communities. *Sleep Breath Schlaf Atm.* 2002;6(2):49–54. doi:10.1007/s11325-002-0049-5

37. Frost & Sullivan. *Hidden Health Crisis Costing America Billions: Underdiagnosing and Undertreating Obstructive Sleep Apnea, Draining Healthcare System.* Commissioned by American Academy of Sleep Medicine; 2016. http://www.aasmnet.org/sleep-apnea-economic-impact.aspx

38. Guilleminault C, Black JE, Palombini L, Ohayon M. A clinical investigation of obstructive sleep apnea syndrome (OSAS) and upper airway resistance syndrome (UARS) patients. *Sleep Med.* 2000;1(1):51–56. doi:10.1016/S1389-9457(99)00011-8

39. Terán-Santos J, Jiménez-Gómez A, Cordero-Guevara J. The association between sleep apnea and the risk of traffic accidents. Cooperative Group Burgos-Santander. *N Engl J Med.* 1999;340(11):847–851. doi:10.1056/NEJM199903183401104

40. Tregear S, Reston J, Schoelles K, Phillips B. Obstructive sleep apnea and risk of motor vehicle crash: Systematic review and meta-analysis. *J Clin Sleep Med.* 2009;5(6):573–581.

41. Davies CR, Harrington JJ. Impact of obstructive sleep apnea on neurocognitive function and impact of continuous positive air pressure. *Sleep Med Clin.* 2016;11(3):287–298. doi:10.1016/j.jsmc.2016.04.006

42. Chen Y-H, Keller JK, Kang J-H, et al. Obstructive sleep apnea and the subsequent risk of depressive disorder: A population-based follow-up study. *J Clin Sleep Med.* 2013;9(5):417–423. doi:10.5664/jcsm.2652

43. Walia HK. Beyond heart health: Consequences of obstructive sleep apnea. *Cleve Clin J Med.* 2019;86(9 Suppl 1):19–25. doi:10.3949/ccjm.86.s1.04

44. Kim H, Yun C-H, Thomas RJ, et al. Obstructive sleep apnea as a risk factor for cerebral white matter change in a middle-aged and older general population. *Sleep.* 2013;36(5):709–715. doi:10.5665/sleep.2632

45. Gelber RP, Redline S, Ross GW, et al. Associations of brain lesions at autopsy with polysomnography features before death. *Neurology.* 2015;84(3):296–303. doi:10.1212/WNL.0000000000001163

46. Osorio RS, Gumb T, Pirraglia E, et al. Sleep-disordered breathing advances cognitive decline in the elderly. *Neurology.* 2015;84(19):1964–1971. doi:10.1212/WNL.0000000000001566

47. Bjornsdottir E, Keenan BT, Eysteinsdottir B, et al. Quality of life among untreated sleep apnea patients compared with the general population and changes after treatment with positive airway pressure. *J Sleep Res.* 2015;24(3):328–338. doi:10.1111/jsr.12262

48. Peppard PE, Young T, Palta M, Skatrud J. Prospective study of the association between sleep-disordered breathing and hypertension. *N Engl J Med.* 2000;342(19):1378–1384.

49. O'Connor GT, Caffo B, Newman AB, et al. Prospective study of sleep-disordered breathing and hypertension: The Sleep Heart Health Study. *Am J Respir Crit Care Med.* 2009;179(12):1159–1164. doi:10.1164/rccm.200712-1809OC

50. Marin JM, Agusti A, Villar I, et al. Association between treated and untreated obstructive sleep apnea and risk of hypertension. *JAMA.* 2012;307(20):2169–2176. doi:10.1001/jama.2012.3418

51. Logan AG, Perlikowski SM, Mente A, et al. High prevalence of unrecognized sleep apnoea in drug-resistant hypertension. *J Hypertens.* 2001;19(12):2271–2277. doi:10.1097/00004872-200112000-00022

52. Mehra R, Benjamin EJ, Shahar E, et al. Association of nocturnal arrhythmias with sleep-disordered breathing: The Sleep Heart Health Study. *Am J Respir Crit Care Med.* 2006;173(8):910–916. doi:10.1164/rccm.200509-1442OC

53. Ng CY, Liu T, Shehata M, et al. Meta-analysis of obstructive sleep apnea as predictor of atrial fibrillation recurrence after catheter ablation. *Am J Cardiol.* 2011;108(1):47–51. doi:10.1016/j.amjcard.2011.02.343

54. Gottlieb DJ, Yenokyan G, Newman AB, et al. Prospective study of obstructive sleep apnea and incident coronary heart disease and heart failure: The Sleep Heart Health Study. *Circulation.* 2010;122(4):352–360. doi:10.1161/CIRCULATIONAHA.109.901801

55. Marin JM, Carrizo SJ, Vicente E, Agusti AGN. Long-term cardiovascular outcomes in men with obstructive sleep apnoea-hypopnoea with or without treatment with continuous positive airway pressure: An observational study. *Lancet.* 2005;365(9464):1046–1053. doi:10.1016/S0140-6736(05)71141-7

56. Al-Delaimy WK, Manson JE, Willett WC, et al. Snoring as a risk factor for type II diabetes mellitus: A prospective study. *Am J Epidemiol.* 2002;155(5):387–393. doi:10.1093/aje/155.5.387

57. Punjabi NM, Shahar E, Redline S, et al. Sleep-disordered breathing, glucose intolerance, and insulin resistance: The Sleep Heart Health Study. *Am J Epidemiol.* 2004;160(6):521–530. doi:10.1093/aje/kwh261

58. Reichmuth KJ, Austin D, Skatrud JB, Young T. Association of sleep apnea and type II diabetes: A population-based study. *Am J Respir Crit Care Med.* 2005;172(12):1590–1595. doi:10.1164/rccm.200504-637OC

59. West SD, Nicoll DJ, Stradling JR. Prevalence of obstructive sleep apnoea in men with type 2 diabetes. *Thorax.* 2006;61(11):945–950. doi:10.1136/thx.2005.057745

60. Marshall NS, Wong KKH, Phillips CL, et al. Is sleep apnea an independent risk factor for prevalent and incident diabetes in the Busselton Health Study? *J Clin Sleep Med.* 2009;5(1):15–20.

61. Peromaa-Haavisto P, Tuomilehto H, Kössi J, et al. Obstructive sleep apnea: The effect of bariatric surgery after 12 months. A prospective multicenter trial. *Sleep Med.* 2017;35:85–90. doi:10.1016/j.sleep.2016.12.017

62. Sullivan CE, Issa FG, Berthon-Jones M, Eves L. Reversal of obstructive sleep apnoea by continuous positive airway pressure applied through the nares. *Lancet.* 1981;1(8225):862–865. doi:10.1016/s0140-6736(81)92140-1

63. Heinzer RC, Stanchina ML, Malhotra A, et al. Lung volume and continuous positive airway pressure requirements in obstructive sleep apnea. *Am J Respir Crit Care Med.* 2005;172(1):114–117. doi:10.1164/rccm.200404-552OC

64. Patil SP, Ayappa IA, Caples SM, et al. Treatment of adult obstructive sleep apnea with positive airway pressure: An American Academy of Sleep Medicine systematic review, meta-analysis, and GRADE assessment. *J Clin Sleep Med.* 2019;15(02):301–334. doi:10.5664/jcsm.7638

65. Antic NA, Catcheside P, Buchan C, et al. The effect of CPAP in normalizing daytime sleepiness, quality of life, and neurocognitive function in patients with moderate to severe OSA. *Sleep.* 2011;34(1):111–119. doi:10.1093/sleep/34.1.111

66. Weaver TE, Mancini C, Maislin G, et al. Continuous positive airway pressure treatment of sleepy patients with milder obstructive sleep apnea: Results of the CPAP Apnea Trial North American Program (CATNAP) randomized clinical trial. *Am J Respir Crit Care Med.* 2012;186(7):677–683. doi:10.1164/rccm.201202-0200OC

67. Weaver TE, Kribbs NB, Pack AI, et al. Night-to-night variability in CPAP use over the first three months of treatment. *Sleep.* 1997;20(4):278–283. doi:10.1093/sleep/20.4.278

68. Barbe F, Duran-Cantolla J, Sanchez-de-la-Torre M, et al. Effect of continuous positive airway pressure on the incidence of hypertension and cardiovascular events in nonsleepy patients with obstructive sleep apnea: A randomized controlled trial. *JAMA.* 2012;307(20):2161–2168.

69. Martínez-García M-A, Capote F, Campos-Rodríguez F, et al. Effect of CPAP on blood pressure in patients with obstructive sleep apnea and resistant hypertension: The HIPARCO randomized clinical trial. *JAMA.* 2013;310(22):2407–2415. doi:10.1001/jama.2013.281250

70. Wolkove N, Baltzan M, Kamel H, et al. Long-term compliance with continuous positive airway pressure in patients with obstructive sleep apnea. *Can Respir J.* 2008;15(7):365–369. doi:10.1155/2008/534372

71. Rotenberg BW, Murariu D, Pang KP. Trends in CPAP adherence over twenty years of data collection: A flattened curve. *J Otolaryngol Head Neck Surg.* 2016;45(1). doi:10.1186/s40463-016-0156-0

72. Cistulli PA, Armitstead J, Pepin J-L, et al. Short-term CPAP adherence in obstructive sleep apnea: A big data analysis using real world data. *Sleep Med.* 2019;59:114–116. doi:10.1016/j.sleep.2019.01.004

73. Kohler M, Smith D, Tippett V, Stradling JR. Predictors of long-term compliance with continuous positive airway pressure. *Thorax.* 2010;65(9):829–832. doi:10.1136/thx.2010.135848

74. Jacobsen AR, Eriksen F, Hansen RW, et al. Determinants for adherence to continuous positive airway pressure therapy in obstructive sleep apnea. *PloS One.* 2017;12(12):e0189614. doi:10.1371/journal.pone.0189614

75. Borel JC, Tamisier R, Dias-Domingos S, et al. Type of mask may impact on continuous positive airway pressure adherence in apneic patients. *PloS One.* 2013;8(5):e64382. doi:10.1371/journal.pone.0064382

76. Richards D, Bartlett DJ, Wong K, et al. Increased adherence to CPAP with a group cognitive behavioral treatment intervention: A randomized trial. *Sleep.* 2007;30(5):635–640. doi:10.1093/sleep/30.5.635

77. Olsen S, Smith SS, Oei TPS, Douglas J. Motivational interviewing (MINT) improves continuous positive airway pressure (CPAP) acceptance and adherence: A randomized controlled trial. *J Consult Clin Psychol.* 2012;80(1):151–163. doi:10.1037/a0026302

78. Foster GD, Borradaile KE, Sanders MH, et al. A randomized study on the effect of weight loss on obstructive sleep apnea among obese patients with type 2 diabetes: The Sleep AHEAD study. *Arch Intern Med.* 2009;169(17):1619–1626. doi:10.1001/archinternmed.2009.266

79. Johansson K, Neovius M, Lagerros YT, et al. Effect of a very low energy diet on moderate and severe obstructive sleep apnoea in obese men: A randomised controlled trial. *BMJ.* 2009;339:b4609. doi:10.1136/bmj.b4609

80. Tuomilehto H, Seppä J, Gylling H, Uusitupa M. Long-term weight loss and maintenance in morbidly obese individuals with obstructive sleep apnea. *Am J Respir Crit Care Med.* 2009;180(2):191. doi:10.1164/ajrccm.180.2.191

81. Kline CE, Crowley EP, Ewing GB, et al. The effect of exercise training on obstructive sleep apnea and sleep quality: A randomized controlled trial. *Sleep.* 2011;34(12):1631–1640. doi:10.5665/sleep.1422

82. Iftikhar IH, Bittencourt L, Youngstedt SD, et al. Comparative efficacy of CPAP, MADs, exercise-training, and dietary weight loss for sleep apnea: A network meta-analysis. *Sleep Med.* 2017;30:7–14. doi:10.1016/j.sleep.2016.06.001

83. Joosten SA, O'Driscoll DM, Berger PJ, Hamilton GS. Supine position related obstructive sleep apnea in adults: Pathogenesis and treatment. *Sleep Med Rev.* 2014;18(1):7–17. doi:10.1016/j.smrv.2013.01.005

84. Benoist L, de Ruiter M, de Lange J, de Vries N. A randomized, controlled trial of positional therapy versus oral appliance therapy for position-dependent sleep apnea. *Sleep Med.* 2017;34:109–117. doi:10.1016/j.sleep.2017.01.024

85. Bignold JJ, Deans-Costi G, Goldsworthy MR, et al. Poor long-term patient compliance with the tennis ball technique for treating positional obstructive sleep apnea. *J Clin Sleep Med.* 2009;5(5):428–430.

86. Levendowski DJ, Seagraves S, Popovic D, Westbrook PR. Assessment of a neck-based treatment and monitoring device for positional obstructive sleep apnea. *J Clin Sleep Med.* 2014;10(8):863–871. doi:10.5664/jcsm.3956

87. van Maanen JP, Meester KAW, Dun LN, et al. The sleep position trainer: A new treatment for positional obstructive sleep apnoea. *Sleep Breath Schlaf Atm.* 2013;17(2):771–779. doi:10.1007/s11325-012-0764-5

88. de Vries GE, Hoekema A, Doff MHJ, et al. Usage of positional therapy in adults with obstructive sleep apnea. *J Clin Sleep Med.* 2015;11(02):131–137. doi:10.5664/jcsm.4458

89. Vanderveken OM, Devolder A, Marklund M, et al. Comparison of a custom-made and a thermoplastic oral appliance for the treatment of mild sleep apnea. *Am J Respir Crit Care Med.* 2008;178(2):197–202. doi:10.1164/rccm.200701-114OC

90. Marklund M, Sahlin C, Stenlund H, et al. Mandibular advancement device in patients with obstructive sleep apnea: Long-term effects on apnea and sleep. *Chest.* 2001;120(1):162–169. doi:10.1378/chest.120.1.162

91. Wiman Eriksson E, Leissner L, et al. A prospective 10-year follow-up polygraphic study of patients treated with a mandibular protruding device. *Sleep Breath Schlaf Atm.* 2015;19(1):393–401. doi:10.1007/s11325-014-1034-5

92. Ramar K, Dort LC, Katz SG, et al. Clinical practice guideline for the treatment of obstructive sleep apnea and snoring with oral appliance therapy: An update for 2015. *J Clin Sleep Med.* 2015;11(7):773–827. doi:10.5664/jcsm.4858

93. Saglam-Aydinatay B, Taner T. Oral appliance therapy in obstructive sleep apnea: Long-term adherence and patients' experiences. *Med Oral Patol Oral Cirugia Bucal.* 2018;23(1):e72–e77. doi:10.4317/medoral.22158

94. Kempfle JS, BuSaba NY, Dobrowski JM, et al. A cost-effectiveness analysis of nasal surgery to increase continuous positive airway pressure adherence in sleep apnea patients with nasal obstruction: Cost-effectiveness of nasal surgery for CPAP. *Laryngoscope.* 2017;127(4):977–983. doi:10.1002/lary.26257

95. Kezirian EJ, Hohenhorst W, de Vries N. Drug-induced sleep endoscopy: The VOTE classification. *Eur Arch Otorhinolaryngol.* 2011;268(8):1233–1236. doi:10.1007/s00405-011-1633-8

96. Van de Heyning PH, Badr MS, Baskin JZ, et al. Implanted upper airway stimulation device for obstructive sleep apnea. *Laryngoscope.* 2012;122(7):1626–1633. doi:10.1002/lary.23301

97. Kezirian EJ, White DP, Malhotra A, et al. Interrater reliability of drug-induced sleep endoscopy. *Arch Otolaryngol Head Neck Surg.* 2010;136(4):393–397. doi:10.1001/archoto.2010.26

98. Chang ET, Certal V, Song SA, et al. Dexmedetomidine versus propofol during drug-induced sleep endoscopy and sedation: A systematic review. *Sleep Breath Schlaf Atm.* 2017;21(3):727–735. doi:10.1007/s11325-017-1465-x

99. Camacho M, Riaz M, Capasso R, et al. The effect of nasal surgery on continuous positive airway pressure device use and therapeutic treatment pressures: A systematic review and meta-analysis. *Sleep.* 2015;38(2):279–286. doi:10.5665/sleep.4414

100. Ishii L, Roxbury C, Godoy A, et al. Does nasal surgery improve OSA in patients with nasal obstruction and OSA? A meta-analysis. *Otolaryngol -Head Neck Surg.* 2015;153(3):326–333. doi:10.1177/0194599815594374

101. Rama AN, Tekwani SH, Kushida CA. Sites of obstruction in obstructive sleep apnea. *Chest.* 2002;122(4):1139–1147. doi:10.1378/chest.122.4.1139

102. Salamanca F, Costantini F, Bianchi A, et al. Identification of obstructive sites and patterns in obstructive sleep apnoea syndrome by sleep endoscopy in 614 patients. *Acta Otorhinolaryngol Ital Organo.* 2013;33(4):261–266.

103. Fujita S, Conway W, Zorick F, Roth T. Surgical correction of anatomic abnormalities in obstructive sleep apnea syndrome: Uvulopalatopharyngoplasty. *Otolaryngol Head Neck Surg.* 1981;89(6):923–934. doi:10.1177/019459988108900609

104. He M, Yin G, Zhan S, et al. Long-term efficacy of uvulopalatopharyngoplasty among adult patients with obstructive sleep apnea: A systematic review and meta-analysis. *Otolaryngol Head Neck Surg.* 2019;161(3):401–411. doi:10.1177/0194599819840356

105. Choi JH, Cho SH, Kim S-N, et al. Predicting outcomes after uvulopalatopharyngoplasty for adult obstructive sleep apnea: A meta-analysis. *Otolaryngol Head Neck Surg.* 2016;155(6):904–913. doi:10.1177/0194599816661481

106. Woodson BT, Toohill RJ. Transpalatal advancement pharyngoplasty for obstructive sleep apnea. *Laryngoscope.* 1993;103(3):269–276. doi:10.1288/00005537-199303000-00006

107. Volner K, Dunn B, Chang ET, et al. Transpalatal advancement pharyngoplasty for obstructive sleep apnea: A systematic review and meta-analysis. *Eur Arch Otorhinolaryngol.* 2017;274(3):1197–1203. doi:10.1007/s00405-016-4121-3

108. Murphey AW, Kandl JA, Nguyen SA, et al. The effect of glossectomy for obstructive sleep apnea: A systematic review and meta-analysis. *Otolaryngol Head Neck Surg.* 2015;153(3):334–342. doi:10.1177/0194599815594347

109. Samutsakorn P, Hirunwiwatkul P, Chaitusaney B, Charakorn N. Lingual tonsillectomy with palatal surgery for the treatment of obstructive sleep apnea in adults: A systematic review and meta-analysis. *Eur Arch Otorhinolaryngol.* 2018;275(4):1005–1013. doi:10.1007/s00405-018-4887-6

110. Song SA, Wei JM, Buttram J, et al. Hyoid surgery alone for obstructive sleep apnea: A systematic review and meta-analysis. *Laryngoscope.* 2016;126(7):1702–1708. doi:10.1002/lary.25847

111. Zaghi S, Holty J-EC, Certal V, et al. Maxillomandibular advancement for treatment of obstructive sleep apnea: A meta-analysis. *JAMA Otolaryngol Head Neck Surg.* 2016;142(1):58–66. doi:10.1001/jamaoto.2015.2678

112. Haapaniemi JJ, Laurikainen EA, Halme P, Antila J. Long-term results of tracheostomy for severe obstructive sleep apnea syndrome. *ORL J Otorhinolaryngol Relat Spec.* 2001;63(3):131–136. doi:10.1159/000055728

113. Camacho M, Certal V, Brietzke SE, et al. Tracheostomy as treatment for adult obstructive sleep apnea: A systematic review and meta-analysis. *Laryngoscope.* 2014;124(3):803–811. doi:10.1002/lary.24433

114. Schwartz AR, Bennett ML, Smith PL, et al. Therapeutic electrical stimulation of the hypoglossal nerve in obstructive sleep apnea. *Arch Otolaryngol Head Neck Surg.* 2001;127(10):1216–1223. doi:10.1001/archotol.127.10.1216

115. Eisele DW, Schwartz AR, Smith PL. Tongue neuromuscular and direct hypoglossal nerve stimulation for obstructive sleep apnea. *Otolaryngol Clin North Am.* 2003;36(3):501–510. doi:10.1016/s0030-6665(02)00178-0

116. Strollo PJ, Soose RJ, Maurer JT, et al. Upper-airway stimulation for obstructive sleep apnea. *N Engl J Med.* 2014;370(2):139–149. doi:10.1056/NEJMoa1308659

# Mechanical Properties, Anatomy, and Control of the Upper Airway

Denise Dewald and Kingman P. Strohl

## 3.1. Introduction

### 3.1.1. Functions of the Pharynx: Airway Patency, Alimentation, and Speech

The human upper airway is a bony, cartilaginous, muscular, and mucosa-lined passageway extending from the nares or lips to the trachea (Figure 3.1). Although our focus in this chapter is its role in the support of respiration, it serves other functions, including warming and humidification of inspired air, olfaction, swallowing, protection from aspiration of food, defense of infection, and, particularly important for humans, speech. Coordination among brainstem neuromuscular control systems also produce coughs, hiccups, aspiration recovery, vomiting, and sneezing.[1]

In human infants and nonhuman mammals of all ages, the epiglottis overlaps the soft palate.[2] In this configuration the larynx abuts the nasopharynx directly, and the oropharynx is limited to the vallecula and is not part of the airway during quiet breathing; air passes directly into the larynx from the nose, and food collection can safely occur in the vallecula without risk of oral or vallecular contents falling into the airway.[3]

The evolution of speech required the soft palate and epiglottis to become uncoupled to allow for easy direction of air through the mouth; this was achieved by hyolaryngeal descent, which occurs during growth and development in humans.[4,5] It is this hyolaryngeal descent that also allows for effortless mouth breathing; in other animals, mouth breathing

**(A) Schematic of the Structures**

**(B) Lateral midsection view**

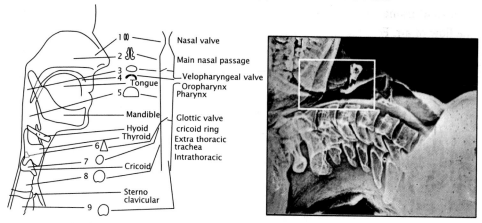

**FIGURE 3.1** This figure serves as an introduction to **(A)** the upper airway structural elements and airway shapes and **(B)** the supine functional region of interest of an airway designed by evolution for behaviors during wakefulness and patency during sleep. The white box shows our region of interest, which includes the major areas of collapse: the soft palate, posterior tongue, muscular pharynx, and distal epiglottis. Figure 3.1A is reproduced with permission of the © ERS 2020.

such as for panting requires that the animal actively pull the larynx down.[3] The descent of the hyolaryngeal complex resulted in the tongue becoming part of the anterior wall of the pharynx in humans, in a constantly shared airway and foodway.[6] The hyolaryngeal apparatus acquired additional degrees of freedom[7] by relinquishing a direct bony connection between the hyoid and skull base; this resulted in a "floating" hyoid bone. Such changes resulted in an increased length and flexibility in a muscular pharynx, making the mature human pharynx profoundly more susceptible to collapse compared to other mammals. Simultaneously, there developed coupling of the central pattern generator for breathing with neuromechanical adjustments to keep the channel open during sleep, as a necessity for sleep health, representing one or more of these mechanisms that fail in obstructive sleep apnea (OSA).

## 3.1.2. Overview of Airway Function

During inspiration, air normally travels through the nose to the nasopharynx, then through the velopharynx (behind the soft palate), the oropharynx (behind the tongue), then behind the epiglottis (in the hypopharynx) and through the larynx before entering the trachea. The narrow regions include the nostrils, the lips, the soft palate, and the larynx, which can act like valves to direct flow.[1]

The depth, width, and complex shape of the airway are determined by many structures. Craniofacial form is a relatively static feature, and the size of the cranial base and the length of the mandible will affect the size of the airway. Noncollapsible structures of the airway include the nose, larynx, and trachea, which are surrounded by a rigid framework of cartilage. However, even these areas can dynamically alter the flow of air. For instance, resistance at the nasal valve influences the downstream pressures on the airway during inspiratory and upstream pressure on expiration; nasal flaring reduces this resistance.[8] The walls of the upper airway are covered with mucosa, and upper airway patency may be influenced by the surface tension of its secretions.[9,10] In the nose, the submucosal vascular network has characteristics of erectile tissue and is capable of influencing airway caliber.[11] Lymphoid tissue in the pharyngeal, palatine, and lingual tonsils may also impinge on the airway. However, the main problem in OSA is a highly deformable pharyngeal wall and lumen. The tube that we call the airway hangs only from the cranial base and mandible; how the muscles of the airway react to the task of supporting the airway will determine the airway lumen shape and size (Figure 3.2). There is a failure of this part of the airway in patients with obstructive sleep apnea syndrome, and the muscles making up the pharynx will be discussed in more detail later in this chapter.

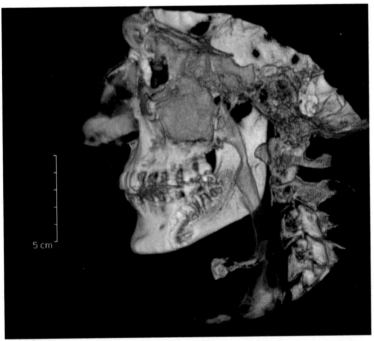

**FIGURE 3.2** This is a representation based on a cone beam computed tomography upright scan in which the air and the skeleton are represented by different colors. Air is depicted in blue and is present in the nose and the sinuses, the nasopharynx, oropharynx, and larynx to the trachea. Note the bony structures of the skull, maxilla, spine, and hyoid. What are the structures around this column of air, and how do they function?

### 3.1.3. Sleep Disordered Obstructed Breathing as a Disease

Sleep is a time of particular vulnerability for an obstructed airway.[12] Neuromuscular systems under both voluntary and involuntary control evolved along with the anatomy to preserve health during sleep.[12,13] A healthy airway stays patent with minimal flow limitation and no snoring during sleep.[14,15] Maintenance of upper airway patency, not its dilation, is the primary objective of these neuromuscular systems. In OSA there is a failure of the systems that maintain upper airway patency. The pathogenesis of OSA involves a complex interplay of the effects of a upper airway closing pressure, deficient pharyngeal motor control, ventilatory instability (loop gain), and predisposition to arousal, alone and/or in combination.[16] The contribution of each in causing repeated obstructive events during sleep in a given individual may vary, emphasizing the importance of defining the causal features in afflicted patients to achieve the goal of individualized, targeted therapy. However, the fundamental event is a collapse of the airway from its mechanical properties. Therefore, neuroanatomy produces an obstruction, but the length, recurrence, position, and sleep stage are other factors that determine clinically significant sleep disordered breathing.

## 3.2. Physical and Mechanical Properties

### 3.2.1. Fluid Mechanics

Air passing from the nares to the lungs traverses a complex upper airway, a conduit in the first step of the cascade for gas exchange and oxygen delivery. The flexible tube is the fundamental unit for understanding the mechanics of the flow of air through it (Figure 3.3A); we can consider the airway as made up of a collection of smaller tubes working as a unit (Figure 3.3C). If energy dissipation through frictional resistance is small, cross-sectional area of the extrathoracic airway (and therefore flow through) will depend on the relative magnitude of driving pressures, transmural pressures, and airway deformability.[17] In the following sections we will describe what this means in terms of the physical properties of flexible tubes.

#### 3.2.1.1. Poiseuille's Law

Poiseuille's law defines the flow (Q) of air through a rigid tube as the pressure gradient along the tube ($\Delta P$) divided by the resistance (R) to flow [$Q = \Delta P/R$]. Resistance is determined by Ohm's law, where [$R = 8\eta l/(\pi r^4)$], where (l) is length of tube, (r) is radius, and ($\eta$) is the viscosity of the gas. Resistance varies linearly with length and viscosity, but radius has a much stronger influence: Resistance varies inversely with $r^4$. Hence a small increase in radius can dramatically decrease the resistance, and a small decrease in radius can dramatically increase the resistance.

(A)    Mechanical Elements in a Tube

(B)         Tube Law

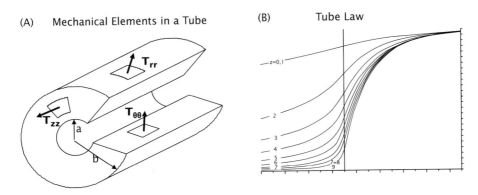

(C)    One can imagine the number of elements determining flow to the trachea

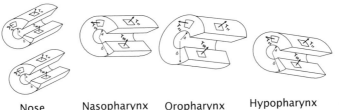

Nose        Nasopharynx    Oropharynx    Hypopharynx

**FIGURE 3.3 (A)** A cutaway cartoon of a thick-walled airway, showing the geometric arrangement in cylindrical coordinates of the tissue stresses in the axial direction ($T_{zz}$), the radial direction ($T_{rr}$), and the circumferential direction ($T_{\theta\theta}$). Shear stresses are not depicted. The internal and external radii are shown as $a$ and $b$ respectively. **(B)** Representation of tube law: how tubes of different diameters and elasticity behave under quasi-static conditions. The x-axis represents transmural pressure, and the vertical line marks a transmural pressure of zero (i.e., pressure inside the tube is equal to pressure outside the tube). The y-axis is the cross-sectional area. The stiffest tubes show little change with changes in transmural pressure, while the more compliant tubes will narrow with increasing negative transmural pressure and expand with increasing positive transmural pressure. **(C)** The concept here is that in the upper airway to the trachea, as represented in Figure 2, there are any number of tubular parts that have independent, local tube laws. Figure 3.3A is reprinted by permission from the American Physiological Society (Strohl, Butler, et al 2012).

### 3.2.1.2. Bernoulli's Principle

Bernoulli's principle describes the changes in a fluid's pressure that occur with changes in its speed; it can be related to Poiseuille's law. As fluid flows through a tube and encounters a narrowing, the speed of the fluid will increase through the area of resistance in order to maintain a constant flow. Its relevance in the airway is that at the end of the narrowing the gas will exert less outward pressure on the airway walls for a limited length after the narrowing, and hence a narrowing of the airway can contribute to airway collapse just distal to it.

### 3.2.1.3. Tube Law

A flowing gas exerts pressure on the inside wall of a tube, pushing it outward, at the same time as the pressure gradient along the tube pushes the gas through the tube.[18]

The outward pressure of the gas accounts for the axial stress, as depicted in Figure 3.3A. Whatever is outside of the tube (such as tissue) is also exerting pressure on the wall of the tube. The difference between the axial pressure of the gas inside the tube and the pressure outside the tube is the transmural pressure, and it will determine if the walls of the tube will move inward or outward. "Tube law" describes the dependence of the cross-sectional area of a flexible tube on the transmural pressure (see Figure 3.3B) and is constructed under static circumstances to predict area at any given circumstance of transmural pressure.[17] It gives us a measure of how stiff or floppy the tube is, with stiff tubes having a relatively flat curve on the graph and floppy tubes having large variations in their cross-sectional areas. Transmural pressure combined with the airway's tube law is a major factor determining the area of the lumen, especially if the airway wall has tissue inhomogeneity and deformability.

### 3.2.1.4. Tissue Pressure

Tissue pressure is the extraluminal pressure adjacent to an airway wall.[19] Tissue pressure in the extrathoracic upper airway is different from both the pleural pressure and atmospheric or barometric pressure. Tissue pressure, as measured in animal models, is known to statically and dynamically affect airway closing properties and is modified by physical attachments or vascular pressures in the airway wall.[20,21] Tension exerted by genioglossus could be envisioned as tissue pressure by exerting a combination of radial stress, $T_{zz}$, on the tongue base, and circumferential stress, $T_{\theta\theta}$, on the lateral pharyngeal airway (see Figure 3.3A). Head and jaw positions under anesthesia alter not only channel angles but also collapsibility.[22] There is also evidence that the extrathoracic airway is influenced by lung volume; the trachea hangs from the upper airway and is subject to stretch when lung volume increases. This "tracheal tug" is an axial stress and would correspond to $T_{zz}$ in Figure 3.3A. As a result of this longitudinal tension, the size and stiffness in the tube change, making it harder to close.[23,24] Intrinsic tension in the longitudinal muscles of the pharynx would produce a similar effect.

### 3.2.1.5. Starling Resistor and $P_{crit}$

The Starling resistor is a model of a collapsible tube that can be used to describe the behavior of the pharyngeal airway.[25] It is a flexible tube that will close if the pressure of the air inside the tube is less than the pressure outside the tube (which in the case of the airway is simply tissue pressure); the pressure in the tissue defines the critical closing pressure, or $P_{crit}$. This tube is positioned between the noncollapsible airway segments of the nose and the trachea (Figure 3.4). In the Starling resistor, the patency of the tube will depend on how the pressures in the upstream segment ($P_{us}$) and downstream segment ($P_{ds}$) relate to the tissue pressure ($P_{crit}$) surrounding the collapsible tube. If $P_{us} > P_{crit}$, air will enter the collapsible portion. Air will flow through the tube unimpeded if downstream $P_{ds} >$

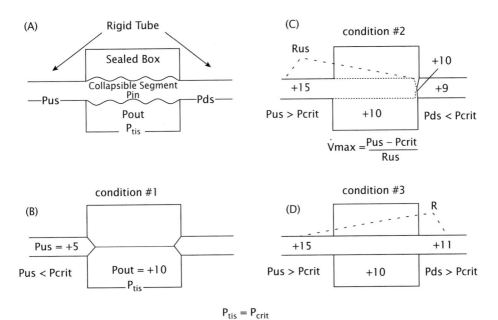

**FIGURE 3.4 (A)** The elements of a collapsible segment (a Starling resistor model) inside a rigid frame with flow from left to right going through rigid tubes at either end. Think of the nose on the left and the trachea on the right. Flow through the tube is determined by a gradient between the upstream pressure (left) during the act of inspiration and the transmural pressure on the collapsible segment—the difference between inside airway pressure ($P_{in}$) and outside tissue pressure ($P_{tis}$) of the collapsible segment. **(B)** When the upstream pressure ($P_{us}$) is lower than $P_{tis}$, the transmural pressure +5 results in closure of the "floppy" segment. $P_{tis}$ is hence the critical closing pressure, or $P_{crit}$. The segment is susceptible to collapse despite any increases in negative pressure in the trachea generated by inspiratory chest wall muscles. In expiration, pressure generated by lung and chest wall recoil is generally higher than the $P_{crit}$, and the airway is open throughout most of expiration. (C) In the flow-limited situation, maximal inspiratory flow will be ($P_{us}$ − $P_{crit}$)/$R_{us}$, where $R_{us}$ is the resistance of the upstream portion of the airway. (D) If $P_{in}$ > $P_{crit}$, the airway will be stable; this can be achieved with the application positive airway pressure. Modified from Chest 110(4). Gold AR, Schwartz AR. The pharyngeal critical pressure. The whys and hows of using nasal continuous positive airway pressure diagnostically. Pages 1077-88, Copyright (1996) with permission from Elsevier.

$P_{crit}$, as at no point along the collapsible section will the tube close. However, if $P_{us}$ > $P_{crit}$ > $P_{ds}$, the situation of flow limitation will occur, such that maximal inspiratory flow will be ($P_{us}$ − $P_{crit}$)/$R_{us}$, where $R_{us}$ is the resistance of the upstream portion of the airway, for instance the nasal valve.[26]

## 3.2.2. Breathing and Functional Mechanics

### 3.2.2.1. Normal Breathing

During quiet breathing, the negative pressures generated by the pump muscles with inspiration expand the lungs, and the positive pressures generated by chest wall and lung recoil push gas out of the lungs with expiration. The driving pressure of inspiratory airflow is the difference between atmospheric pressure at the entrance at the lips and nose to the pressures in the chest, as determined by the lungs, diaphragm, and chest wall (rib-cage and muscles of the thorax and abdominal wall).[27] Pressure drops will occur as air passes through areas of narrowing, and these will be accompanied by eddies of convective acceleration, such as when air goes from the parallel channels of the nares into the nasopharynx.[17]

In humans, steady flow is defined operationally by the absence of snoring during sleep, and flows are taken to be quasi-steady state, in which case the dynamic characteristics of the airway walls (their effective mass) appears to have a negligible influence.[28] There are known instances where balance is achieved. Such is apparent in the human neonate who has a very small and fairly stable airway in the first few months, even with a high respiratory frequency; its airway's mechanical properties become even more stable with growth and development over the first 2 to 3 years of life.[29] This ability to change and adjust with growth and development operationally defines healthy adult humans who do not snore. In OSA, such stability is altered.

## 3.2.2.2. When Does the Airway Actually Close?

It is interesting to consider the moment of truth: exactly when during the respiratory cycle does the airway collapse? For this there are limited data. In concept, it may vary by individual, sleep state, and position, or even within a night. The aforementioned Starling resistor and Bernoulli-like closure with reduced wall pressure distal to a narrowing is based on the assumption that closure occurs at the instant of inspiration. However, it is known that an airway during a central (nonobstructive) apnea will close.[30,31] This central apnea is a prolonged expiratory event, so it is not unreasonable to postulate that airway closure may also occur at the end of expiration, a prolongation of which occurs in the decline of respiratory drive that leads to an obstructive event.[32] Indeed, a prolonged expiratory time quantitatively increases the risk of severe OSA in patients with the overlap syndrome of chronic obstructive pulmonary disease with OSA.[33] The response to continuous positive pressure is not helpful, as it opens the airway indiscriminately during the entire respiratory cycle.[34] However, with bilevel positive airway pressure treatment, increasing the expiratory pressure is more effective at maintaining airway patency than increasing the inspiratory pressure.[35] It takes more mechanical work to reopen an airway once it has closed than it does to just keep it open.[36,37] Once full closure occurs, surface tension forces make it very difficult to reopen, which is a rationale for the need for an arousal to activate many muscles. Indeed, simply lubricating the airway to decrease the surface tension required for reopening has been found to decrease the apnea–hypopnea index (AHI).[9] In summary, it takes less work to keep the airway open than to reopen it once it is closed.

Hence a feedback control for hypoglossal nerve stimulation based on respiratory phase need not be very precise, as long as the airway is kept from completely closing. Indeed, attempting to time stimulation physiologically with inspiration is difficult, as normally the upper airway muscles activate prior to the diaphragm; timing stimulation with the chest wall muscles already producing a negative pressure in the chest or a chest movement means that genioglossus will be playing "catch up" with the other upper airway muscles.[38] In anesthetized animals in a sealed upper airway there occur volume increases in the upper airway before and during inspiratory tidal volume generated by the chest wall muscles.[39,40] In expiration, stimulation would open the airway widely and relaxation back to the resting state is slow enough so as not to close before inspiration. In inspiration, stimulation opens the airway wider or activation spans across expiration.[41] Keeping the vulnerable portion of the airway open enough is the goal.

### 3.2.2.3. Forces on the Airway

Upper airway muscles act on the airway through their attachments to the skull, mandible, tongue, hyoid bone, thyroid and cricoid cartilages, and other upper airway muscles. Coordination of the upper airway muscles with the diaphragm and chest wall muscles is crucial for the maintenance of upper airway patency during sleep. There are complicated interrelationships between these muscles and structures, and these interrelationships affect airway patency.[22,42,43] In humans such coupling is also used for the specialized function of speech, the evolution of which may have compromised the coordination and muscle orientations needed for upper airway patency during sleep.

The upper airway tissues deform secondary to inhomogeneous axial and perpendicular forces. For instance, tracheal traction or complex musculature coupling in the airway wall can interact to make the airway stiff. Regional or segmental deposits of deformable fatty tissue (liquid at body temperature) cause resting luminal areas to change.[44] Certain deposits may deform but not change substantially the tube law of the segment, but a lumen could approach or even reach full closure.[45] On the other hand, a structure like the anterior pharyngeal wall may collect tissue but not substantially affect the airway. Here might lie the effects of position or gravitational forces. The tolerance for such loading is in terms of sleep disordered breathing is not known.

Finite element models of the upper airway,[46,47] which attempt to explain observed behavior by breaking the airway down into small segments, are incomplete with regard to the anatomic interactions that occur across the upper airway segments, each of which also contributes regionally to airway size and stiffness. One region of the pharynx (e.g., oropharynx) may influence the collapsibility of "the tube" at another region (e.g., the velopharynx). For example, displacement of the tongue hydrostat during inspiration is coupled to displacements in the nasopharynx or epiglottis, and this cannot be described by simple tube law ideas, unless models can incorporate variation in axial length or tension. Axial coupling has application to flow limitation, particularly negative effort dependence, a commonly observed phenomenon of reduced airflow with increased inspiratory driving pressure seen in flow profiles in OSA patients during sleep.[48]

## 3.2.3. Critical Closing Pressure ($P_{crit}$) and OSA

The practical application of the Starling resistor model to OSA was the measurement of critical closing pressure ($P_{crit}$). Raising the upstream pressure ($P_{us}$) in the nasal mask relieves recurrent obstructive events by maintaining the downstream pressure ($P_{ds}$) above tissue pressure ($P_{crit}$) (Figure 3.4D). The actual positive pressure delivered to the collapsible airway will vary according to the resistance of the proximal nasal airway. $P_{crit}$ can be easily measured in people in the sleep lab by using a positive airway pressure (PAP) device capable of rapid pressure drops, and measuring the airflow through a nasal mask when pressures delivered by it are manipulated.[25] The patient's PAP is started at a point where there is no flow limitation, and it is then lowered several times for 2-3 breaths so that a graph of maximal flow at any given upstream pressure ($P_{us}$) is generated. The curve can then be extrapolated to a flow of zero, and that will be the point where the applied pressure results in airway closure (Figure 3.5), which is the critical closing pressure ($P_{crit}$).[49] Such closing pressures do not represent a total airway volume of zero, since only a portion of the upper airway may be closed. While this is a simplification of airway resistance responses to transmural pressure, there is ample evidence that $P_{crit}$ is a useful estimator of airway stability and that it is correlated loosely with airway closure during sleep.[25] Rapid drops are used to create the passive $P_{crit}$ curve, which is thought to reflect the "anatomy" at rest, as the speed with which they are done does not allow time for neuromuscular compensation. This value has been incorporated into the physiologic phenotyping of OSA

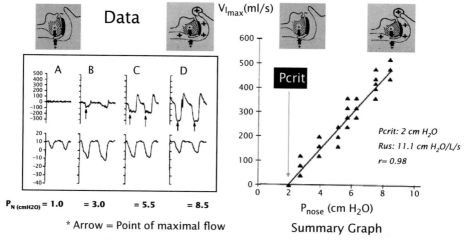

**FIGURE 3.5** (Left) The effect of increasing upstream pressure on maximal inspiratory flow in a patient with OSA. When the pressure in the nasal mask is ~1 cmH$_2$O, the airway is closed, as indicated by no flow in the presence of two inspiratory efforts. $P_{crit}$ is 1.2 cmH$_2$O. At 3 and 5.5 cmH$_2$O there is flow limitation, while at 8.5 cmH$_2$O flow is highest (no flow limitation or snoring) while esophageal pressure is lowest (i.e., the lowest resistance). (Right) The upstream pressure at which the airway is closed would be the closing pressure. In this instance transmural pressure is in the direction of closing the airway, and the closing pressure (or $P_{crit}$) is positive. Figure is modified from Chest 110(4). Gold AR, Schwartz AR. The pharyngeal critical pressure. The whys and hows of using nasal continuous positive airway pressure diagnostically. Pages 1077-88, Copyright (1996) with permission from Elsevier.

patients as representing the anatomic functionality[16,50] and is used in models where upper airway closure might occur in the presence of respiratory control instability.[51]

One can do slower pressure drops that allow time for neuromuscular compensation mechanisms to activate, and create an active $P_{crit}$ curve. The neuromuscular contribution to airway collapsibility is to move the intercept ($P_{crit}$) to the left, and the channel becomes harder to close.[52]

Patients with OSA during sleep generally have $P_{crit}$ values close to or above atmospheric pressure, whereas patients with upper airway resistance or simple snoring have more distinctly negative mean values, meaning that a negative pressure must be applied to close the airway (Figure 3.6A). Such observations form the basis for thinking that an

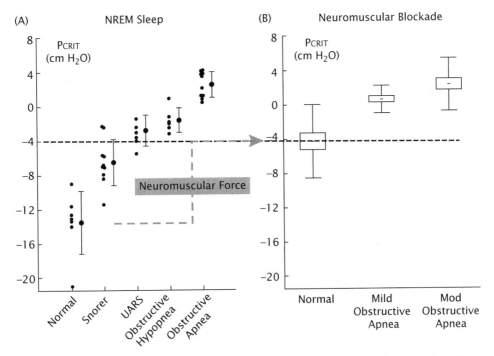

**FIGURE 3.6 (A)** Shown are values of $P_{crit}$ during natural sleep for different clinical presentations. Those with OSA have $P_{crit}$ values at or above atmospheric pressure; those who are normal breathing during sleep or with upper airway resistance or simple snoring have more negative mean values, meaning that a negative pressure must be applied to close the airway. **(B)** In a second dataset obtained in individuals who had received anesthesia with neuromuscular blockade, $P_{crit}$ became distinctively more positive (unstable) in those without sleep disordered breathing ("normal"). Less of an effect by anesthesia with neuromuscular blockade was seen in subjects with OSA; $P_{crit}$ values in in those subjects were similar to the unanesthetized, sleep state. This result suggests that muscular activity plays an important role in airway stability during sleep in normal individuals. Figure 3.6A is reprinted from Gleadhill IC, Schwartz AR, Schubert N, Wise RA, Permutt S, Smith PL. Upper airway collapsibility in snorers and in patients with obstructive hypopnea and apnea. Am Rev Respir Dis. 143(6):Pages 1300-3, 1991, with permission of the American Thoracic Society. Copyright © 2020 American Thoracic Society. Figure 3.6B is adapted from *Journal of Applied Physiology* 82(4):1319-1326. Isono S, Remmers JE, Tanaka A, Sho Y, Sato J, Nishino T. Anatomy of pharynx in patients with obstructive sleep apnea and in normal subjects. 1997, with permission of the American Physiological Society.

airway with abnormal anatomy will need counterbalancing mechanisms to maintain patency during wakefulness.

Airway stability in health has an active process lost in even mild OSA, given the data shown in Figure 3.6B. Data were obtained in individuals undergoing anesthesia with neuromuscular blockade, in whom the severity of sleep apnea was known. When one compares studies in sleep with those in anesthesia with neuromuscular blockade, an absence of muscle tone is associated with more marked worsening of $P_{crit}$ in those without OSA than those with OSA. Hence, much of the difference in anatomic functionality between these two groups appears to come from neuromuscular forces that are absent in OSA.

This suggests to us that the main driver for OSA is the withdrawal of some active mechanism that maintains a balance, much as it does for the neonate which has the challenge of a small airway. While the healthy adult airway also appears to gain some additional stability from non-neuromuscular contributions (which may include ligament and elastic tissue orientation, surface tension between tongue and palate, and potentially other possibilities), it is important to note that in those with mild and moderate OSA the differences in $P_{crit}$ are not so great once neuromuscular compensation is removed. This is important when one thinks of therapy, because subtle changes in size or resting tone or coordination among upper airway muscles could make a big difference.

Furthermore, not only is the critical closing pressure different among normal subjects and patients with OSA, but the shape of the pressure–area curve for the velopharynx differs between normal subjects and patients with moderate and severe OSA, being steeper in slope near $P_{crit}$ in patients with sleep disordered breathing[53] (Figure 3.7). In addition, the maximal flow in the plateau part of the curve is lower in OSA than in those without sleep disordered breathing. This suggests that there is a smaller air channel; it also suggests that this smaller size is sufficient for breathing at higher upstream pressures. In this same study there was a significant correlation across segments as velopharyngeal and oropharyngeal $P_{crit}$ show association, as least in anesthetized subjects.[53] This is an important observation in regard to the interdependence of upper airway segments: structural changes or neuromuscular adaptations in one segment are likely over time to change other segments. An alternate explanation is that the concept of airway segments is a contrived one, and that the structural features that predispose to upper airway stability span the entire pharyngeal airway.

Other measures of airway mechanics could complement the metric of $P_{crit}$—for example, airway resistance in segments of the upper airway and the presence or absence of flow limitation during sleep.[54] Imaging studies could give some indication of the cross-sectional size of the airway to produce a more comprehensive view of upper airway mechanical properties.[11] All these measures may explain the occurrence of one obstruction during sleep but not necessarily the number or consequent severity of apnea.[55] Other factors like unstable chemosensor reactivity ("loop gain") and muscle recruitment

NORMALS     MODERATE OSA     SEVERE OSA

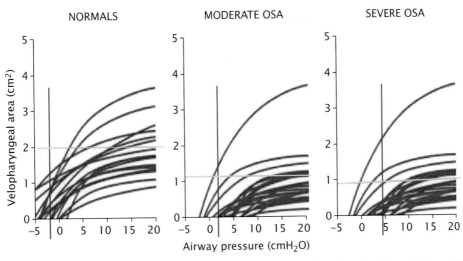

**FIGURE 3.7** Curves for the calculation of $P_{crit}$ in anesthetized individuals who are healthy and those with known levels of OSA. The x-axis shows pressure starting with subatmospheric values (–5 cmH$_2$O). The y-axis shows the velopharyngeal area. Each curve represents a single individual. The vertical line represents the mean $P_{crit}$ and the horizontal line is the mean area, which would be correlated to flow. Adapted from *Journal of Applied Physiology* 82(4):1319-1326. Isono S, Remmers JE, Tanaka A, Sho Y, Sato J, Nishino T. Anatomy of pharynx in patients with obstructive sleep apnea and normal subjects. 1997, with permission of the American Physiological Society.

contribute to the variance in apnea occurrence in non–rapid-eye-movement (NREM) and rapid-eye-movement (REM) sleep.

In health we assume that the upper airway is evolutionarily developed to be open (enough) during sleep to permit adequate gas exchange, but in snoring and in disease like OSA, there is an imbalance tipping the scale to mechanical instability. This keeping the airway open is a hidden talent, unlike its functionality for speech or swallowing. Our mechanical concepts for breathing during sleep will depend on its purpose and acknowledge its limitations, especially if it is based on static imaging or assumptions of linearity and independence of segments. Promoting airway patency and structural integrity is muscle tone or activation, with some stiffening contribution by tracheal traction with the increase in lung volume.

# 3.3. The Peculiar Aspects of Pharyngeal Anatomy

## 3.3.1. Conceptualization

The most simplistic conceptualization of hypoglossal nerve stimulation as a treatment for OSA is that it opens the airway by pulling the tongue out of it. Stimulation of the medial division of the hypoglossal nerve targets the genioglossus, which connects the genial tubercle and the hyoid bone, and fans upward and forms a large bulk of the tongue muscle. Stimulation forcefully moves the hyoid bone anteriorly,[56] carrying the base of the tongue with it and out of the airway. However, simply opening the oropharynx by pulling the tongue forward is not sufficient to treat OSA.[57] Instead, the effectiveness of the treatment appears to depend on how the hyoid–tongue movement increases tension on the surrounding pharynx, and particularly on the soft palate.[57,58] This section will present a broader view of the musculature of the upper airway and provide an argument that OSA represents a failure of the integrated system of upper airway muscles involved in the many functions of the shared airway and foodway.

Many of the muscles of the pharynx could potentially keep the airway open during breathing. How well the system works in an energy-efficient manner depends on the coordination and relative activation matching with the anatomy. Such concepts are followed in considerations of mechanics during swallowing and breathing. In swallowing, these muscles must also protect the glottis while simultaneously facilitating the transfer of oral and vallecular contents into the esophagus. In breathing, the pharyngeal muscles must support the larynx (and, by extension, the hyoid bone and tongue base) against the downward pull of the aspirational pump created by the diaphragm and chest wall muscles. Indeed, we hypothesize that the original impetus for the evolution of the muscular mammalian pharynx was to stabilize the glottis from this downward pull; the chest wall pump of reptiles (and presumably that of our premammalian ancestors) does exert a pull on the glottis but not much because reptilian lungs have much higher compliance than mammalian lungs.[59] Airflow resistance and frictional losses are presumably low as well. In OSA there is a profound failure of pharyngeal function, leading to excessive respiratory movement of the hyolaryngeal apparatus,[60] a characteristically low-lying hyoid,[61,62] as well as a higher prevalence of subclinical swallowing dysfunction and increased risk of pneumonia.[63,64]

## 3.3.2. Pharyngeal Support

The human pharynx is basically a muscular tube that hangs from the skull base and mandible and attaches to the thyroid and cricoid cartilages as well as the entryway to the esophagus. The skull base is the only truly solid support of the pharynx; while the thyroid/ cricoid cartilage complex is circumferentially stable, it can move up or down depending on the tension of the muscles on either side of it and the extent of tracheal traction, which in turn depends on pleural forces and lung volume. It should be emphasized that there are no attachments of the pharynx to the spinal column; indeed, the entire pharynx can be moved to the side in order to access the spine for cervical spinal fusion surgery. The dorsolateral walls of the pharynx consist of longitudinal muscles and constrictor muscles, and there are potential spaces around them, which makes their collapse possible. The anterior wall is formed by the soft palate, tongue base with its supporting hyoid bone, and epiglottis. All of these structures—dorsolateral walls and anterior structures—may be involved in airway embarrassment.

### 3.3.2.1. Longitudinal Muscles

The longitudinal support between the skull base and thyroid cartilage is critical in understanding lateral pharyngeal wall collapsibility. Tension from the trachea on the pharyngeal muscles decreases airway collapsibility.[23] Mechanically, it is the longitudinally oriented muscles that would participate in this force vector, and likely play a significant role in airway stability versus collapsibility.[65] This concept can be illustrated by picturing a rectangular sail: The amount of longitudinal tension on it will determine how far the wind will make it billow out. Forces exerted at the anterior attachments of this muscular sleeve—the soft palate, jaw, tongue, and hyoid bone—can modify the pharynx by altering pharyngeal wall tension. Hence these attachments affect wall collapsibility, as well as lumen shape and diameter. It is this transfer of forces that is likely responsible for the effectiveness of hypoglossal nerve stimulation. To return to the sail analogy, this would be like pulling on the corner of a loose sail to increase the tautness of the sail.

The bulk of the longitudinal walls is formed by the palatopharyngeus and stylopharyngeus (Figure 3.8). The palatopharyngeus originates from the palatine aponeurosis of the soft palate; the stylopharyngeus originates from the styloid process and enters

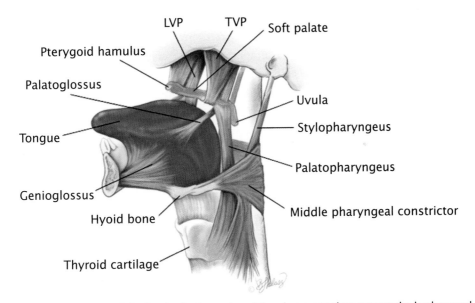

**FIGURE 3.8** Depiction of the longitudinal muscles of the pharynx as they support the hyolaryngeal complex from the skull base. The combined action of tensor veli palatini (TVP), levator veli palatini (LVP), palatopharyngeus, and stylopharyngeus are situated to provide counter-tension to the downward vector force exerted by diaphragmatic excursion (aka "tracheal tug"), as well as to provide longitudinal support of the pharyngeal walls against collapse. Deficient activity of these muscles would be expected to cause downward migration of the hyolaryngeal complex, as well as an increased collapsibility of the pharyngeal walls. Activity of these muscles would also be expected to provide lateral spreading of the airway. Many of the muscles of the tongue, hyoid, and pharynx has been omitted for clarity. Note that the superior pharyngeal constrictor may provide additional support from the skull base via its attachment to the pterygoid plate and hamulus. Part of the mandible has been removed to expose the geniohyoid and genioglossus. Conceptualization by Denise Dewald, MD. Artwork and copyright by Beth Halasz, BFA, MFA

the pharyngeal musculature via the dorsolateral pharyngeal wall in the upper portion of the middle pharyngeal constrictor. Both insert into the thyroid cartilage and spread out widely within the pharyngeal aponeurosis of the hypopharynx, with some fibers inserting into the mucosa around the epiglottis.[66–68] Tensor veli palatini (TVP) and levator veli palatini (LVP) form the longitudinal support of the nasopharynx; these muscles originate from the skull base in an oblique anterior-posterior direction, and also attach to the eustachian tube. They insert into the palatine aponeurosis, the fibrous core of the soft palate which attaches to the end of the hard palate. TVP courses around and inserts into the pterygoid hamulus, a hook-like extension of the hard palate, and firmly supports the anterior soft palate.[69] The support of the palatine aponeurosis from the skull base by TVP and LVP provides a firm base of support for the palatopharyngeus, which will enhance the ability of the palatopharyngeus to open up the lateral recesses of the pharynx.

The palatopharyngeus plays a pivotal role in elevating the larynx during swallowing.[69] For this action, the hyolaryngeal complex is pulled anteriorly to open up the foodway, and the larynx is pulled upward and against the tongue base to protect the glottis from incursion.[70–72] On the other hand, the role of the stylopharyngeus in swallowing is not completely clear; experimental disabling of this muscle in dogs and horses does not disturb this function.[73,74] However, the stylopharyngeus has been shown to play a critical role in maintaining airway stability in exercising horses,[75] and a loss of tone in the stylopharyngeus during sleep has been implicated in dorsolateral wall collapse in OSA.[76] Indeed, neurostimulation of the stylopharyngeus via the glossopharyngeal nerve in animals showed greater airway dilation than stimulation of the hypoglossal nerve.[77] Hence, the stylopharyngeus may play an underrecognized, even primary, role in maintaining airway patency and stability in both wakefulness and sleep.

### 3.3.2.2. The Soft Palate
Hypoglossal nerve stimulation effectiveness may depend in part on its effects on the soft palate; this has attracted attention to linkages between the tongue and the velopharynx. The soft palate consists of four paired muscles (LVP, TVP, palatopharyngeus, and palatoglossus) and the musculus uvulae, all of which attach to the palatine aponeurosis.[69] We and others proposed that the palatoglossus is coupling the anterior movement of the tongue to anterior movement of the soft palate, thereby improving velopharyngeal airway patency during hypoglossal nerve stimulation.[56,58,78] While the anatomic dissections of the palatoglossus make it an attractive candidate, support for this supposed function is limited. This rather small muscle originates in the palatine aponeurosis and inserts into the tongue laterally and joins with other tongue muscle as it courses toward the tip of the tongue; it elevates the posterior tongue and assists in closure of the fauces.[69] An alternative is the palatopharyngeus, a much larger muscle that functions to pull the soft palate downward.[69] It could be involved in the coupling of tongue movement to anterior movement of the soft palate via its interconnections with the superior pharyngeal constrictor, which has an insertion in the tongue. The soft palate plays a significant role in airway

obstruction,[65] probably directly or indirectly, in almost all patients with OSA.[79–82] The reader is directed to a review of the muscular and soft tissue palatal anatomy as it relates the phenotypic variations that generate the shape and collapsibility of the retropalatal airway.[65]

### 3.3.2.3. Constrictor Muscles and Linkages

There are three sets of constrictor muscles in the pharynx: the superior, middle, and inferior. All of these constrictor muscles attach to the pharyngeal raphe, which spans from the pharyngeal tubercle on the skull base to the cricoid cartilage.[69] These muscles have significant longitudinal components to them as well as horizontal/circumferential ones, and are in places extensively intertwined with the aforementioned longitudinal muscles.[67,83] Tension in the constrictor muscles will significantly *decrease* airway collapsibility, particularly at smaller diameters when the horizontal fibers reach the extreme of their effective length–tension relationships.[84,85] Hence, tension transmitted to these muscles may not necessarily close the airway, as the name might suggest.

As far as hypoglossal nerve stimulation is concerned, the authors know of no research that has studied its effect on these other muscles. However, there are two linkages between the tongue and the constrictors that should be noted. The first is the glossopharyngeus muscle, a slip of the superior pharyngeal constrictor that inserts into the tongue. This might be important because the superior constrictor muscle coordinates with and is closely intertwined with the muscles of the soft palate, as all these muscles work together to regulate the velopharynx. As a result, forces on the tongue can be transmitted through this glossopharyngeal portion of the superior constrictor to the soft palate and related structures.[86] A second linkage is the hyoid bone itself; the middle pharyngeal constrictor attaches to the hyoid bone, and hence would receive direct tension from the hypoglossal nerve stimulation as the hyoid is pulled forward. It should be noted that the middle pharyngeal constrictor has a direct linkage to the stylopharyngeus, and hence forward hyoid movement could create tension on this longitudinal pharyngeal muscle. Understanding this linkage is important in determining the effectiveness of hypoglossal nerve stimulation.

## 3.3.3. Muscles and Airway Shape: A Thought Experiment

The normal human airway has an oval shape, with its long axis oriented coronally.[87] This configuration has also been reported in cats that have been used in neurostimulation experiments.[87,88] People with OSA, however, have an airway that is circular or has its long axis oriented in the anteroposterior direction.[87,89] Snorers and people with mild OSA lie in between these extremes (Figure 3.9). The question is: Why is there this tube geometry? Arguments proposed to date emphasize passive anatomy, such as fat or tissue mass. However, one may propose an alternative view based on muscle orientation and function.

We note that the anteroposterior orientation of the airway in OSA is more pronounced in the retroglossal and low retropalatal levels, consistent with the increased

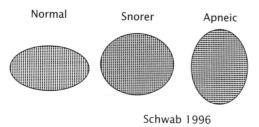

Schwab 1996

**FIGURE 3.9** Shape of the upper airway in three groups of patients. Here the shape changes are emphasized, and the interpretation of these shape differences is crucial in understanding the pathogenesis of OSA. For more discussion see the text. Reprinted by permission from *Sleep*, Schwab RJ. Properties of tissues surrounding the upper airway. 19 (10 Suppl):S170-174 with the permission of Oxford University Press.

basal tone of the genioglossus found in awake subjects with OSA.[90] Hence, increased activation of the genioglossus in the awake OSA patient could explain this shape. The high retropalatal and nasopharyngeal regions, however, are circular in OSA as well. This suggests that the shape changes throughout the airway, starting with the muscles that are anchoring the airway from the skull, mainly TVP, LVP, palatopharyngeus (via soft palate linkages in the palatine aponeurosis with TVP and LVP), and stylopharyngeus.

One can make a reasonable argument that the shape of the airway is secondary to reduced muscle tension in these longitudinal muscles, rather than primarily due to collections of fat. It may be that the laxity of these muscles is what allows fat to collect around the pharyngeal walls. Considering how the stylopharyngeus muscle attaches to the dorsolateral pharyngeal wall at the level of the upper portion of the middle pharyngeal constrictor—which is at the level of the tongue—the airway shape in the retroglossal region would suggest that there is abnormally low tone of this muscle in OSA, even in wakefulness. The presence of adequate tone in the stylopharyngeus and palatopharyngeus would tend to expand the airway walls in a lateral direction, leading to the shape seen in the normal airway. Interestingly, the stylopharyngeus and palatopharyngeus both attach to the tonsillar capsule;[68,91] if these muscles are responsible for keeping the tonsils out of the airway in children, this could link deficient muscular activity in pediatric OSA to adult OSA airway shapes. Indeed, the early fiberoptic studies of OSA reported "partial or total invagination of the posterolateral pharyngeal walls" that accompanied the loss of electromyographic (EMG) activity in the middle pharyngeal constrictor/stylopharyngeus electrode, *despite* persistence of genioglossus activity.[76] The authors posited that a lack of activity of the stylopharyngeus and the middle pharyngeal constrictor could explain the collapse of these walls.[76] Furthermore, the stylopharyngeus EMG showed inspiratory bursts of muscle activity in normal subjects even during phasic REM sleep. The question then is whether the genioglossal activation we have been studying for many years is actually compensating for deficient muscle tone elsewhere, for instance in the longitudinal pharyngeal muscles.

### 3.3.4. Nerve Stimulation as an Airway Rescue Maneuver

The tongue's primary evolutionary purpose in mammals and their land-dwelling ancestors is as a feeding appendage.[92] This calls into question the supposition that the genioglossus is supposed to stay active during sleep. EMG studies also call this supposition into question. Healthy subjects show decreased genioglossus activity during sleep, as well as lower levels of genioglossus activity while awake during quiet breathing compared with subjects with OSA.[90] During REM sleep, the genioglossus EMG activity nearly ceases in normal individuals.[93] The genioglossus is activated during stress in normal animals in order to dilate the airway,[94,95] but sleep is not supposed to be a stressful situation requiring airway dilation. In contrast, subjects with OSA show increased activity of genioglossus while awake (suggesting a neuromuscular compensatory strategy),[96] with variable ability to maintain this compensation during sleep, and decreased activity at the start of an obstructive apnea.[97–99] Support of airway patency with nasal continuous positive airway pressure (CPAP) is associated with a marked decrease in the activity of the genioglossus during sleep, down to levels comparable to those seen in normal individuals.[100] If OSA is characterized by a generalized loss of structural pharyngeal muscle tone, activation of the genioglossus seems to be an attempt to compensate for it: The genioglossus pulls the lax airway forward in an attempt to increase the tension on its walls, and thereby decrease collapsibility and maintain patency. Theoretically, then, hypoglossal nerve stimulation compensates for a weakness in pharyngeal tone in OSA by attempting to keep genioglossus "awake" during sleep. Hence it would make sense that the ability of hypoglossal nerve stimulation to benefit an individual patient will depend on (1) the extent to which the patient's own genioglossus activity is maintained during sleep and (2) the extent to which tension on the soft tissue linkages between the tongue and the pharynx can open the airway. The soft palate function may be important since nasal breathing is the preferred breathing route during sleep in a normal airway,[101] and the soft palate is commonly involved in OSA.[79,80]

The critical element for sleep is to have airway stability and sufficient patency, and active dilation is not necessary in health. Active dilation is needed to increase airway capacity during exertion, or in recovery after closure, for instance during a swallow. The stimulated genioglossus has an action on the hyoid bone that serves to salvage an impaired pharyngeal airway.

## 3.4. Neuromuscular Control

There are three main elements of breathing regulation that are relevant to the outcomes of hypoglossal nerve stimulation. These are: (1) the general elements in the brainstem that are involved in feedback control of respiration, (2) the distribution of neuromuscular drive, and (3) the outcomes of this drive. This literature is extensive.[102–105] This chapter is not an exhaustive summary but is designed to emphasize the issues of neuromuscular control that inform us of opportunities to reconsider how an active neuromuscular system keeps the airway open during sleep in health and how it does not work in OSA.

# 3.4.1. Evolution

An interesting place to start is with an evolutionary viewpoint. Evolution and comparative zoology can inform us regarding the original purpose of muscles and structures, and provide us on insights on how they fit into our unique physiology. We study other animals because they are often simpler and more easily manipulated versions of the elements we have inherited as a species.

## 3.4.1.1. Gill Arches and the Evolution of the System for Human Sleep

Fish without jaws use branchial (intrinsic gill arch) muscles and their associated nerves (cranial nerves [CN] V and VII) to drive a weak pump to move water through an orifice and over respiratory exchange structures. Fish with jaws evolved a much more effective suction-based pump by using the hyoid arch as a hinge or lever, stabilized by the skull, to provide power for jaw opening. This hypobranchial pump was derived from spino-occipital somites that migrated forward through the branchial arches, the hyoid, and to the lower jaw, and were innervated by CN XII; fish use this active jaw-opening pump to augment flow during exertion and hypoxia, as well as for suction feeding. Hence, our tongue muscles started out as an exertional pump and the tongue was repurposed into a food-handling appendage with the transition to terrestrial life.[92] CN IX and X were involved in chemoreception and mechanoreception.[7,92] Breathing air required an outpouching of the pharyngeal endoderm and the development of a glottis (controlled by CN X), and coordination with the respiratory pump and with swallowing. Feeding mammalian infants with milk required the development of a series of valves and constricting muscles (soft palate and constrictor muscles) to maintain the airway during suckling and to ensure complete clearance of liquids with swallowing (also controlled mainly by CN X). Hence, at some point in our evolution, CN V, VII, IX, X, XII, and spinal nerves became involved in respiration and were required to participate in central pattern generators to maintain upper airway patency during sleep maybe more than wakefulness, where proprioceptive feedback is present. The muscles derived from these primordial anlagen are more often studied in orofacial behaviors as food and fluid ingestion, coughing, and sneezing, and for human speech. In most respiratory and critical care reviews, the upper airway muscles are classified as accessory respiratory muscles because they do not directly drive movement of air in and out of the lungs. They hold a hidden role when one considers healthy breathing during sleep.

## 3.4.1.2. Respiratory Pattern Generation

A rhythm generator, called the respiratory pattern generator in fish and central pattern generator (CPG) in mammals, organizes the distribution of drive for respiration. This is located in the medulla[103,104] and in mammals consists of three tangled mechanisms: (1) glutamatergic synaptic traffic, amplified by (2) intrinsic bursting in one or more points in the brainstem and opposed by (3) reciprocal inhibition.[106] There are phases of brainstem respiratory output—inspiratory, post-inspiratory, and expiratory (also including a pre-inspiratory component under low frequencies)—patterns that are represented in most respiratory-bursting neuronal pools. This control system also coordinates upper airway functions with those of the diaphragm and chest wall during sleep to maintain patency. It reconfigures and recombines to allow breathing to remain robust despite changes in posture, state, and head position, and interruptions by a swallow or cough. How it does this and then how it might fail to maintain patency are basic issues in understanding the pathogenesis of OSA syndromes. In addition, the CPG has connections to cardio-vascular sympathetic and parasympathetic nuclei regulating blood pressure and heart rate.[102] Thus, the brainstem organizes the first step in oxygen acquisition and delivery to tissues and the integration of breathing with metabolism and oxygen delivery, regulating its response to afferent signals, or altering its patterns with behavioral acts. The functional need for a CPG between humans and lampreys is similar.[107]

## 3.4.2. Controlling Ventilatory Function

### 3.4.2.1. Airway Muscle Response to Changing Conditions

Generating and controlling respiratory motor activity during normal eupneic breathing in vivo are distributed bilaterally in the pons and medulla oblongata. The medulla has bilateral ventral respiratory columns of respiratory neurons, interacting within the columns and interconnected with several pontine nuclei. The output of these circuits is transmitted through premotor networks to motor nuclei (Figure 3.10). The reader is directed to contemporary reviews providing detailed discussion of circuits, motor nuclei, afferent inputs, and cortical connections in the brainstem.[104]

### 3.4.2.2. Coordination of Activation Patterns

In humans, we see only the outputs of upper airway muscles (such as EMG activity) and have to interpret this to provide an insight into a central process operating in the control of breathing. The brainstem nuclei of the cranial nerves are projected to the muscles and are responsible for signaling all their actions. These muscles exhibit all muscle phenotypes, including both fast- and slow-twitch fibers. Animal studies identify some as fatigue-resistant as well as fatigue-susceptible, sculpted for the purposes of that species. Nonrespiratory muscles are capable of changing the "phenotype" as this is probably the case in human upper airway muscles.[108] Neural activation changes with chemical and nonchemical reflexes directed to the brainstem, with projections to muscles that influence airway size and shape.[109] Temporally, upper airway muscles are activated in humans before the onset of diaphragm inspiration,[110] consistent with a role in regulation of flow.

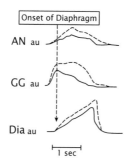

FIGURE 3.10 The respiratory control system distributes drive from the brain to the muscles that act on the upper airway, diaphragm, and chest wall, which in turn alter gas exchange, as sensed by receptors such as the carotid body or the brainstem, and feedback from irritant and mechano-receptors in the muscles and lung. NTS, nucleus tractus solitarius; VMS, ventral medullary surface; DRG, dorsal medullary surface; KF, Kolliker-Fuse; CB, carotid body; AB, aortic body; GG, genioglossus; ICs, intercostal muscles; DIA, diaphragm.

The EMG activation in Figure 3.11 illustrates the moving-time average of the nasalis muscle that dilates the alae nasi, genioglossus, and diaphragm, showing a coordination of the activation profiles through CN VII, CN XII, and phrenic motor neuron pools.

The abrupt onset, earlier peak activation, and decline in activation pattern is present in the upper airway motor pools with respiration. The decline before entering expiration is a result of vagally mediated inhibition of inspiration at the brainstem level, an action that is more prominent in the upper airway muscles than in the diaphragm. The nonchemical response to loading is to increase activation at any given level of chemoreception, and

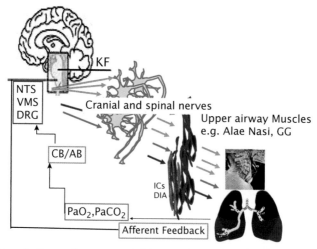

FIGURE 3.11 Shown is the moving average (arbitrary units = au) in the alae nasi (AN), genioglossus (GG), and diaphragm (Dia) measured during wakefulness in a seated human under conditions of mild hypercapnia (~50 mmHg of end-tidal $CO_2$) during rebreathing without (solid line) and with (dashed line) an imposed respiratory resistance of 15 $cmH_2O/l/s$. There is preactivation and with loading an increase in EMG measured drive in all signals.

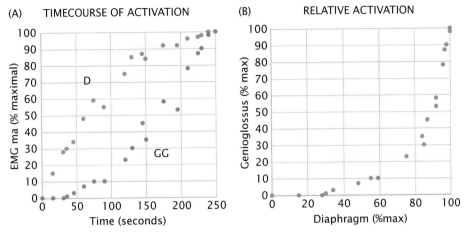

**FIGURE 3.12 (A)** Time course of increases in EMG activation of the diaphragm (D) and genioglossus (GG), expressed as percentage of maximal activation in an anesthetized animal. At the start the inspired gas was changed from 100% oxygen (producing apnea) to 7% carbon oxide/93% oxygen. There is a delay in the increases in genioglossal activity. **(B)** Plot of the data in **A**, indicating a different recruitment in the genioglossus and diaphragm EMG.

is composed of both a reduction in lung inflation and negative pressure in respiratory airways.

Another feature of contrast between diaphragmatic and genioglossal muscle activation is a curious difference in the response to chemoreception.[111–113] Figure 3.12 illustrates the difference in responses when an anesthetized, vagotomized animal is exposed to high carbon dioxide levels after being put in a state of induced central apnea by ventilation with 100% oxygen. Both the diaphragm and genioglossus reach maximal activation, but the diaphragm responds quickly, while there is a lag before the genioglossus activates. This curvilinear relationship is present in the recovery from chemostimulation and in the production of apnea by hyperventilation.

Alterations in the relative activation of upper airway and chest wall muscles also occur in the setting of reflexes from afferents, such as those in the esophagus, the sciatic nerve, and blood pressure sensors in the carotid body and the aortic arch.[114,115] Sciatic nerve stimulation will augment the respiratory and particularly inspiratory drive to all muscles (potentially in preparation for running), but unfortunately does not reduce upper airway resistance in the anesthetized rabbit.[116] This is in contrast to the effect of hypoglossal nerve stimulation in the same model in which resistance is reduced without altering respiratory drive.[117]

### 3.4.2.3. Respiratory Patterning and Sleep
In preclinical models and neurophysiologic and neuropharmacological studies, the nuclei that innervate upper airway muscles have connections to brainstem circuits also involved in swallowing and speech, to cortical control, and to behavioral state-controlling

neurons in the midbrain and hypothalamus. Turning to quiet wakefulness and the different stages of sleep, there is a change in breathing frequency and depth as the metabolic rate declines. There is a lengthening of both inspiratory and expiratory phases, and differences exist among individuals.[12]

One must not only consider the generation of a single breath but also the patterning of respiratory cycles over time that represent the moment-to-moment adjustments in motor control of the diaphragm, the intercostal and abdominal muscles, and the upper airway muscles.[113,118] Physiologic conditions in which breathing regulation changes during sleep produce vulnerable times for sleep disordered breathing.[119,120] There are the transitions from wake to sleep and the transitions from NREM to REM sleep. In the latter there is a confounding interaction between the higher brain centers and the brainstem overriding the somewhat cortically uncoupled state in NREM sleep, where breathing is regular.[115,121] In REM sleep, control of breathing and upper airway muscles is more erratic, and healthy subjects will normally exhibit a limited number of central and obstructive events.[12]

Sleep is associated with a reduction in metabolism, so ventilatory needs for carbon dioxide excretion and oxygen delivery diminish. In general, upper airway resistance increases in most healthy humans, but snoring and/or flow resistance are absent or at least relatively infrequent. An increase in upper airway resistance is enhanced in snorers and OSA patients.[12] The greater the fall in ventilation in the transition from wakefulness to sleep, the more likely that sleep disordered breathing will occur in NREM sleep; microarousals with repeat transitions to sleep amplify this instability.[122] If the upper airway is prone to snoring and collapse, these events of decreased respiratory drive will manifest as obstructive in nature.

## 3.4.2.4. Not Solely the Genioglossus

There are 22 pairs of muscles, other than the genioglossi, being controlled through the brainstem nuclei from the trigeminal to the hypoglossal nerves.[123–127] These muscles also are classified in various different ways—for instance, phasic versus tonic (i.e., those that burst with each inspiration vs. those with constant activity through the respiratory cycle), protruders versus retractors, dilators versus constrictors, or those with or without state dependence (i.e., degree of change in activity at sleep onset).[128,129] Some muscles have phasic expiratory activity, which is related to regulating the expiration rate or assisting in maintaining airway stability during exhalation.[130,131] Pharyngeal muscles may have subtle effects on the airway, as evolution would tend to optimize the system to use the least energy for regular, constant breathing.

Muscles declared to be airway opening or closing based on their anatomy are often activated simultaneously, rather than reciprocally, and such an action can stiffen the airway walls and enlarge the airway lumen more than expected from that activation of the opening muscle alone.[7] Some muscles narrow and stiffen the airway walls,[132] playing a role as airway stabilizers. This occurs throughout the path to and from the lungs.[1] Hence, in sleep the airway primarily needs stability to prevent airway collapse; dilation may be more important for exertion, whether during wakeful activity or to reopen a closed airway.

### 3.4.2.5. The Obstructive Apnea

The diminishment of respiratory control of upper airway muscles is directly associated with an obstructive apnea.[133] The genioglossus has received much investigative attention because EMG recording is safe and informative of brainstem control. Shown in Figure 3.13 is a recording of genioglossal EMG activity before, during, and after an obstructive apnea. In this recording the onset of the obstructive apnea is marked by a reduced EMG activation in the context of a general reduction in drive. Also noted is a change in the onset of activation in that the start of the apnea displays a burst of EMG activity **after** the onset of the inspiratory swing of negative pressure; this is in contrast with the normal anticipatory pre-inspiratory activation shown in Figure 3.11. Recovery occurs after a period of increasing EMG activation and a movement of the onset of the EMG burst to before the onset of the fall in esophageal pressure.

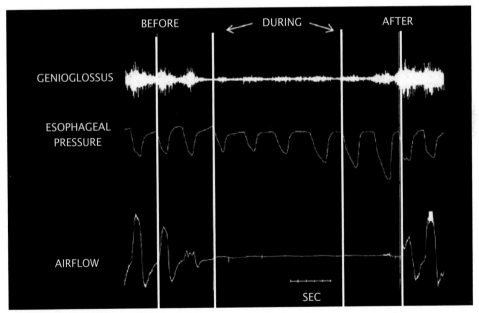

**FIGURE 3.13** The raw genioglossal EMG, airflow at the nose and mouth and esophageal pressure over the course of an obstructive apnea. At the start of the event there is a reduction in both tonic and phasic EMG activity, along with a reduced flow-limited breath and unchanged negative pressure swing. The absence of airflow on the next effort occurs in the setting of an even greater reduction in tonic and phasic activity, and notably a change in the timing of the small, phasic genioglossal EMG activation, which now occurs AFTER the negative deflection of the esophageal pressure. As the apnea progresses, negative pressures swings increase and the recruitment of phasic activation begins to precede the esophageal effort. The termination of an apnea is accompanied by a burst of genioglossal activity.

The genioglossus data are so emphasized in the literature that some believe that the genioglossus is the only muscle that is pathogenetic. In fact, a pattern of a reduction in activation prior to an obstructive apnea (as shown in Figure 3.13) is present in other upper airway muscles such as the alae nasi, TVP, and stylopharyngeus.[38] Indeed, recruitment of muscle activity is a compensatory event, as overweight/obese subjects without apnea are found to have a two- to three-fold higher genioglossal responsiveness than overweight/obese patients with apnea and normal-weight control subjects.[134] The degree of anatomic compromise ($P_{crit}$) was modest. The conclusion is such that there is a degree of enhanced drive to maintain upper airway patency, and in those with OSA that is lost with sleep. These observations support the concept of targeting the central control of upper airway activation as a therapy pathway.

## 3.4.3. Treatment Opportunities Through Neurochemistry

Information about the neurochemistry of state-dependent control of upper airway muscles has accumulated from preclinical models and has spawned approaches to attempt to treat OSA pharmacologically by targeting different aspects of OSA, including loop gain, arousals, and muscle responsiveness. Focusing on brainstem control during sleep, there occurs a sleep-dependent withdrawal of excitation from motor neurons or an active, sleep-related inhibition of motor neurons, such that breathing rate and depth, and cardiovascular tone, generally fall in the transition from wake to NREM sleep (the alpha–theta transition).[102]

One line of research is based on the knowledge that reflex circuits involved in loop gain could be targeted to treat OSA[135]. In this heuristic, the number of pauses in breathing can be reduced by pharmacological manipulation in the afferent ganglions that project to the central pattern generator. In this case one is not fixing the muscles but rather making the central respiratory generator less susceptible to the feedback perturbations (e.g., afferent aspect of loop gain) that reduce drive. Such reflex central apneas in rats could be decreased by dronabinol, an exogenous nonselective cannabinoid type 1 and type 2 (CB1 and CB2) receptor agonist, when dronabinol was injected into the nodose ganglion (inferior ganglion of the vagus nerve). However, dronabinol was ineffective when injected intracerebroventricularly, suggesting that its actions are mediated via suppression at the vagal nerve.[136–139] A pilot one-night study indicated that dronabinol, used off-label, could attenuate human apneas.[140] In a group of patients with a baseline AHI of ~26 per hour, dronabinol was associated with a 35% drop in AHI, improved self-reported sleepiness, and greater overall treatment satisfaction.

Another pharmacological approach is aimed at "waking up" the tongue during sleep. Rodent-derived descriptions of CN XII inputs and outputs comparing wake to NREM and REM sleep identified putative circuits and receptor targets on the pathways controlling upper airway muscles, summarized in a review article.[141] The researchers demonstrated that withdrawal of norepinephrine was responsible for the fall in genioglossus

EMG activity in NREM sleep and the enhancement of cholinergic tone was responsible for the fall in genioglossus EMG tone in REM sleep.

Single-agent studies using desipramine, a high-affinity norepinephrine reuptake inhibitor but a less potent anticholinergic, were not successful in significantly reducing the AHI.[142,143] Hence, the thinking has evolved that two neurotransmitter targets might be needed: noradrenergic reuptake inhibitors (NRIs) and muscarinic receptor antagonists (MRAs). NRIs increase tone in norepinephrine in NREM sleep and lighten but not completely suppress sleep. MRAs can increase sleepiness, and in REM sleep increase genioglossal tone, but suppress REM somewhat.

The combination of atomoxetine (NRI) and oxybutynin (MRA) lowered AHI by 63%, without significant effects by either drug alone.[144] The arousal index remained high and unchanged, while the duration of events was reduced. Probably most important was that the study also measured genioglossus EMG activity and showed that the rate of change in recruitment in the EMG was higher with the drugs than in control situations.[144] This is consistent with a central brainstem effect.

A second laboratory targeting the same pathways measured other EMG responses before and after administration of reboxetine (NRI) and hyoscine butylbromide (MRA) in healthy subjects.[145] Surprisingly, genioglossus muscle EMG activation fell with sleep onset with the drug combination compared to placebo, but tensor palatini EMG activity decreased less with sleep onset with the drugs. In addition, there was evidence for improved upper airway patency by the presence of reduced pharyngeal pressure swings and airway resistance and better respiratory load compensation. These findings show the feasibility of methodologic approaches to understanding pharmacological actions on upper airway function in healthy and OSA subjects.

To summarize this section on neuromuscular control: The upper airway is under active control by a CPG and reflex systems that are derived evolutionarily from an ancient system of muscles that coordinated pumps and valves to move air or fluid/food through a shared pharynx. This role of this neural control system is to keep the upper airway reasonably open during quiet wakefulness and sleep. The bulky genioglossus moves food into, within, and from the mouth and must be kept out of the airway, and other muscles help to do that. The circuits can be exploited, as illustrated by the interventions directed at neurotransmitters and neural circuits that improve OSA.

# 3.5. Considering Hypoglossal Nerve Stimulation

## 3.5.1. Effects on Anterior Pharyngeal Wall

Given this body of physiologic information, we now have a framework to talk about how OSA might be treated by hypoglossal nerve stimulation. However, the remainder of this book will address many details on this therapy. Our approach will be to relate this therapy

(A)    No Stimulation    (B)    Stimulation

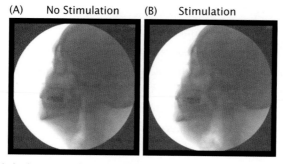

**FIGURE 3.14** Lateral shadow image from a cone beam computed tomography image of a patient **(A)** at rest and **(B)** during the height of hypoglossal nerve stimulation, using the home therapy setting. The concave line from the chin to the lower neck is transformed into a convex pattern by outward movement of the anterior pharyngeal wall.

to upper airway function. We are not aware of imaging of the effects of hypoglossal nerve stimulation during natural sleep, but a number of observations in patients awake and under drug-induced sedation endoscopy are consistent with actions on the size of the oropharyngeal and velopharyngeal regions.[78] On endoscopic visualization, there occurs a forward movement of the tongue and palate, by *unilateral* stimulation of the hypoglossal nerve.[56] Hypoglossal nerve stimulation produces an upward and forward movement of the hyoid and shortening of the tongue length.[78] The action on the velopharynx could occur through multiple mechanisms, through attachments of the palatoglossus to the tongue, the glossopharyngeal slip of the superior pharyngeal constrictor, and attachments to the hyoid bone and force transmitted to the middle constrictor and its associated muscles, in addition to opening the hypopharynx through the hyo-epiglottic ligament and of course the oropharynx. In addition, there is an outward movement of the anterior pharyngeal wall (Figure 3.14). Therefore, the action of hypoglossal nerve stimulation is also to push the tissue away from the posterior pharynx.

## 3.5.2. The Force Produced by Hypoglossal Nerve Stimulation

So how much force does hypoglossal nerve stimulation produce in its action? Our preliminary data suggest that it is substantial (Figure 3.15). We employed a novel, newly constructed set of 22 pressure sensor slips placed in a lower mouthguard, providing average "force" measure in arbitrary units. A subject with an implanted hypoglossal nerve stimulator was tasked to produce maximal force by tongue protrusion, followed by submaximal efforts at 50%, 25%, and 75% of maximal (as determined subjectively), followed by a maximal sustained protrusion. This voluntary activation was performed by the patient before and after measurements of force with nerve stimulation regulated by the implanted device in which the stimulation strength was changed. The patient had used a range of 1.0 to 1.2 mA as therapeutic at home. As illustrated, the force produced by hypoglossal nerve stimulation is in a range of 40% to 70% maximal.

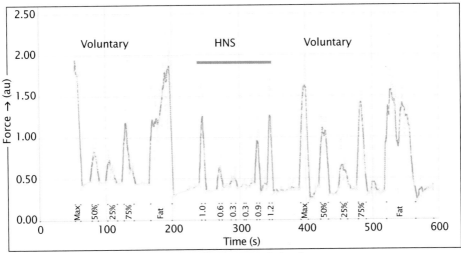

1.0 is the therapeutic level

**FIGURE 3.15** Estimates of force generated by hypoglossal nerve stimulation. Shown on the vertical axis is relative mean force (in arbitrary units) of 22 wafer sensors placed on a lower mouthguard. Values of force are shown during tongue protrusions in the seated posture initially with a maximal voluntary effort (Max), and then 50%, 25%, 75% of maximal force, according to the patient, followed by a maximal protrusion held over time, a fatiguing task (Fat.). The hypoglossal nerve stimulations are at different voltage settings, with 1.0 being the therapeutic level at home, followed by different settings ending with 1.2 volts. The last five are the same voluntary efforts as described above, performed before the stimulation values. Hypoglossal nerve stimulation (HNS) at the level used therapeutically in this patient appears to produce a force that is >50% of the maximal voluntary force. Data collected courtesy of CleveMed, Cleveland, OH, using the INFORM technology.

## 3.5.3. An Integrative Model of the Action of Hypoglossal Nerve Stimulation

The significance of these data is that the therapeutic range of stimulation produces a force that is quite high, substantially above a load that if sustained over time could be fatiguing.[146] This is a supraphysiologic level of activation. Indeed, there is evidence that in OSA itself there can be fatigue of the genioglossus muscle.[147,148] There are no formal reports of muscle fatigue with hypoglossal nerve stimulation, probably because the duty cycle is short enough to permit recovery and/or the load of an open airway is relatively low. One of us (KPS) had a patient report that the effectiveness of the intermittent stimulation seems to wane over several hours, and recover after an hour or so of rest. In the context of this chapter, our conclusion is that current therapy is like using a sledgehammer to open a rusty airway, and fortunately a fatigue response is not common, as patients mostly appear to get sufficient rest for it to maintain effectiveness.

In a healthy airway this level of activation is not needed, as the neuromuscular system maintains patency via tuning the output through the anatomy and the activation of this muscle network. This concept is shown in Figure 3.16. As the upper airway drive falls with sleep onset, patency can be challenged. If there is an appropriate neuromechanical function, airway patency is maintained. Appropriate airway function may not be acquired by

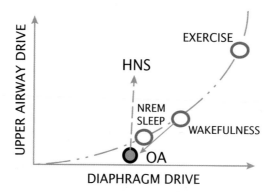

**FIGURE 3.16** This graph indicates the relationship between diaphragmatic drive (x-axis) and upper airway patency (y-axis). This relationship is curvilinear so that from wakefulness patency increases with diaphragm activation during exercise, and in the transition to NREM the fall in drive and patency is proportional and the airway remains patent. In an obstructive apnea (OA) there is a dysfunction in that the airway collapses while diaphragmatic activation persists. The role of hypoglossal nerve stimulation (HNS) is to use its force to open the airway, and it does so without a change in diaphragmatic drive.

anatomic surgery, as the effect of sleep is to downregulate efferent drive and the intensity of afferent input.[149] With variations in drive there are instances where the activation of upper airway drive is insufficient to maintain patency if basal anatomic functioning is vulnerable. Thus, there is a need to "boost" this drive to open the airway for diaphragm drive to produce adequate minute ventilation. The current technology produces a dramatic level of force through hypoglossal nerve stimulation to get around the failure of this system.

## 3.6. Summary and Future Directions

Knowing the upper airway is fundamental for understanding current and trending therapy with neurostimulation. Hypoglossal nerve stimulation has led the field to reconsider its knowledge and understanding of the mechanical properties of the upper airway that promote health as defined by maintenance of upper airway patency during sleep, and the static and dynamic causes for airflow insufficiency producing snoring, and obstructive hypopneas and apnea.

A first step in sleep health, in upper airway terms, is to identify and understand where and how a particular section of the upper airway (e.g. velopharynx, oropharynx, or hypopharynx) is held open while it hangs from the skull and mandible. This may account for the reports of more "curable" outcomes achieved by adjusting the bony structures using maxillomandibular advancement surgery. In contrast, surgical approaches to the soft tissue anatomy and oral appliances are not as predictable as one would like. Surgical implants for neural control are at present second-line therapy but have quite interesting and selective inclusion criteria. Now we have some scientific rationale for pharmacological therapy directed at the brainstem circuits that appear to be involved in upper airway dysfunction during sleep, and its stages. The current medical therapy is not proven as yet, but, in some patients, upper airway patency is better maintained.

What muscles other than the genioglossus are important? Put another way, why do we have all these other muscles in the soft palate and pharynx if not for breathing well during sleep? Anatomy texts have only rarely considered the forces needed for maintenance of the pharyngeal airway when they assign likely functions to muscles based on their attachments. We have much to understand about how these muscles coordinate with the anatomy to form a functional apparatus adjustable for human respiration, feeding, and speech in wakefulness, and stability during sleep. Finally, the upper airway exhibits adaptations and changes in its neuroanatomic functions with posture, growth, development, and probably diet and activity as well. If OSA is caused by the loss of such coordination, it may be useful to approach current and future therapy with an intent to rehabilitate and restore this function.

# References

1. Proctor DF. The naso-oro-pharyngo-laryngeal airway. *Eur J Respir Dis Suppl.* 1983;128 (Pt 1):89–96.
2. Guilleminault C, Huang YS. From oral facial dysfunction to dysmorphism and the onset of pediatric OSA. *Sleep Med Rev.* 2018;40:203–214.
3. Crompton AW, Musinsky C, Bonaparte JR, Bhullar B-A, Owerkowicz T. Evolution of the mammalian fauces region and the origin of suckling. *J Mammal Evol.* (submitted).
4. Dharmarathna I, Miles A, Allen J. Twenty years of quantitative instrumental measures of swallowing in children: A systematic review. *Eur J Pediatr.* 2020;179(2):203–223.
5. Lo Bue A, Salvaggio A, Insalaco G. Obstructive sleep apnea in developmental age: A narrative review. *Eur J Pediatr.* 2020;179(3):357–365.
6. Laitman JT, Reidenberg JS. The evolution and development of human swallowing: The most important function we least appreciate. *Otolaryngol Clin North Am.* 2013;46(6):923–935.
7. Taylor EW, Leite CAC, McKenzxie DJ, Wang T. Control of respiration in fish, amphibians, and reptiles. *Brazil J Med Biol Res.* 2010;43:409–424.
8. Strohl KP, O'Cain CF, Slutsky AS. Alae nasi activation and nasal resistance in healthy subjects. *J Appl Physiol Respir Environ Exerc Physiol.* 1982;52(6):1432–1437.
9. Jokic R, Klimaszewski A, Mink J, Fitzpatrick MF. Surface tension forces in sleep apnea: The role of a soft tissue lubricant: A randomized double-blind, placebo-controlled trial. *Am J Respir Crit Care Med.* 1998;157(5 Pt 1):1522–1525.
10. Kirkness JP, Madronio M, Stavrinou R, et al. Relationship between surface tension of upper airway lining liquid and upper airway collapsibility during sleep in obstructive sleep apnea hypopnea syndrome. *J Appl Physiol.* 2003;95(5):1761–1766.
11. Bilston LE, Gandevia SC. Biomechanical properties of the human upper airway and their effect on its behavior during breathing and in obstructive sleep apnea. *J Appl Physiol.* 2014;116(3):314–324.
12. Dempsey JA, Veasey SC, Morgan BJ, O'Donnell CP. Pathophysiology of sleep apnea. *Physiol Rev.* 2010;90(1):47–112.
13. Remmers JE. Sleeping and breathing. *Chest.* 1990;97(3 Suppl):77S–80S.
14. Pamidi S, Redline S, Rapoport D, et al. An official American Thoracic Society workshop report: Noninvasive identification of inspiratory flow limitation in sleep studies. *Ann Am Thorac Soc.* 2017;14(7):1076–1085.

15. Palombini LO, Tufik S, Rapoport DM, et al. Inspiratory flow limitation in a normal population of adults in Sao Paulo, Brazil. *Sleep.* 2013;36(11):1663–1668.

16. Eckert DJ, White DP, Jordan AS, et al. Defining phenotypic causes of obstructive sleep apnea: Identification of novel therapeutic targets. *Am J Respir Crit Care Med.* 2013;188(8):996–1004.

17. Strohl KP, Butler JP, Malhotra A. Mechanical properties of the upper airway. *Compr Physiol.* 2012;2(3):1853–1872.

18. Macklem PT. Respiratory mechanics. *Ann Rev Physiol.* 1978;40:157–184.

19. Amatoury J, Kairaitis K, Wheatley JR, et al. Peripharyngeal tissue deformation, stress distributions, and hyoid bone movement in response to mandibular advancement. *J Appl Physiol.* 2015;118(3):282–291.

20. Kairaitis K, Stavrinou R, Parikh R, et al. Mandibular advancement decreases pressures in the tissues surrounding the upper airway in rabbits. *J Appl Physiol.* 2006;100(1):349–356.

21. Kairaitis K, Verma M, Fish V, et al. Pharyngeal muscle contraction modifies peri-pharyngeal tissue pressure in rabbits. *Respir Physiol Neurobiol.* 2009;166(2):95–101.

22. Isono S, Tanaka A, Nishino T. Dynamic interaction between the tongue and soft palate during obstructive apnea in anesthetized patients with sleep-disordered breathing. *J Appl Physiol.* 2003;95(6):2257–2264.

23. Kairaitis K, Byth K, Parikh R, et al. Tracheal traction effects on upper airway patency in rabbits: The role of tissue pressure. *Sleep.* 2007;30(2):179–186.

24. Van de Graaff WB. Thoracic traction on the trachea: Mechanisms and magnitude. *J Appl Physiol.* 1991;70(3):1328–1336.

25. Gold AR, Schwartz AR. The pharyngeal critical pressure: The whys and hows of using nasal continuous positive airway pressure diagnostically. *Chest.* 1996;110(4):1077–1088.

26. Hillman DR, Platt PR, Eastwood PR. The upper airway during anaesthesia. *Br J Anaesth.* 2003;91(1):31–39.

27. Mead J. Respiration: Pulmonary mechanics. *Ann Rev Physiol.* 1973;35:169–192.

28. Drain CB. Physiology of respiratory system related to anesthesia. *CRNA.* 1996;7(4):163–180.

29. Isono S, Tanaka A, Ishikawa T, Nishino T. Developmental changes in collapsibility of the passive pharynx during infancy. *Am J Respir Crit Care Med.* 2000;162(3 Pt 1):832–836.

30. Badr MS. Effect of ventilatory drive on upper airway patency in humans during NREM sleep. *Respir Physiol.* 1996;103(1):1–10.

31. Sankri-Tarbichi AG, Rowley JA, Badr MS. Expiratory pharyngeal narrowing during central hypocapnic hypopnea. *Am J Respir Crit Care Med.* 2009;179(4):313–319.

32. Hudgel DW, Martin RJ, Johnson B, Hill P. Mechanics of the respiratory system and breathing pattern during sleep in normal humans. *J Appl Physiol Respir Environ Exerc Physiol.* 1984;56(1):133–137.

33. Wiriyaporn D, Wang L, Aboussouan LS. Expiratory time constant and sleep apnea severity in the overlap syndrome. *J Clin Sleep Med.* 2016;12(3):327–332.

34. Sanders MH, Montserrat JM, Farre R, Givelber RJ. Positive pressure therapy: A perspective on evidence-based outcomes and methods of application. *Proc Am Thoracic Soc.* 2008;5(2):161–172.

35. Okuyama M, Kato S, Sato S, et al. Dynamic behaviour of the soft palate during nasal positive pressure ventilation under anaesthesia and paralysis: Comparison between patients with and without obstructive sleep-disordered breathing. *Br J Anaesth.* 2018;120(1):181–187.

36. Olson LG, Strohl KP. Airway secretions influence upper airway patency in the rabbit. *Am Rev Respir Dis.* 1988;137(6):1379–1381.

37. Olson LG, Strohl KP. Non-muscular factors in upper airway patency in the rabbit. *Respir Physiol.* 1988;71(2):147–155.

38. Suratt PM, McTier R, Wilhoit SC. Alae nasi electromyographic activity and timing in obstructive sleep apnea. *J Appl Physiol.* 1985;58(4):1252–1256.

39. Fouke JM, Teeter JP, Strohl KP. Pressure-volume behavior of the upper airway. *J Appl Physiol.* 1986;61(3):912–918.

40. Teeter JP, Strohl KP, Fouke JM. Comparison of volume changes in the upper airway and thorax. *J Appl Physiol.* 1987;62(1):284–290.

41. Gottfried SB, Strohl KP, Van de Graaff W, et al. Effects of phrenic stimulation on upper airway resistance in anesthetized dogs. *J Appl Physiol Respir Environ Exerc Physiol.* 1983;55(2):419–426.

42. Isono S, Tanaka A, Sho Y, et al. Advancement of the mandible improves velopharyngeal airway patency. *J Appl Physiol.* 1995;79(6):2132–2138.

43. Van de Graaff WB, Gottfried SB, Mitra J, et al. Respiratory function of hyoid muscles and hyoid arch. *J Appl Physiol.* 1984;57(1):197–204.

44. Douglas NJ. Upper airway imaging. *Clin Physics Physiol Measure.* 1990;11(Suppl A):117–119.

45. Kairaitis K, Howitt L, Wheatley JR, Amis TC. Mass loading of the upper airway extraluminal tissue space in rabbits: Effects on tissue pressure and pharyngeal airway lumen geometry. *J Appl Physiol.* 2009;106(3):887–892.

46. Carrigy NB, Carey JP, Martin AR, et al. Simulation of muscle and adipose tissue deformation in the passive human pharynx. *Comput Meth Biomechanics Biomed Eng.* 2016;19(7):780–788.

47. Dhaliwal SS, Hesabgar SM, Haddad SMH, et al. Constructing a patient-specific computer model of the upper airway in sleep apnea patients. *Laryngoscope.* 2018;128(1):277–282.

48. Wellman A, Genta PR, Owens RL, et al. Test of the Starling resistor model in the human upper airway during sleep. *J Appl Physiol.* 2014;117(12):1478–1485.

49. Pham LV, Schwartz AR. The pathogenesis of obstructive sleep apnea. *J Thorac Dis.* 2015;7(8):1358–1372.

50. Bamagoos AA, Cistulli PA, Sutherland K, et al. Polysomnographic endotyping to select obstructive sleep apnea patients for oral appliances. *Ann Am Thoracic Soc.* 2019;16(11):1422–1431.

51. Longobardo GS, Evangelisti CJ, Cherniack NS. Analysis of the interplay between neurochemical control of respiration and upper airway mechanics producing upper airway obstruction during sleep in humans. *Exp Physiol.* 2008;93(2):271–287.

52. Patil SP, Schneider H, Marx JJ, et al. Neuromechanical control of upper airway patency during sleep. *J Appl Physiol.* 2007;102(2):547–556.

53. Isono S, Remmers JE, Tanaka A, et al. Anatomy of pharynx in patients with obstructive sleep apnea and in normal subjects. *J Appl Physiol.* 1997;82(4):1319–1326.

54. Hosselet JJ, Norman RG, Ayappa I, Rapoport DM. Detection of flow limitation with a nasal cannula/pressure transducer system. *Am J Respir Crit Care Med.* 1998;157(5 Pt 1):1461–1467.

55. Kirkness JP, McGinley BM, Sgambati FP, et al. Developing quantitative physiological phenotypes of sleep apnea for epidemiological studies. *Conference proceedings: Annual International Conference of the IEEE Engineering in Medicine and Biology Society IEEE Engineering in Medicine and Biology Society Annual Conference.* 2011;2011:8319–8322.

56. ElShebiny T, Venkat D, Strohl K, et al. Hyoid arch displacement with hypoglossal nerve stimulation. *Am J Respir Crit Care Med.* 2017;196(6):790–792.

57. Vanderveken OM, Maurer JT, Hohenhorst W, et al. Evaluation of drug-induced sleep endoscopy as a patient selection tool for implanted upper airway stimulation for obstructive sleep apnea. *J Clin Sleep Med.* 2013;9(5):433–438.

58. Heiser C, Edenharter G, Bas M, et al. Palatoglossus coupling in selective upper airway stimulation. *Laryngoscope.* 2017;127(10):E378–E383.

59. Perry SF, Similowski T, Klein W, Codd JR. The evolutionary origin of the mammalian diaphragm. *Respir Physiol Neurobiol.* 2010;171(1):1–16.

60. Tong J, Juge L, Burke PG, et al. Respiratory-related displacement of the trachea in obstructive sleep apnea. *J Appl Physiol.* 2019;127(5):1307–1316.

61. deBerry-Borowiecki B, Kukwa A, Blanks RH. Cephalometric analysis for diagnosis and treatment of obstructive sleep apnea. *Laryngoscope.* 1988;98(2):226–234.

62. Yamashiro Y, Kryger M. Is laryngeal descent associated with increased risk for obstructive sleep apnea? *Chest.* 2012;141(6):1407–1413.

63. Levring Jaghagen E, Franklin KA, Isberg A. Snoring, sleep apnoea and swallowing dysfunction: A videoradiographic study. *Dentomaxillofac Radiol.* 2003;32(5):311–316.

64. Su VY, Liu CJ, Wang HK, et al. Sleep apnea and risk of pneumonia: A nationwide population-based study. *CMAJ.* 2014;186(6):415–421.

65. Olszewska E, Woodson BT. Palatal anatomy for sleep apnea surgery. *Laryngoscope Invest Otolaryngol.* 2019;4(1):181–187.

66. Sumida K, Yamashita K, Kitamura S. Gross anatomical study of the human palatopharyngeus muscle throughout its entire course from origin to insertion. *Clin Anat.* 2012;25(3):314–323.

67. Sakamoto Y. Classification of pharyngeal muscles based on innervations from glossopharyngeal and vagus nerves in human. *Surg Radiol Anat.* 2009;31(10):755–761.

68. Meng H, Murakami G, Suzuki D, Miyamoto S. Anatomical variations in stylopharyngeus muscle insertions suggest interindividual and left/right differences in pharyngeal clearance function of elderly patients: A cadaveric study. *Dysphagia.* 2008;23(3):251–257.

69. Standring S. *Gray's Anatomy: The Anatomical Basis of Clinical Practice.* 41st ed. New York: Elsevier Limited; 2016.

70. Logemann JA, Kahrilas PJ, Cheng J, et al. Closure mechanisms of laryngeal vestibule during swallow. *Am J Physiol.* 1992;262(2 Pt 1):G338–344.

71. Kahrilas PJ, Lin S, Rademaker AW, Logemann JA. Impaired deglutitive airway protection: A videofluoroscopic analysis of severity and mechanism. *Gastroenterology.* 1997;113(5):1457–1464.

72. Dodds WJ, Stewart ET, Logemann JA. Physiology and radiology of the normal oral and pharyngeal phases of swallowing. *AJR Am J Roentgenol.* 1990;154(5):953–963.

73. Klebe EA, Holcombe SJ, Rosenstein D, et al. The effect of bilateral glossopharyngeal nerve anaesthesia on swallowing in horses. *Equine Vet J.* 2005;37(1):65–69.

74. Venker-van Haagen AJ, Hartman W, Wolvekamp WT. Contributions of the glossopharyngeal nerve and the pharyngeal branch of the vagus nerve to the swallowing process in dogs. *Am J Vet Res.* 1986;47(6):1300–1307.

75. Tessier C, Holcombe SJ, Derksen FJ, et al. Effects of stylopharyngeus muscle dysfunction on the nasopharynx in exercising horses. *Equine Vet J.* 2004;36(4):318–323.

76. Guilleminault C, Hill MW, Simmons FB, Dement WC. Obstructive sleep apnea: Electromyographic and fiberoptic studies. *Exp Neurol.* 1978;62(1):48–67.

77. Kuna ST. Effects of pharyngeal muscle activation on airway size and configuration. *Am J Respir Crit Care Med.* 2001;164(7):1236–1241.

78. Safiruddin F, Vanderveken OM, de Vries N, et al. Effect of upper-airway stimulation for obstructive sleep apnoea on airway dimensions. *Eur Respir J.* 2015;45(1):129–138.

79. Blumen M, Bequignon E, Chabolle F. Drug-induced sleep endoscopy: A new gold standard for evaluating OSAS? Part II: Results. *Eur Ann Otorhinolaryngol Head Neck Dis.* 2017;134(2):109–115.

80. Okuno K, Sasao Y, Nohara K, et al. Endoscopy evaluation to predict oral appliance outcomes in obstructive sleep apnoea. *Eur Respir J.* 2016;47(5):1410–1419.

81. Kavcic P, Koren A, Koritnik B, et al. Sleep magnetic resonance imaging with electroencephalogram in obstructive sleep apnea syndrome. *Laryngoscope.* 2015;125(6):1485–1490.

82. Huon LK, Liu SY, Shih TT, et al. Dynamic upper airway collapse observed from sleep MRI: BMI-matched severe and mild OSA patients. *Eur Arch Otorhinolaryngol.* 2016;273(11):4021–4026.

83. Sakamoto Y. Gross anatomical observations of attachments of the middle pharyngeal constrictor. *Clin Anat.* 2014;27(4):603–609.

84. Kuna ST, Smickley JS, Vanoye CR. Respiratory-related pharyngeal constrictor muscle activity in normal human adults. *Am J Respir Crit Care Med.* 1997;155(6):1991–1999.

85. Kuna ST, Vanoye CR. Respiratory-related pharyngeal constrictor muscle activity in decerebrate cats. *J Appl Physiol.* 1997;83(5):1588–1594.

86. Sakamoto Y. Spatial relationship between the palatopharyngeus and the superior constrictor of the pharynx. *Surg Radiol Anat.* 2015;37(6):649–655.

87. Schwab RJ, Gefter WB, Hoffman EA, et al. Dynamic upper airway imaging during awake respiration in normal subjects and patients with sleep disordered breathing. *Am Rev Respir Dis.* 1993;148(5):1385–1400.

88. Kuna ST. Regional effects of selective pharyngeal muscle activation on airway shape. *Am J Respir Crit Care Med.* 2004;169(9):1063–1069.

89. Schwab RJ. Properties of tissues surrounding the upper airway. *Sleep.* 1996;19(10 Suppl):S170–S174.

90. Fogel RB, Malhotra A, Pillar G, et al. Genioglossal activation in patients with obstructive sleep apnea versus control subjects. Mechanisms of muscle control. *Am J Respir Crit Care Med.* 2001;164(11):2025–2030.

91. Rood SR, Langdon H, Klueber K, Greenberg E. Muscular anatomy of the tonsil and tonsillar bed: A reexamination. *Otolaryngol Head Neck Surg.* 1979;87(4):401–408.

92. Liem KF, Walker WF. *Functional Anatomy of the Vertebrates: An Evolutionary Perspective.* 3rd ed. Fort Worth, TX: Harcourt College Publishers; 2001.

93. Sauerland EK, Harper RM. The human tongue during sleep: Electromyographic activity of the genioglossus muscle. *Exp Neurol.* 1976;51(1):160–170.

94. Brouillette RT, Thach BT. Control of genioglossus muscle inspiratory activity. *J Appl Physiol Respir Environ Exerc Physiol.* 1980;49(5):801–808.

95. Mathew OP, Abu-Osba YK, Thach BT. Genioglossus muscle responses to upper airway pressure changes: Afferent pathways. *J Appl Physiol Respir Environ Exerc Physiol.* 1982;52(2):445–450.

96. Mezzanotte WS, Tangel DJ, White DP. Waking genioglossal electromyogram in sleep apnea patients versus normal controls (a neuromuscular compensatory mechanism). *J Clin Invest.* 1992;89(5):1571–1579.

97. Katz ES, White DP. Genioglossus activity during sleep in normal control subjects and children with obstructive sleep apnea. *Am J Respir Crit Care Med.* 2004;170(5):553–560.

98. Katz ES, White DP. Genioglossus activity in children with obstructive sleep apnea during wakefulness and sleep onset. *Am J Respir Crit Care Med.* 2003;168(6):664–670.

99. Mezzanotte WS, Tangel DJ, White DP. Influence of sleep onset on upper-airway muscle activity in apnea patients versus normal controls. *Am J Respir Crit Care Med.* 1996;153(6 Pt 1):1880–1887.

100. Strohl KP, Redline S. Nasal CPAP therapy, upper airway muscle activation, and obstructive sleep apnea. *Am Rev Respir Dis.* 1986;134(3):555–558.

101. Fitzpatrick MF, Driver HS, Chatha N, et al. Partitioning of inhaled ventilation between the nasal and oral routes during sleep in normal subjects. *J Appl Physiol.* 2003;94(3):883–890.

102. Benarroch EE. Control of the cardiovascular and respiratory systems during sleep. *Autonom Neurosci Basic Clin.* 2019;218:54–63.

103. Feldman JL, Kam K. Facing the challenge of mammalian neural microcircuits: Taking a few breaths may help. *J Physiol.* 2015;593(1):3–23.

104. Ikeda K, Kawakami K, Onimaru H, et al. The respiratory control mechanisms in the brainstem and spinal cord: Integrative views of the neuroanatomy and neurophysiology. *J Physiol Sci.* 2017;67(1):45–62.

105. Inoue T, Nakayama K, Ihara Y, et al. Coordinated control of the tongue during suckling-like activity and respiration. *J Oral Sci.* 2017;59(2):183–188.

106. Ramirez JM, Baertsch NA. The dynamic basis of respiratory rhythm generation: One breath at a time. *Ann Rev Neurosci.* 2018;41:475–499.

107. Missaghi K, Le Gal JP, Gray PA, Dubuc R. The neural control of respiration in lampreys. *Respir Physiol Neurobiol.* 2016;234:14–25.

108. van Lunteren E, Strohl KP. The muscles of the upper airways. *Clin Chest Med.* 1986;7(2):171–188.

109. Haxhiu MA, Cherniack NS, Mitra J, et al. Nonvagal modulation of hypoglossal neural activity. *Respiration.* 1992;59(2):65–71.

110. Strohl KP, Hensley MJ, Hallett M, et al. Activation of upper airway muscles before onset of inspiration in normal humans. *J Appl Physiol Respir Environ Exerc Physiol.* 1980;49(4):638–642.

111. Haxhiu MA, van Lunteren E, Mitra J, Cherniack NS. Comparison of the response of diaphragm and upper airway dilating muscle activity in sleeping cats. *Respir Physiology.* 1987;70(2):183–193.

112. Haxhiu MA, Mitra J, van Lunteren E, et al. Hypoglossal and phrenic responses to cholinergic agents applied to ventral medullary surface. *Am J Physiol.* 1984;247(6 Pt 2):R939–R944.

113. Weiner D, Mitra J, Salamone J, Cherniack NS. Effect of chemical stimuli on nerves supplying upper airway muscles. *J Appl Physiol Respir Environ Exerc Physiol.* 1982;52(3):530–536.

114. Horner RL. Neural control of the upper airway: Integrative physiological mechanisms and relevance for sleep disordered breathing. *Compr Physiol.* 2012;2(1):479–535.

115. Horner RL, Hughes SW, Malhotra A. State-dependent and reflex drives to the upper airway: Basic physiology with clinical implications. *J Appl Physiol.* 2014;116(3):325–336.

116. Schiefer M, Gamble J, Strohl KP. Sciatic nerve stimulation and its effects on upper airway resistance in the anesthetized rabbit model relevant to sleep apnea. *J Appl Physiol.* 2018;125(3):763–769.

117. Benderro GF, Gamble J, Schiefer MA, et al. Hypoglossal nerve stimulation in a pre-clinical anesthetized rabbit model relevant to OSA. *Respir Physiol Neurobiol.* 2018;250:31–38.

118. Salamone JA, Strohl KP, Weiner DM, et al. Cranial and phrenic nerve responses to changes in systemic blood pressure. *J Appl Physiol Respir Environ Exerc Physiol.* 1983;55(1 Pt 1):61–68.

119. Longobardo GS, Gothe B, Goldman MD, Cherniack NS. Sleep apnea considered as a control system instability. *Respir Physiol.* 1982;50(3):311–333.

120. Younes M. Role of respiratory control mechanisms in the pathogenesis of obstructive sleep disorders. *J Appl Physiol.* 2008;105(5):1389–1405.

121. Phillipson EA. Control of breathing during sleep. *Am Rev Respir Dis.* 1978;118(5):909–939.

122. Yamauchi M, Fujita Y, Kumamoto M, et al. Nonrapid eye movement-predominant obstructive sleep apnea: Detection and mechanism. *J Clin Sleep Med.* 2015;11(9):987–993.

123. Remmers JE, Lahiri S. Regulating the ventilatory pump: A splendid control system prone to fail during sleep. *Am J Respir Crit Care Med.* 1998;157(4 Pt 2):S95–S100.

124. Remmers JE, Launois S, Feroah T, Whitelaw WA. Mechanics of the pharynx in patients with obstructive sleep apnea. *Prog Clin Biol Res.* 1990;345:261–271.

125. Kubin L, Tojima H, Davies RO, Pack AI. Serotonergic excitatory drive to hypoglossal motoneuron in the decerebrate cat. *Neurosci Lett.* 1992;139:243–248.

126. Kubin L, Reignier C, Tojima H, et al. Changes in serotonin level in the hypoglossal nucleus region during carbachol-induced atonia. *Brain Res.* 1994;645(1–2):291–302.

127. Kubin L, Kimura H, Tojima H, et al. Suppression of hypoglossal motoneurons during the carbachol-induced atonia of REM sleep is not caused by fast synaptic inhibition. *Brain Res.* 1993;611(2):300–312.

128. Saboisky JP, Jordan AS, Eckert DJ, et al. Recruitment and rate-coding strategies of the human genioglossus muscle. *J Appl Physiol.* 2010;109(6):1939–1949.

129. Saboisky JP, Chamberlin NL, Malhotra A. Potential therapeutic targets in obstructive sleep apnoea. *Expert Opin Ther Targets.* 2009;13(7):795–809.

130. Kuna ST. Respiratory-related activation and mechanical effects of the pharyngeal constrictor muscles. *Respir Physiol.* 2000;119(2–3):155–161.

131. O'Halloran KD, Herman JK, Bisgard GE. Respiratory-related pharyngeal constrictor muscle activity in awake goats. *Respir Physiol.* 1999;116(1):9–23.

132. Kuna ST, Vanoye CR. Mechanical effects of pharyngeal constrictor activation on pharyngeal airway function. *J Appl Physiol.* 1999;86(1):411–417.

133. Remmers JE, deGroot WJ, Sauerland EK, Anch AM. Pathogenesis of upper airway occlusion during sleep. *J Appl Physiol Respir Environ Exerc Physiol.* 1978;44(6):931–938.

134. Sands SA, Eckert DJ, Jordan AS, et al. Enhanced upper-airway muscle responsiveness is a distinct feature of overweight/obese individuals without sleep apnea. *Am J Respir Crit Care Med.* 2014;190(8):930–937.

135. Carley DW, Prasad B, Reid KJ, et al. Pharmacotherapy of apnea by cannabimimetic enhancement, the PACE clinical trial: Effects of dronabinol in obstructive sleep apnea. *Sleep.* 2018;41(1):zsx184.

136. Calik MW, Carley DW. Cannabinoid type 1 and type 2 receptor antagonists prevent attenuation of serotonin-induced reflex apneas by dronabinol in Sprague-Dawley rats. *PLoS One.* 2014;9(10):e111412.

137. Calik MW, Carley DW. Intracerebroventricular injections of dronabinol, a cannabinoid receptor agonist, does not attenuate serotonin-induced apnea in Sprague-Dawley rats. *J Negat Results Biomed.* 2016;15:8.

138. Calik MW, Carley DW. Effects of cannabinoid agonists and antagonists on sleep and breathing in Sprague-Dawley Rats. *Sleep.* 2017;40(9):zsx112.

139. Radulovacki M, Pavlovic S, Saponjic J, Carley DW. Modulation of reflex and sleep related apnea by pedunculopontine tegmental and intertrigeminal neurons. *Respir Physiol Neurobiol.* 2004;143(2–3):293–306.

140. Prasad B, Radulovacki MG, Carley DW. Proof of concept trial of dronabinol in obstructive sleep apnea. *Front Psychiatry.* 2013;4:1.

141. Horner RL, Grace KP, Wellman A. A resource of potential drug targets and strategic decision-making for obstructive sleep apnoea pharmacotherapy. *Respirology.* 2017;22(5):861–873.

142. Taranto-Montemurro L, Sands SA, Edwards BA, et al. Desipramine improves upper airway collapsibility and reduces OSA severity in patients with minimal muscle compensation. *Eur Respir J.* 2016;48(5):1340–1350.

143. Taranto-Montemurro L, Edwards BA, Sands SA, et al. Desipramine increases genioglossus activity and reduces upper airway collapsibility during non-REM sleep in healthy subjects. *Am J Respir Crit Care Med.* 2016;194(7):878–885.

144. Taranto-Montemurro L, Messineo L, Sands SA, et al. The combination of atomoxetine and oxybutynin greatly reduces obstructive sleep apnea severity: A randomized, placebo-controlled, double-blind crossover trial. *Am J Respir Crit Care Med.* 2019;199(10):1267–1276.

145. Lim R, Carberry JC, Wellman A, et al. Reboxetine and hyoscine butylbromide improve upper airway function during nonrapid eye movement and suppress rapid eye movement sleep in healthy individuals. *Sleep.* 2019;42(4):zsy261.

146. Derenne JP, Macklem PT, Roussos C. The respiratory muscles: Mechanics, control, and pathophysiology. Part III. *Am Rev Respir Dis.* 1978;118(3):581–601.

147. Li WY, Gakwaya S, Saey D, Series F. Assessment of tongue mechanical properties using different contraction tasks. *J Appl Physiol.* 2017;123(1):116–125.

148. Mortimore IL, Bennett SP, Douglas NJ. Tongue protrusion strength and fatiguability: Relationship to apnoea/hypopnoea index and age. *J Sleep Res.* 2000;9(4):389–393.

149. Strohl M, Strohl K, Palomo JM, Ponsky D. Hypoglossal nerve stimulation rescue surgery after multiple multilevel procedures for obstructive sleep apnea. *Am J Otolaryngol.* 2016;37(1):51–53.

# Clinical Protocol in the Multidisciplinary Setting

Jonathan Waxman, Kerolos Shenouda, Ho-sheng Lin, and Safwan Badr

## 4.1. Introduction

The pathogenesis of obstructive sleep apnea (OSA) is related to numerous interacting processes that directly or indirectly alter upper airway patency, including anatomic abnormalities, impaired pharyngeal dilator muscle function, sleep stability and arousal threshold, ventilatory control stability, autonomic dysfunction, and genetic factors.[1] Given the complex multifactorial pathophysiology of OSA, as well as an increasing awareness of its immense societal impact, the diagnosis and management of OSA is a multidisciplinary endeavor and frequently involves multiple medical and nonmedical practitioners employing multiple treatment modalities. While the majority of OSA patients initially present to primary care physicians, sleep medicine specialists, pulmonologists, or otolaryngologists, reports of OSA in the outpatient setting may arise from over 100 other surgical and nonsurgical specialists, including neurologists, cardiologists, and psychiatrists.[2] In particular, the role of the otolaryngologist has long been established in the care of OSA patients, as Fujita et al. described the treatment of OSA with uvulopalatopharyngoplasty (UPPP) in 1981, the same year that Sullivan et al. first described continuous positive airway pressure (CPAP).

The therapeutic options for OSA are diverse and include exercise training[3] and weight loss;[4] positional therapy;[5] myofunctional therapy;[6] oral appliance therapy; CPAP; single-level or multilevel nasal, oropharyngeal, or hypopharyngeal surgery; and most recently upper airway stimulation therapy. The type of therapy a patient ultimately chooses depends on several factors, such as disease severity, medical comorbidities, symptoms, anthropometric measurements, site and pattern of airway collapse, patient preference, and the type of physician to whom the patient initially presents. The most efficacious treatment for OSA is CPAP;[7] for this reason, CPAP remains the gold standard and first-line treatment modality. Unfortunately, many people are unable to tolerate CPAP, and low rates of adherence have persisted for the past two decades despite behavioral intervention and patient coaching efforts.[8] For patients who fail CPAP or prefer an alternative, the use of an oral appliance or mandibular advancement device custom made by a dentist may be beneficial.[9] While not as effective as CPAP in decreasing the apnea–hypopnea index (AHI), mandibular advancement devices can improve daytime sleepiness, energy levels, and vigilance and are as effective as CPAP at reducing the risk of cardiovascular mortality. However, like CPAP, long-term adherence is low,[10] and their use is limited to those with adequate dentition, good mandibular protrusion, and mild to moderate OSA, and individuals who are not morbidly obese.[7] Therefore, for many individuals who are unable to use CPAP, surgical treatment is the best next step.

OSA surgery aims to restore airway patency by removing or displacing obstructing tissue along the upper airway or by increasing the size of the airway via reconstructive techniques. The recognition that obstruction may occur at more than one anatomic level has led to multilevel surgical approaches in which more than one surgical procedure is performed at the nasal, soft palate, oropharyngeal, and/or hypopharyngeal levels.[11] Historically, tracheostomy was the primary surgical modality to treat OSA; while effective, it is now reserved for individuals who fail medical management and are not suitable candidates for other surgical options.[12] Nasal surgery, such as septoplasty and inferior turbinate reduction, has an inconsistent impact on AHI but may improve quality of life and CPAP adherence.[13] The most common surgical procedure for OSA is UPPP. However, studies have demonstrated poor outcomes for UPPP in isolation when used to treat OSA in all but a select group of patients. Consequently, variations of UPPP, as well as palatopharyngeal reconstructive procedures, have been introduced.[14,15] Several palatal reconstructive procedures have been proposed for lateral pharyngeal wall collapse, such as lateral pharyngoplasty and expansion sphincter pharyngoplasty. Other procedures described to address specific shortcomings of UPPP and improve outcomes include anterior palatoplasty, uvulopalatal flap, z-palatoplasty, and relocation pharyngoplasty. Surgical techniques designed to address obstruction at the level of the tongue base include radiofrequency, coblation, and transoral robotic tongue base reduction, genioglossus advancement, and hyoid suspension. For patients who are refractory to other surgical modalities, maxillomandibular advancement may be an effective option, although it is a highly invasive procedure with significant risks.[16] Frequently, more than one of these surgeries are performed in a single-stage or multistaged manner to achieve correction of anatomic abnormalities at multiple levels of the upper airway. The effect of different surgical techniques on OSA is inconsistent, and the comparative and differential impact of these procedures has not been fully studied.[17] Moreover, it is unclear which patients will benefit the most from surgery or from which type of surgery.

A recent novel therapy for OSA is electrical stimulation of the hypoglossal nerve, also known as upper airway stimulation (UAStim). By stimulating the hypoglossal nerve during sleep continuously or in synchrony with respiration, tongue muscle activity is increased to protrude and stiffen the tongue, preventing it from prolapsing into the pharynx. There is evidence that UAStim has a multilevel mechanism of action, as its therapeutic effect is evident at both the level of the palate and tongue base.[18,19] Recent studies have demonstrated that UAStim is effective;[20,21] however, optimal patient selection strategies and predictors of success are not yet well defined.

While each patient's journey is unique and guidelines should be patient-oriented, given the complex nature of OSA and its relationship to the healthcare system, a well-defined clinical protocol delineating each step in the diagnosis and treatment of OSA can help clinicians, as well as patients, navigate clinical boundaries and different treatment settings. In this chapter we describe a multidisciplinary evidence-based clinical protocol for the diagnosis and management of OSA for patients who plan to undergo UAStim therapy. A flowchart of the proposed clinical protocol is depicted in Figure 4.1.

At the time of this writing, there are three available UAStim systems for which clinical data have been published:

Inspire II Upper Airway Stimulation device (Inspire Medical Systems, Inc, Maple Grove, MN)[22]
aura6000 targeted hypoglossal neurostimulation device (LivaNova, PLC, London, England)[23]
Genio dual-sided hypoglossal nerve stimulation system (Nyxoah S.A., Belgium)[24]

Currently, only the Inspire II device has been approved by the U.S. Food and Drug Administration (FDA). Therefore, most of the work cited in this chapter focuses on this device.

## 4.2. Initial Evaluation

A common evaluation and treatment model for OSA involves referral by a primary care provider to a sleep specialist physician. At this time, there is insufficient evidence to support screening for OSA in asymptomatic individuals, and validated screening tools to predict which asymptomatic patients should receive further testing for OSA is lacking.[25] Moreover, the American Academy of Sleep Medicine (AASM) strongly recommends that screening tools should not be used to diagnose OSA in adults without objective testing. There are currently no validated screening instruments oriented specifically toward individuals who may benefit from UAStim.

In some cases, the initial workup for OSA is performed by a primary care provider or by a specialist other than a sleep physician. In any scenario, the diagnostic

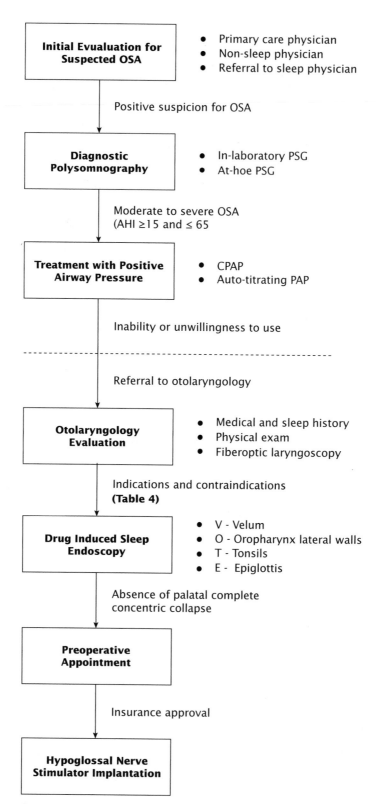

**FIGURE 4.1** Clinical protocol for UAStim therapy

workup for OSA and eventual consideration for UAStim therapy begins with a sleep history and physical examination, including an assessment of anthropometric variables.[26] Information gathered from the patient or bedpartner should include presence of snoring, witnessed apneas, choking or gasping during sleep, and excessive daytime sleepiness. The severity of daytime sleepiness may be assessed using the Epworth Sleepiness Scale, the most commonly used subjective assessment of sleepiness.[27]

A thorough medical history should identify any conditions associated with an increased risk for OSA, including obesity, hypertension, stroke, diabetes, congestive heart failure, atrial fibrillation, pulmonary hypertension, chronic obstructive pulmonary disease, and asthma. A thorough sleep history should include the presence of other sleep disorders, such as insomnia or restless leg syndrome.

Physical examination should include the respiratory, cardiovascular, and neurologic systems. In particular, patients should be assessed for obesity and physical characteristics suggestive of upper airway narrowing. Findings that may suggest OSA are listed in Box 4.1.

Specific criteria related to UAStim and possible exclusion from implantation may be considered at this point. Inclusion and exclusion criteria from clinical studies published for three UAStim systems are listed in Table 4.1 and may provide guidance regarding which patients should continue along the UAStim treatment pathway. The phase II and III studies for the Inspire II system excluded patients with neuromuscular diseases, neurologic disorders, pulmonary diseases, severe cardiac dysfunction, uncontrolled hypertension, psychiatric disease, and other sleep disorders. Also, the Inspire II device is currently indicated for adults 22 years of age and older; however, UAStim therapy for children with Down syndrome is currently under investigation.[28,29] In addition, when the Inspire II device was evaluated in morbidly obese patients with OSA during the phase II study, there was a greater likelihood of failure.[30] Consequently, individuals with a body mass index (BMI) greater than 32 kg/m$^2$ may not be ideal candidates for UAStim therapy. However, recent data demonstrate that patients with a BMI greater than 32 kg/m$^2$ may be successfully treated with UAStim therapy.[31,32]

# 4.3. Polysomnography

Following evaluation for suspected OSA, objective testing is obtained to diagnose and assess the severity and type of sleep apnea. The standard diagnostic test for OSA is in-laboratory attended polysomnography (PSG), also referred to as type I PSG. Type I PSG typically takes place at a sleep laboratory where the patient sleeps overnight while physiologic signals, including electroencephalography, electro-oculography, chin electromyography, electrocardiography, airflow, respiratory effort, and pulse oximetry, are continuously monitored by a sleep laboratory technician or technologist.

## BOX 4.1 Conditions Associated with an Increased Risk of OSA

**High-Risk Factors for OSA**

Obesity (BMI >35 kg/m$^2$)

Congestive heart failure

Atrial fibrillation

Hypertension refractory to treatment

Type 2 diabetes

Nocturnal dysrhythmias

Stroke

Pulmonary hypertension

**Signs**

BMI $\geq$ 30 kg/m$^2$

Modified Mallampati score of 3 or 4

Retrognathia

Lateral peritonsillar narrowing

Macroglossia

Tonsillar hypertrophy

Elongated/enlarged uvula

High-arched or narrow hard palate

Nasal polyps, deviated septum, or turbinate hypertrophy

Overjet

**Symptoms**

Snoring

Witnessed apneas

Choking or gasping during sleep

Excessive daytime sleepiness

Nonrefreshing sleep

Sleep fragmentation

Maintenance insomnia

Nocturia

Morning headaches

Decreased concentration

Memory loss

Irritability

Decreased libido

Data from references 1 and 2.

**TABLE 4.1 Inclusion and Exclusion Criteria of Clinical Trials for Available UAStim Systems**

| System | Inclusion Criteria | Exclusion Criteria |
|---|---|---|
| Inspire II[65] | 1. Adults<br>2. AHI ≥ 20 and ≤ 50, central apneas + mixed apneas < 25%<br>3. BMI ≤ 32 kg/m² | 1. Pronounced anatomic abnormalities preventing effective use or assessment of upper airway stimulation (e.g., tonsil size 3 or 4)<br>2. Complete retropalatal concentric collapse observed during DISE<br>3. Neuromuscular disease<br>4. Hypoglossal nerve palsy<br>5. Severe restrictive or obstructive pulmonary disease<br>6. Moderate to severe pulmonary arterial hypertension<br>7. Severe valvular heart disease<br>8. New York Heart Association class III or IV heart failure<br>9. Recent myocardial infarction or severe cardiac arrhythmias within the past 6 months<br>10. Persistent uncontrolled hypertension despite medication use<br>11. Active psychiatric disease<br>12. Coexisting nonrespiratory sleep disorders |
| aura6000[23] | 1. Adults<br>2. AHI ≥ 20, central apneas <10%<br>3. BMI ≤ 37 kg/m² | 1. Clinically enlarged tonsils (3⁺ or 4⁺)<br>2. Modified Mallampati IV<br>3. Presence of nasal obstruction<br>4. Syndromic craniofacial abnormalities<br>5. Epiglottic obstruction<br>6. Evidence of positional OSA (as judged from baseline polysomnography as >50% reduction in AHI between supine and nonsupine positions)<br>7. Other active implanted medical devices |
| Genio[24] | 1. 21–75 years of age<br>2. AHI ≥ 20 and ≤ 60, central apnea index + mixed AHI <10<br>3. BMI <32 kg/m² | 1. Participants with chemical abuse history within the previous 3 years<br>2. Unable to provide or incapable of providing informed written consent<br>3. Unwilling to return or incapable of returning for all follow-up visits and sleep studies, including evaluation procedures and filling out questionnaires<br>4. Presence of another active implantable medical device, specifically pacemaker or implantable cardioverter-defibrillator<br>5. Participants who are or have been implanted with a hypoglossal nerve stimulation device<br>6. Diagnosed coagulopathy or taking anticoagulant medications that cannot be temporarily be bridged or stopped to allow surgery to take place<br>7. Shift workers<br>8. Pregnant or plan to become pregnant within the next 12 months or breastfeeding<br>9. Patient with life expectancy <12 months<br>10. Surgical resection or radiation therapy for cancer or congenital malformations in the larynx, tongue, or throat<br>11. Hypoglossal nerve palsy or patients with degenerative neurologic disorder<br>12. Previous surgery on the soft tissue of the upper airway performed within 12 weeks of scheduled implant<br>13. Obvious fixed upper airway obstructions<br>14. Any chronic medical illness or condition that contraindicates a surgical procedure under general anesthesia<br>15. Participants with prior surgery to the mandible and/or maxilla<br>16. Presence of CCC of the soft palate on endoscopy<br>17. Any functional or structural problem that would impair the ability of a hypoglossal nerve stimulator to treat OSA<br>18. Medications such as opiates that may affect sleep, alertness, or breathing |

Due to the relatively high cost and time requirement of type I PSG, the modified home-based, or type III, PSG was introduced that records sleep data while a patient sleeps at home. A type III PSG records two respiratory signals (e.g., respiratory movement and airflow), a cardiac signal (e.g., heart rate or electrocardiography), and pulse oximetry. AASM guidelines recommend home testing as an alternative to in-laboratory testing for patients with a high pretest probability of moderate to severe OSA without comorbidities or other sleep disorders or when in-laboratory PSG is not possible due to immobility, safety, or critical illness.[33]

Noninferiority of type III PSG to type I PSG has been demonstrated in random-ized clinical trials.[34] However, the cost-effectiveness for both payers and providers has not been established and may only apply to a subset of patients.[35,36] Nevertheless, home testing for OSA is increasingly popular and may be employed by primary care phys-icians and specialists other than sleep physicians. There is high-level evidence that sug-gests the clinical equivalence of primary care and specialist models for the diagnosis and care of OSA patients,[37] and the involvement of non-sleep physicians at this stage may help to compensate for the lack of availability of sleep laboratories and sleep specialists.[38] However, other comparative effectiveness studies have shown improved outcomes for OSA patients associated with AASM accreditation and Sleep Medicine certification status of physicians and sleep centers.[39] When initially evaluated by a non-sleep specialist, a pa-tient should be referred to a sleep physician for a type I PSG (1) when there is a mismatch between clinical and type III PSG findings, (2) when a sleep disorder other than OSA is suspected, or (3) when there are severe or multiple comorbidities.

Many clinical parameters related to respiratory, cardiac, neurologic, and move-ment status during sleep are derived from PSG and used in scoring a sleep study.[40] For the diagnosis of OSA, the most commonly used PSG-derived metric is the apnea–hypopnea index (AHI), which reflects the number of apnea and hypopnea events per hour of sleep. An apnea is defined as a >90% drop from baseline in a respiratory signal for ≥10 seconds. An apnea is considered obstructive if there is continued or increased inspiratory effort throughout the period of the apnea. The AASM-recommended definition of a hypopnea is a drop in peak signal excursion of a respiratory signal by ≥30% of the pre-event baseline for ≥10 seconds with an associ-ated oxygen desaturation of ≥3% from baseline. However, there are other definitions of hypopnea that may be employed. For instance, in clinical trials that have inves-tigated UAStim systems, the hypopnea score was based on a 30% airflow reduction with a 4% oxygen desaturation.[23,24,41] Importantly, varying hypopnea definitions may affect OSA diagnosis and cardiovascular associations.[42] In addition, the duration as well as the frequency of disordered breathing events may have an impact on mortality risk;[43] however, event duration is not currently included in the classification of OSA severity. Despite some controversy and a developing understanding of the impact of sleep parameters on OSA severity, OSA is defined as mild for an AHI between 5 and 15, moderate for an AHI between 15 and 30, and severe for an AHI >30. There may be significant night-to-night variability of OSA and, consequently, variability of AHI, especially in patients with mild OSA.[44,45] Nevertheless, the AHI obtained from a single night in-laboratory or home-based PSG is frequently used to diagnose OSA and determine initial eligibility for UAStim therapy.

When in-laboratory testing is performed, patients with uncomplicated OSA may undergo a split-night diagnostic protocol during which CPAP titration is performed following a diagnosis of OSA during the same night. This is recommended only when moderate to severe OSA is observed during the PSG for ≥2 hours and ≥3 hours are available for CPAP titration.[46] While considered to provide adequate accuracy for the diagnosis of OSA, the cost-effectiveness of split-night PSG has been questioned.[47]

The results of PSG mark a second point in the clinical protocol to determine if a patient may proceed with UAStim therapy. Based on data from the Inspire II feasibility study, the device is currently indicated for individuals with an AHI from 15 to 65 with <25% central apneas.[30] However, the ability to predict success based on AHI is modest at best,[48] and there is some evidence of UAStim therapy success for patients with an AHI outside this range.[32] Further study is required to reconsider the AHI indications for UAStim therapy.

# 4.4. Treatment with Positive Airway Pressure

Once a technically adequate in-laboratory or home-based PSG has been obtained and a diagnosis of OSA is made, treatment with CPAP should be initiated. Although not curative, CPAP is effective in suppressing disordered breathing and may improve daytime sleepiness,[49] cardiovascular function,[50] cognitive function,[51] and quality of life.[52] Even suboptimal adherence to CPAP may significantly improve sleepiness;[53] however, other studies demonstrate a decrease in daytime performance with just a single night of CPAP withdrawal in otherwise compliant patients.[54]

CPAP adherence is commonly defined as using the device for ≥4 hours per night for ≥70% of the nights monitored. Unfortunately, despite low morbidity and high effectiveness, CPAP adherence is <40% and has remained low for the past two decades.[8] Common barriers to usage include patients' uncertainty about their OSA diagnosis and need for CPAP, feeling ashamed of needing CPAP, difficulties in using the mask and traveling with CPAP, claustrophobia and anxiety, nasal congestion, dry throat, and eye irritation.[55] If patients have a negative experience with CPAP very early in their usage, they are unlikely to continue long-term usage.[56]

While CPAP delivers a continuous level of airway pressure determined by in-laboratory titration, patients may alternatively be started on home-based auto-titrating PAP (APAP), which employs algorithms to detect the onset of abnormal breathing and adaptively titrate and control pressure levels throughout the night. An APAP device can be used to titrate to a constant pressure level or may be left in auto-titrating mode. APAP was introduced to improve conventional CPAP by reducing the cost of attended titration studies, reduce average pressure exposure, and increase adherence. AASM guidelines recommend either APAP or CPAP for ongoing treatment of OSA; however, the results of comparative meta-analyses are mixed,[57,58] and the cost-effectiveness of APAP has not been conclusively established.[59] Furthermore, APAP may not be as effective as CPAP in reducing major OSA-associated cardiovascular risk factors.[60] This may be due to residual abnormal breathing events during APAP resulting from imperfect detection algorithms.[61] Further comparative studies are needed as the technology continues to improve.

For patients who are unable or unwilling to use CPAP, alternative therapies may be offered, including weight loss, positional therapy, oral appliance therapy, or surgery.[26] Referral to a medical weight loss program may be beneficial for patients regardless of the treatment modality they choose, and should be considered on a case-by-case basis. Patients contemplating surgical treatment for OSA, including UAStim therapy, should be referred to an otolaryngologist with expertise in sleep surgery.

# 4.5. Referral to Otolaryngology

All patients referred to otolaryngology for evaluation of UAStim therapy should undergo a thorough medical and sleep history to determine eligibility. Weight, height, and BMI should be obtained. A complete head and neck physical examination should be performed with a focus on anatomic factors that might predispose to upper airway collapse, such as tonsil size, palatal length and presence of redundant palatal tissue, macroglossia, and tongue position (rated with the Friedman classification and modified Mallampati classification). Flexible fiberoptic laryngoscopy should be performed to visualize and evaluate the nasopharynx, oropharynx, hypopharynx, and supraglottic larynx for narrowing of the airway space. At this point, surgical options other than UAStim may be recommended to patients with anatomic factors that may interfere with the assessment or successful function of UAStim—for example, size 3 or 4 tonsils.

Patients who are thus far eligible for UAStim therapy must next undergo drug-induced sleep endoscopy (DISE) prior to surgery to determine the type and pattern of upper airway collapse. During DISE, collapse of the upper airway is directly visualized in the operating room with fiberoptic endoscopy under conditions of sedation thought to mimic natural sleep. The most common sedative drugs used during DISE are propofol, midazolam, and dexmedetomidine. The following is a description of how a DISE may be performed. During DISE, no other sedating medications such as benzodiazepines or ketamine should be administered. Glycopyrrolate may be administered preoperatively to reduce secretions. Once in the operating room, a nasal cannula is placed between the lips and the patient is oxygenated at 2 to 4 L/min. The inside of the nose is anesthetized with topical 4% lidocaine and oxymetazoline. Propofol is administered by an anesthesiologist with an infusion pump and is titrated slowly upward until the patient falls asleep and starts to snore. Once the patient appears to be asleep, a flexible pediatric bronchoscope is advanced through the patient's nose and structures of the nasopharynx, oropharynx, hypopharynx, and supraglottic larynx are evaluated and patterns of collapse are recorded.

There are numerous classification systems to describe the location and pattern of upper airway collapse observed during DISE, none of which is universally accepted.[62] Several include information that could be used to screen for UAStim eligibility and are listed in Table 4.2. The most common classification system discussed in the literature is the Velum, Oropharyngeal walls, Tonsils, Epiglottis (VOTE) system.[63] The system was designed on the premise that the most common structures involved in upper airway collapse are the velum, the oropharyngeal lateral walls, the tonsils, and the epiglottis. During DISE, the degree of obstruction at each region is assigned a value of 0 to 2 (0 = no obstruction, 1 = partial obstruction, and 2 = total obstruction). Also, the configuration of airway collapse (i.e., anteroposterior, lateral, or concentric) is recorded for each region. Velopharyngeal obstruction may be related to soft palate, uvula, or lateral pharyngeal wall tissue and may demonstrate any configuration. Lateral collapse of the oropharyngeal lateral walls may involve the palatine tonsils or the lateral pharyngeal wall tissues. Tongue base collapse may occur in an anteroposterior configuration. Obstruction at the level of the epiglottis may be in an anteroposterior or lateral configuration. In many patients, upper airway collapse is not limited to a single region; rather, collapse is commonly observed at multiple anatomic regions, which may be captured by the VOTE system.

During the phase II study for the Inspire II system, seven participants underwent DISE prior to implantation. The three patients who responded to UAStim did not have complete concentric collapse (CCC) at the level of the soft palate, and all four patients who did not respond to UAStim had CCC at the level of the soft palate.[30] A subsequent study of 21 patients with moderate to severe OSA who underwent DISE prior to implantation with the Inspire II system demonstrated a significant decrease in AHI in patients without palatal CCC and no significant decrease in AHI in patients with palatal CCC.[64] The authors concluded that the absence of CCC at the level of the palate could predict therapeutic success of UAStim and that DISE should be used as a patient selection tool for UAStim. Consequently, the phase III clinical trial (Stimulation Therapy for Apnea Reduction [STAR] trial) for the Inspire II system excluded patients with palatal CCC observed during DISE using the VOTE system.[65] CCC is also now considered a contraindication to implantation.

A post-hoc analysis of the STAR trial data found that of the 170 participants without palatal CCC who were included, 96% had multilevel collapse.[66] The velum and tongue base were the most common sites of obstruction. In addition, UAStim responders at 12 months had lower baseline VOTE scores compared to nonresponders. Nonresponders had a higher proportion of complete anteroposterior or lateral collapse at the level of the velum and epiglottis.

Following DISE, the surgeon should have all the information required to determine final eligibility for UAStim therapy. At this point in the clinical protocol, patients without

**TABLE 4.2  DISE Classification Systems That May Be Used to Screen for UAStim Eligibility**

| Author, year | Classification | Description/Rating System |
|---|---|---|
| Iwanaga, 2003[68] | Soft palate | Uvula and soft palate come into contact with the posterior pharyngeal wall |
| | Circumferential palatal | Full-circumference soft palatal airway obstruction involving the posterior and lateral pharyngeal walls |
| | Tonsillar | Palatine tonsils come into contact in the midline during expiration |
| | Root of tongue | Soft palatal plus and tongue base obstruction |
| | Mixed | Obstruction purely at the root of the tongue |
| Kezirian, 2011[63] | Velum<br>Oropharynx lateral walls<br>Tongue base<br>Epiglottis | Each structure receives a rating for degree of obstruction (0 = no obstruction [<50%], 1 = partial obstruction [50–75%], 2 = complete obstruction [>75%]) and configuration of obstruction (anteroposterior [AP], lateral, concentric)[a] |
| Vicini, 2012[69] | Nose | 1 = 0–25%, 2 = 25–50%, 3 = 50–75%, 4 = 75–100% |
| | Oropharynx/retropalatal | 1 = 0–25%, 2 = 25–50%, 3 = 50–75%, 4 = 75–100% |
| | Hypopharynx/base of tongue | 1 = 0–25%, 2 = 25–50%, 3 = 50–75%, 4 = 75–100% |
| | Larynx | Positive/negative collapse |
| Koo, 2013[70] | Retropalatal<br>  Palate (AP diameter)<br>  LPW (lateral diameter)<br>  Tonsil (contributing structure)<br>Retrolingual<br>  Tongue base (AP diameter)<br>  Lateral pharyngeal wall (lateral diameter)<br>  Epiglottis (contributing structure) | Each structure receives a rating for degree of obstruction (0 = no obstruction [<50%], 1 = partial obstruction [50–75%], 2 = complete obstruction [>75%]) |
| Herzog, 2015[71] | Pharyngeal collapse at velum level | I° = no collapse, II° = lateral collapse (<50%), III° = lateral collapse (>50%), IV° = circular collapse (<50%), V° = circular collapse (>50%) |
| | Uvula/palate contact to posterior pharyngeal wall | I° = no contact, II° = contact of the tip of the uvula, III° = contact of half of the uvula, IV° = contact of the base of the uvula/palate |
| | Dorsal movement of the tongue base | I° = vallecula completely visible, II° = vallecula partially visible, III° = vallecula not visible, IV° = contact to the posterior pharyngeal wall |
| | Pharyngeal collapse at tongue base level | I° = no collapse, II° = lateral collapse (<50%), III° = lateral collapse (>50%), IV° = circular collapse (<50%), V° = circular collapse (>50%) |
| Carrasco-Llatas, 2017[72] | Velum<br>Oropharynx lateral walls<br>Tongue base<br>Epiglottis | Each structure receives a rating for degree of obstruction (0 = no obstruction [<50%], 1 = partial obstruction [50–75%], 2 = complete obstruction [>75%]) and configuration of obstruction (AP, lateral, concentric)[b] |
| Veer, 2016[62] | Palate | P1 = no obstruction, P2 = AP obstruction, P3 = circumferential collapse |
| | Tonsils | T1 = no obstruction, T2 = <50% obstruction, T3 = >50% obstruction |

**TABLE 4.2 Continued**

| Author, year | Classification | Description/Rating System |
|---|---|---|
| | Lateral pharyngeal wall | L1 = no obstruction, L2 = <50% obstruction, L3 = >50% obstruction |
| | Tongue base | Tb1 = no obstruction, Tb2 = <50% obstruction, Tb3 = >50% obstruction |
| | Epiglottis | E1 = no trap door phenomenon, E2 = collapses down on the glottis aperture during inspiration |

[a] Structure/configurations that cannot be visualized include oropharynx lateral walls/AP, tongue base/lateral, oropharynx lateral walls/concentric, tongue base/concentric, and epiglottis/concentric.
[b] Structure/configurations that cannot be visualized include oropharynx lateral walls/AP, oropharynx lateral walls/concentric, and epiglottis/concentric.

palatal CCC may be offered UAStim implantation. The complete set of indications and contraindications for the Inspire II system is listed in Box 4.2.

# 4.6. Insurance Coverage

The last step prior to surgery is to obtain insurance authorization. Access to insurance coverage for the Inspire II device, the only device currently approved by the FDA, has significantly improved in recent years. While there is currently no Medicare national coverage policy for UAStim implantation, there are some policies at the local or regional level. The Inspire system is currently included in the Government Services Administration Federal Supply Schedule, which makes it available to active military members, veterans, and their beneficiaries at select Veterans Administration hospitals. According to current 2020 information provided by the Inspire website (https://professionals.inspiresleep.com/reimbursement), some 35 private health plans, including 4 nationwide plans and at least 30 statewide plans, currently cover the Inspire II device.

Many patients who meet the eligibility requirements for UAStim therapy will be covered by their insurance; however, significant challenges remain. Many payers consider UAStim therapy experimental or investigational and are reluctant to share the large upfront costs of implantation. For many patients with private insurance, prior authorization may be initially denied and require appeal, resulting in significant delays in treatment. A recent study that investigated the impact of insurance status on delivery of care for UAStim therapy found that compared to patients with private insurance, Medicare patients had a shorter mean wait time to surgery and fewer insurance-related treatment delays.[67] In this study, almost half of patients with private insurance were initially denied prior authorization. Ultimately, 21.1% of patients with private insurance were denied treatment, whereas only 6.4% of patients with Medicare coverage were denied treatment. Additional cost-effectiveness studies and studies comparing short- and long-term outcomes of UAStim treatment to CPAP are likely required before there is widespread coverage of UAStim by private insurers.

---

### BOX 4.2 Indications and Contraindications for Inspire II Implantation

**Indications**

- Age >22 years
- AHI ≥ 15 and ≤ 65
- BMI < 32 m/kg$^2$
- Inability or unwillingness to use CPAP
- Free of CCC at the level of the palate

**Contraindications**

- Central + mixed apneas >25% of total AHI
- Concentric collapse at the level of the palate
- Preexisting conditions that have compromised neurologic control of the upper airway
- Patients who are unable to or do not have the necessary assistance to operate Inspire therapy
- Patients who are pregnant or plan to become pregnant
- Patients who will require magnetic resonance imaging
- Patients with an implantable device that may be susceptible to unintended interaction with the Inspire system

---

# References

1. Dempsey JA, Veasey SC, Morgan BJ, O'Donnell CP. Pathophysiology of sleep apnea. *Physiol Rev.* 2010;90(1):47–112. doi:10.1152/physrev.00043.2008
2. Namen AM, Chatterjee A, Huang KE, et al. Recognition of sleep apnea is increasing: Analysis of trends in two large, representative databases of outpatient practice. *Ann Am Thorac Soc.* 2016;13(11):2027–2034. doi:10.1513/AnnalsATS.201603-152OC
3. Aiello KD, Caughey WG, Nelluri B, et al. Effect of exercise training on sleep apnea: A systematic review and meta-analysis. *Respir Med.* 2016;116:85–92. doi:10.1016/j.rmed.2016.05.015
4. Joosten SA, Khoo JK, Edwards BA, et al. Improvement in obstructive sleep apnea with weight loss is dependent on body position during sleep. *Sleep.* 2017;40(5). doi:10.1093/sleep/zsx047
5. Yingjuan M, Siang WH, Leong Alvin TK, Poh HP. Positional therapy for positional obstructive sleep apnea. *Sleep Med Clin.* 2019;14(1):119–133. doi:10.1016/j.jsmc.2018.10.003
6. Camacho M, Certal V, Abdullatif J, et al. Myofunctional therapy to treat obstructive sleep apnea: A systematic review and meta-analysis. *Sleep.* 2015;38(5):669–675. doi:10.5665/sleep.4652
7. Iftikhar IH, Bittencourt L, Youngstedt SD, et al. Comparative efficacy of CPAP, MADs, exercise-training, and dietary weight loss for sleep apnea: A network meta-analysis. *Sleep Med.* 2017;30:7–14. doi:10.1016/j.sleep.2016.06.001
8. Rotenberg BW, Murariu D, Pang KP. Trends in CPAP adherence over twenty years of data collection: A flattened curve. *J Otolaryngol Head Neck Surg.* 2016;45(1):43. doi:10.1186/s40463-016-0156-0

9. Ramar K, Dort LC, Katz SG, et al. Clinical practice guideline for the treatment of obstructive sleep apnea and snoring with oral appliance therapy: An update for 2015. *J Clin Sleep Med*. 2015;11(7):773–827. doi:10.5664/jcsm.4858

10. Saglam-Aydinatay B, Taner T. Oral appliance therapy in obstructive sleep apnea: Long-term adherence and patients experiences. *Med Oral Patol Oral Cirugia Bucal*. 2018;23(1):e72–e77. doi:10.4317/medoral.22158

11. Lin H-C, Friedman M, Chang H-W, Gurpinar B. The efficacy of multilevel surgery of the upper airway in adults with obstructive sleep apnea/hypopnea syndrome. *Laryngoscope*. 2008;118(5):902–908. doi:10.1097/MLG.0b013e31816422ea

12. Camacho M, Certal V, Brietzke SE, et al. Tracheostomy as treatment for adult obstructive sleep apnea: A systematic review and meta-analysis. *Laryngoscope*. 2014;124(3):803–811. doi:10.1002/lary.24433

13. Johnson DM, Soose RJ. Updated nasal surgery for obstructive sleep apnea. *Adv Otorhinolaryngol*. 2017;80:66–73. doi:10.1159/000470868

14. Aurora RN, Casey KR, Kristo D, et al. Practice parameters for the surgical modifications of the upper airway for obstructive sleep apnea in adults. *Sleep*. 2010;33(10):1408–1413.

15. Pang KP, Plaza G, Baptista J PM, et al. Palate surgery for obstructive sleep apnea: A 17-year meta-analysis. *Eur Arch Otorhinolaryngol*. 2018;275(7):1697–1707. doi:10.1007/s00405-018-5015-3

16. Zaghi S, Holty J-EC, Certal V, et al. Maxillomandibular advancement for treatment of obstructive sleep apnea: A meta-analysis. *JAMA Otolaryngol Head Neck Surg*. 2016;142(1):58–66. doi:10.1001/jamaoto.2015.2678

17. Caples SM, Rowley JA, Prinsell JR, et al. Surgical modifications of the upper airway for obstructive sleep apnea in adults: A systematic review and meta-analysis. *Sleep*. 2010;33(10):1396–1407.

18. Safiruddin F, Vanderveken OM, Vries N de, et al. Effect of upper-airway stimulation for obstructive sleep apnoea on airway dimensions. *Eur Respir J*. 2015;45(1):129–138. doi:10.1183/09031936.00059414

19. Heiser C, Edenharter G, Bas M, et al. Palatoglossus coupling in selective upper airway stimulation. *Laryngoscope*. 2017;127(10):E378–E383. doi:10.1002/lary.26487

20. Boon M, Huntley C, Steffen A, et al. Upper airway stimulation for obstructive sleep apnea: Results from the ADHERE registry. *Otolaryngol Head Neck Surg*. 2018;159(2):379–385. doi:10.1177/0194599818764896

21. Woodson BT, Strohl KP, Soose RJ, et al. Upper airway stimulation for obstructive sleep apnea: 5-year outcomes. *Otolaryngol Head Neck Surg*. 2018;159(1):194–202. doi:10.1177/0194599818762383

22. Maurer JT, Van de Heyning P, Lin H-S, et al. Operative technique of upper airway stimulation: An implantable treatment of obstructive sleep apnea. *Oper Tech Otolaryngol Head Neck Surg*. 2012;23(3):227–233. doi:10.1016/j.otot.2012.07.002

23. Friedman M, Jacobowitz O, Hwang MS, et al. Targeted hypoglossal nerve stimulation for the treatment of obstructive sleep apnea: Six-month results. *Laryngoscope*. 2016;126(11):2618–2623. doi:10.1002/lary.25909

24. Eastwood PR, Barnes M, MacKay SG, et al. Bilateral hypoglossal nerve stimulation for treatment of adult obstructive sleep apnea. *Eur Respir J*. 2020;55:1901320. doi:10.1183/13993003.01320-2019

25. US Preventive Services Task Force, Bibbins-Domingo K, Grossman DC, et al. Screening for obstructive sleep apnea in adults: US Preventive Services Task Force recommendation statement. *JAMA*. 2017;317(4):407–414. doi:10.1001/jama.2016.20325

26. Epstein LJ, Kristo D, Strollo PJ Jr, et al. Clinical guideline for the evaluation, management and long-term care of obstructive sleep apnea in adults. *J Clin Sleep Med*. 2009;5(3):263–276.

27. Johns MW. A new method for measuring daytime sleepiness: The Epworth sleepiness scale. *Sleep*. 1991;14(6):540–545.

28. Diercks GR, Wentland C, Keamy D, et al. Hypoglossal nerve stimulation in adolescents with Down syndrome and obstructive sleep apnea. *JAMA Otolaryngol Head Neck Surg*. 2018;144(1):37–42. doi:10.1001/jamaoto.2017.1871

29. Caloway CL, Diercks GR, Keamy D, et al. Update on hypoglossal nerve stimulation in children with Down syndrome and obstructive sleep apnea. *Laryngoscope*. 2020;130(4):E263–E267. doi:10.1002/lary.28138

30. Van de Heyning PH, Badr MS, Baskin JZ, et al. Implanted upper airway stimulation device for obstructive sleep apnea. *Laryngoscope*. 2012;122(7):1626–1633. doi:10.1002/lary.23301

31. Huntley C, Steffen A, Doghramji K, et al. Upper airway stimulation in patients with obstructive sleep apnea and an elevated body mass index: A multi-institutional review. *Laryngoscope*. 2018;128(10):2425–2428. doi:10.1002/lary.27426

32. Sarber KM, Chang KW, Ishman SL, et al. Hypoglossal nerve stimulator outcomes for patients outside the U.S.: FDA recommendations. *Laryngoscope*. 2020;130(4):866–872. doi:10.1002/lary.28175

33. Collop NA, Anderson WM, Boehlecke B, et al. Clinical guidelines for the use of unattended portable monitors in the diagnosis of obstructive sleep apnea in adult patients. Portable Monitoring Task Force of the American Academy of Sleep Medicine. *J Clin Sleep Med*. 2007;3(7):737–747.

34. Corral J, Sánchez-Quiroga M-Á, Carmona-Bernal C, et al. Conventional polysomnography is not necessary for the management of most patients with suspected obstructive sleep apnea. Noninferiority, randomized controlled trial. *Am J Respir Crit Care Med*. 2017;196(9):1181–1190. doi:10.1164/rccm.201612-2497OC

35. Kim RD, Kapur VK, Redline-Bruch J, et al. An economic evaluation of home versus laboratory-based diagnosis of obstructive sleep apnea. *Sleep*. 2015;38(7):1027–1037. doi:10.5665/sleep.4804

36. Kundel V, Shah N. Impact of portable sleep testing. *Sleep Med Clin*. 2017;12(1):137–147. doi:10.1016/j.jsmc.2016.10.006

37. Kunisaki KM, Greer N, Khalil W, et al. Provider types and outcomes in obstructive sleep apnea case finding and treatment: A systematic review. *Ann Intern Med*. 2018;168(3):195–202. doi:10.7326/M17-2511

38. Ouayoun MC, Chabolle F, De Vito A, et al. International consensus (ICON) on the ENT role in diagnosis of obstructive sleep apnea syndrome. *Eur Ann Otorhinolaryngol Head Neck Dis*. 2018;135(1S):S3–S6. doi:10.1016/j.anorl.2017.12.012

39. Parthasarathy S, Subramanian S, Quan SF. A multicenter prospective comparative effectiveness study of the effect of physician certification and center accreditation on patient-centered outcomes in obstructive sleep apnea. *J Clin Sleep Med*. 2014;10(3):243–249. doi:10.5664/jcsm.3518

40. Berry RB, Brooks R, Gamaldo C, et al. AASM scoring manual updates for 2017 (version 2.4). *J Clin Sleep Med*. 2017;13(5):665–666. doi:10.5664/jcsm.6576

41. Woodson BT, Soose RJ, Gillespie MB, et al. Three-year outcomes of cranial nerve stimulation for obstructive sleep apnea: The STAR trial. *Otolaryngol Head Neck Surg*. 2016;154(1):181–188. doi:10.1177/0194599815616618

42. Won CHJ, Qin L, Selim B, Yaggi HK. Varying hypopnea definitions affect obstructive sleep apnea severity classification and association with cardiovascular disease. *J Clin Sleep Med*. 2018;14(12):1987–1994. doi:10.5664/jcsm.7520

43. Butler MP, Emch JT, Rueschman M, et al. Apnea–hypopnea event duration predicts mortality in men and women in the Sleep Heart Health Study. *Am J Respir Crit Care Med*. 2019;199(7):903–912. doi:10.1164/rccm.201804-0758OC

44. Stöberl AS, Schwarz EI, Haile SR, et al. Night-to-night variability of obstructive sleep apnea. *J Sleep Res*. 2017;26(6):782–788. doi:10.1111/jsr.12558

45. Sforza E, Roche F, Chapelle C, Pichot V. Internight variability of apnea–hypopnea index in obstructive sleep apnea using ambulatory polysomnography. *Front Physiol*. 2019;10:849. doi:10.3389/fphys.2019.00849

46. Kapur VK, Auckley DH, Chowdhuri S, et al. Clinical practice guideline for diagnostic testing for adult obstructive sleep apnea: An American Academy of Sleep Medicine clinical practice guideline. *J Clin Sleep Med*. 2017;13(03):479–504. doi:10.5664/jcsm.6506

47. Deutsch PA, Simmons MS, Wallace JM. Cost-effectiveness of split-night polysomnography and home studies in the evaluation of obstructive sleep apnea syndrome. *J Clin Sleep Med*. 2006;2(2):145–153.

48. Steffen A, Frenzel H, Wollenberg B, König IR. Patient selection for upper airway stimulation: Is concentric collapse in sleep endoscopy predictable? *Sleep Breath Schlaf Atm*. 2015;19(4):1373–1376. doi:10.1007/s11325-015-1277-9

49. Battan G, Kumar S, Panwar A, et al. Effect of CPAP therapy in improving daytime sleepiness in Indian patients with moderate and severe OSA. *J Clin Diagn Res*. 2016;10(11):OC14–OC16. doi:10.7860/JCDR/2016/23800.8876

50. Feldstein CA. Blood pressure effects of CPAP in nonresistant and resistant hypertension associated with OSA: A systematic review of randomized clinical trials. *Clin Exp Hypertens.* 2016;38(4):337–346. doi:10.3109/10641963.2016.1148156

51. Wang G, Goebel JR, Li C, et al. Therapeutic effects of CPAP on cognitive impairments associated with OSA. *J Neurol.* [E-pub before print, May 2019]. doi:10.1007/s00415-019-09381-2

52. Kuhn E, Schwarz EI, Bratton DJ, et al. Effects of CPAP and mandibular advancement devices on health-related quality of life in OSA: A systematic review and meta-analysis. *Chest.* 2017;151(4):786–794. doi:10.1016/j.chest.2017.01.020

53. Gaisl T, Rejmer P, Thiel S, et al. Effects of suboptimal adherence of CPAP-therapy on symptoms of obstructive sleep apnea: A randomised, double-blind, controlled trial. *Eur Respir J.* 2020;55(3):1901526. doi:10.1183/13993003.01526-2019

54. Filtness AJ, Reyner LA, Horne JA. One night's CPAP withdrawal in otherwise compliant OSA patients: Marked driving impairment but good awareness of increased sleepiness. *Sleep Breath Schlaf Atm.* 2012;16:865–871. doi:10.1007/s11325-011-0588-8

55. Broström A, Nilsen P, Johansson P, et al. Putative facilitators and barriers for adherence to CPAP treatment in patients with obstructive sleep apnea syndrome: A qualitative content analysis. *Sleep Med.* 2010;11(2):126–130. doi:10.1016/j.sleep.2009.04.010

56. Van Ryswyk E, Anderson CS, Antic NA, et al. Predictors of long-term adherence to continuous positive airway pressure in patients with obstructive sleep apnea and cardiovascular disease. *Sleep.* 2019;42(10). doi:10.1093/sleep/zsz152

57. Xu T, Li T, Wei D, et al. Effect of automatic versus fixed continuous positive airway pressure for the treatment of obstructive sleep apnea: An up-to-date meta-analysis. *Sleep Breath Schlaf Atm.* 2012;16(4):1017–1026. doi:10.1007/s11325-011-0626-6

58. Ip S, D'Ambrosio C, Patel K, et al. Auto-titrating versus fixed continuous positive airway pressure for the treatment of obstructive sleep apnea: A systematic review with meta-analyses. *Syst Rev.* 2012;1(1):20. doi:10.1186/2046-4053-1-20

59. Hertegonne K, Bauters F. The value of auto-adjustable CPAP devices in pressure titration and treatment of patients with obstructive sleep apnea syndrome. *Sleep Med Rev.* 2010;14(2):115–119. doi:10.1016/j.smrv.2009.07.001

60. Pépin JL, Tamisier R, Baguet JP, et al. Fixed-pressure CPAP versus auto-adjusting CPAP: Comparison of efficacy on blood pressure in obstructive sleep apnoea, a randomised clinical trial. *Thorax.* 2016;71(8):726–733. doi:10.1136/thoraxjnl-2015-207700

61. Denotti AL, Wong KKH, Dungan GC 2nd, et al. Residual sleep disordered breathing during auto-titrating positive airway pressure therapy. *Eur Respir J.* 2012;39:1391–1397. doi:10.1183/09031936.00093811

62. Dijemeni E, D'Amone G, Gbati I. Drug-induced sedation endoscopy (DISE) classification systems: A systematic review and meta-analysis. *Sleep Breath Schlaf Atm.* 2017;21(4):983–994. doi:10.1007/s11325-017-1521-6

63. Kezirian EJ, Hohenhorst W, de Vries N. Drug-induced sleep endoscopy: The VOTE classification. *Eur Arch Otorhinolaryngol.* 2011;268(8):1233–1236. doi:10.1007/s00405-011-1633-8

64. Vanderveken OM, Maurer JT, Hohenhorst W, et al. Evaluation of drug-induced sleep endoscopy as a patient selection tool for implanted upper airway stimulation for obstructive sleep apnea. *J Clin Sleep Med.* 2013;9(5):433–438. doi:10.5664/jcsm.2658

65. Strollo PJ, Soose RJ, Maurer JT, et al. Upper-airway stimulation for obstructive sleep apnea. *N Engl J Med.* 2014;370(2):139–149. doi:10.1056/NEJMoa1308659

66. Ong AA, Murphey AW, Nguyen SA, et al. Efficacy of upper airway stimulation on collapse patterns observed during drug-induced sedation endoscopy. *Otolaryngol Head Neck Surg.* 2016;154(5):970–977. doi:10.1177/0194599816636835

67. Patel J, Topf MC, Huntley C, Boon M. Does insurance status impact delivery of care with upper airway stimulation for OSA? *Ann Otol Rhinol Laryngol.* 2020;129(2):128–134. doi:10.1177/0003489419878454

68. Iwanaga K, Hasegawa K, Shibata N, et al. Endoscopic examination of obstructive sleep apnea syndrome patients during drug-induced sleep. *Acta Otolaryngol Suppl.* 2003;(550):36–40. doi:10.1080/0365523031000055

69. Vicini C, De Vito A, Benazzo M, et al. The nose oropharynx hypopharynx and larynx (NOHL) classification: A new system of diagnostic standardized examination for OSAHS patients. *Eur Arch Otorhinolaryngol.* 2012;269(4):1297–1300. doi:10.1007/s00405-012-1965-z

70. Koo SK, Choi JW, Myung NS, et al. Analysis of obstruction site in obstructive sleep apnea syndrome patients by drug-induced sleep endoscopy. *Am J Otolaryngol*. 2013;34(6):626–630. doi:10.1016/j.amjoto.2013.07.013

71. Herzog M, Kellner P, Plößl S, et al. Drug-induced sleep endoscopy and simulated snoring in patients with sleep-disordered breathing: Agreement of anatomic changes in the upper airway. *Eur Arch Otorhinolaryngol*. 2015;272(9):2541–2550. doi:10.1007/s00405-015-3559-z

72. Carrasco-Llatas M, Zerpa-Zerpa V, Dalmau-Galofre J. Reliability of drug-induced sedation endoscopy: Interobserver agreement. *Sleep Breath Schlaf Atm*. 2017;21(1):173–179. doi:10.1007/s11325-016-1426-9

# Criteria for Patient Selection

Sara W. Liu and Alan Kominsky

## 5.1. Introduction

Positive airway pressure (PAP) remains the gold standard for treatment of obstructive sleep apnea (OSA). Although the benefits and outcomes of PAP therapy have been well demonstrated, there are many patients who struggle to maintain compliance with the therapy because of intolerance to the pressure or the interfaces. For some of these patients, a mandibular advance device (oral appliance) may be an option. However, these devices can be limited by patient compliance, comfort with the device, and presence of healthy dentition. In addition, although data suggest that dental devices can decrease the severity of OSA regardless of apnea–hypopnea index (AHI), the efficacy of a mandibular advancement device is lower in patients with higher baseline AHI.[1] In these patients, hypoglossal nerve stimulation can be considered.

One of the most important factors to achieve treatment success with upper airway stimulation is careful patient selection. Several patient characteristics must be considered before implanting the upper airway stimulation device. The selection criteria were determined through a number of studies during initial clinical trials that compared the characteristics of patients who were successfully treated with upper airway stimulation (responders) with those were not successfully treated (nonresponders).[2,3] These considerations are of prognostic value when determining patient candidacy for upper airway stimulation. Currently, the hypoglossal nerve stimulator device is approved by the U.S. Food and Drug Administration (FDA) for treatment of moderate to severe OSA in nonobese patients who do not tolerate PAP therapy.

---

### FDA Exclusion Criteria

- Body mass index (BMI) > 35 kg/m$^2$
- AHI < 15 or ≥ 65
- Complete concentric collapse at soft palate on drug-induced sleep endoscopy (DISE)
- Central apnea index > 25% of total AHI

### Other Contraindications and Considerations

- Neuromuscular disease
- Severe cardiopulmonary disease
- Active debilitating psychiatric disease
- Need for frequent magnetic resonance imaging (MRI) scans
- Pregnancy or intent to become pregnant
- Minimum age of 22
- Onset or maintenance insomnia; other comorbid sleep conditions

---

# 5.2. Anthropometric Considerations

During patient workup and selection, the main anthropometric parameter that must be assessed in this population is obesity. In initial trials of the hypoglossal nerve stimulator, BMI < 35 kg/m$^2$ was proposed as the upper limit for patient selection. Twenty-one subjects were implanted during part one of the trial, and data analysis showed that BMI ≤ 32 kg/m$^2$ was a significant predictor of therapy response.[2] This can be explained by considering the pathophysiology of OSA in obese individuals.

The causal association between increased BMI and prevalence of OSA is well known and has been well established in the literature. Obesity can affect upper airway collapsibility through both mechanical effects on pharyngeal soft tissue and via airway neuromuscular control.[4-6] Anatomic alterations that occur with obesity can predispose to airway obstruction while sleeping by increasing adiposity in the pharynx and torso. This is believed to contribute to OSA through several mechanisms:

1. An increase in soft tissue in the neck and pharynx can narrow the lumen of the upper airway.[5]
2. Obesity (central obesity in particular) is associated with lung volume reductions, which is hypothesized to decrease longitudinal tracheal traction, which increases pharyngeal collapse.
3. Perhaps most relevant to hypoglossal nerve stimulation, upper airway collapsibility is higher in obese individuals compared with nonobese individuals, and anterior displacement of the mandible does not proportionately increase airway diameter.[7,8] This

is perhaps the reason for the decreased therapy response of the hypoglossal nerve stimulator device in obese individuals.

A cohort study of the Adherence and Outcome of Upper Airway Stimulation for O SA International Registry (ADHERE registry, an ongoing international, multicenter prospective observational study of patients who have undergone hypoglossal nerve stimulator implantation) further confirmed that increased BMI is a predictor of therapy failure. Each unit decrease of BMI was found to be associated with 8.5% increased odds of having a successful response to therapy, as defined by the Sher criteria ($\geq$ 50% reduction in AHI to AHI $\leq$ 20).[9] Although there exists anecdotal therapy success reported at higher BMI, this study corroborated current recommendations against implanting patients with BMI > 32 kg/m².

# 5.3. Clinical

There are several clinical considerations that must be made while taking a history for a hypoglossal nerve stimulator candidate. Currently, the device is FDA approved for patients with a minimum age of 22; there is no upper age limit at present. Pregnant individuals, or those planning to become pregnant, are excluded from device implantation. Prospective observational studies have shown more favorable AHI response in female patients.[9] This difference, however, should not influence patient selection based on gender, and both males and females should be considered for hypoglossal nerve stimulation.

As mentioned previously, the patient should have trialed and failed PAP. "Failure" is typically defined as an inability or unwillingness to use PAP. It is assumed that the usual clinical measures have been taken to optimize PAP use, such as mask and pressure changes, use of bilevel PAP devices, and acclimatization sessions, among others. Although not a requirement, a mandibular advancement device or a dental sleep appliance should also be considered, particularly in patients with mild to moderate OSA.[1,10] However, patients who have already failed such a device or those for whom it is not an appropriate therapy may be candidates for the hypoglossal neve stimulator.

Prior sleep surgery does not preclude success with hypoglossal nerve stimulation. Implantation of the hypoglossal nerve stimulator provided significant improvement in postoperative AHI and nadir oxyhemoglobin saturation, with prior airway surgery showing no statistically significant difference compared to a control population.[11] Considerations should be made regarding prior head and neck surgery or radiation therapy that resulted in limited or altered tongue protrusion or movement, which may affect the success of the therapy. This must be evaluated on an individual patient basis. Other conditions related to mandible or tongue size can be considered; however, there are no current published data on anatomic variability and its effect on upper airway stimulation.

A careful medical history should be obtained. Patients with neuromuscular disorders, such as cranial nerve XII palsy or other motor neuron pathologies that would interfere with device function, should be excluded. In addition, individuals with severe cardiopulmonary disorders, active severe or debilitating psychiatric disease, and other comorbid nonrespiratory sleep disorders should be excluded from device implantation, as all these conditions may affect device function and therapy or bias polysomnogram results. Patients must also be able to operate the device remote control or have reliable assistance to do so. Other sleep disorders will be discussed in more detail in a later section.

Another clinical consideration is the need for future magnetic resonance imaging (MRI) scans. Older versions of the Inspire device are incompatible with MRI; however, the newest model allows for patients to undergo MRI of the head and/or extremities with a 1.5T magnet (see Chapter 12).

The presence of delayed sleep onset latency or sleep maintenance insomnia should be considered during the patient selection process; in this patient population, the device is less likely to be successfully used. The device provides a delay after turning it on to allow for sleep onset; however, the patient must be able to initiate and maintain sleep within the given time period of the device delay. Patients who are easily aroused during sleep ("light sleepers") may experience frequent awakenings from the tongue protrusion or stimulus sensation discomfort, which can require postoperative device titration with an awake endoscopy. Patients with a preexisting diagnosis of insomnia were found to require awake endoscopy with device reconfiguration at a significantly higher rate than those without insomnia.[12] As sleep habits and pathologies can affect the success of hypoglossal nerve stimulation, a thorough history of the patient's sleep patterns should be obtained during the selection process.

## 5.4. Upper Airway

The upper airway anatomy of candidates should be assessed via physical examination and flexible fiberoptic nasopharyngoscopy in an outpatient clinic setting during the initial evaluation and workup. Prior to the advent of upper airway stimulation for the treatment of OSA, options for surgical intervention included soft tissue upper airway modifications (nasal surgery, uvulopalatopharyngoplasty, lingual tonsil reduction, tonsillectomy, arytenoid reduction, epiglottoplasty, genioglossus advancement, hyoid suspension, etc.), orthognathic procedures (maxillomandibular advancement, mandibular distraction, maxillary expansion), or the definitive gold standard for cure, a tracheostomy.[13] All of these procedures aim to improve upper airway patency to decrease collapse or anatomic obstruction during sleep or, in the case of a tracheostomy, bypass the upper airway entirely. Upper airway stimulation has not supplanted these options as they still have utility in appropriately selected individuals with OSA.

The nasal airway should be assessed with anterior rhinoscopy for anatomic nasal obstruction due to severe nasal septal deviation, nasal polyp burden, or turbinate hypertrophy. Nasal valve competency should be evaluated with the modified Cottle maneuver. It is important to evaluate whether the patient's nasal airway is contributing to the OSA or is contributing to decreased compliance with PAP therapy.[14] Reduced nasal airway patency can occur concurrently with sleep disordered breathing. Although there are no published data to suggest that improved nasal airway patency corrects OSA, it is generally accepted that correction of significant nasal obstruction should be considered as part of comprehensive upper airway surgical therapy for OSA.

The soft palate and oropharynx should be assessed in clinic when examining a patient with OSA. Classifications such as the Friedman tongue position and Mallampati score can be used to predict the severity of OSA by acting as a surrogate for evaluating oropharyngeal crowding; it shows some correlation to upper airway collapse.[15-17] The tonsils should also be assessed on physical exam. Tonsillar hypertrophy can indicate increased lateral oropharyngeal obstruction. This pattern of obstruction is unlikely to resolve with forward protrusion of the tongue with the hypoglossal nerve stimulator. In this patient population, a tonsillectomy prior to evaluating candidacy for the hypoglossal nerve stimulator may be a reasonable consideration.[18]

Flexible fiberoptic nasopharyngoscopy should be used in addition to physical exam to evaluate these anatomic structures. Ultimately, although the anatomy of the upper airway in an upright and awake patient can be helpful in the initial workup of the patient selection process, DISE must also be performed to truly evaluate upper airway collapse during sleep.[19,20] This will be discussed further in the DISE section.

Radiographic imaging to obtain measurements of the upper airway in OSA has been used for research purposes but has not proved to play a role in the clinical setting. Both 2D and 3D imaging have been explored, including x-ray, computed tomographic (CT) imaging, MRI, and dynamic MRI. Numerous studies have identified dimensions or measurements that are associated with increased airway collapse or severity of OSA.[21-27] Barrera et al. demonstrated larger tongue volume, longer mandibular plane–hyoid distance, and smaller posterior airway space on lateral cephalometry and MRI in individuals with OSA compared to controls.[22] A meta-analysis of craniofacial anatomy seen on lateral cephalograms showed several significant measurements associated with OSA when compared to control subjects, including position and length of mandible, maxillary length, soft palate area, upper airway length, and tongue area.[23] However, these measurements have yet to be validated in the setting of determining response with a hypoglossal nerve stimulator, although this may be an area for future research in determining appropriate candidacy for the device.

# 5.5. Polysomnography

Following a thorough history and physical exam, the next step in the patient selection process is a sleep study. Attended polysomnography (PSG), which is performed in a sleep laboratory, is the gold standard for diagnosing OSA and establishing its severity. However, for the purposes of patient selection, home sleep studies may suffice—although they tend to underestimate the severity of the condition. In addition, patient selection and efficacy assessments in the preclinical studies that led to the FDA indication of the device were based on attended PSG. The parameters measured in a typical PSG include electrocardiography, electroencephalography, electro-oculography, chin and limb electromyography, respiratory airflow assessment through a nasal pressure transducer and an oronasal thermal airflow sensor, respiratory effort (via chest and abdominal wall movement), and continuous pulse oximetry (Figure 5.1).

For the purposes of the hypoglossal nerve stimulator, the AHI, which is a marker for OSA severity and which established the diagnosis, is used to determine if a patient is a candidate for the device. Preclinical trials for the hypoglossal nerve stimulator included patients with an AHI $\geq$ 25 per hour. It was then determined from this cohort of patients that an AHI $\leq$ 50 per hour was significantly associated with response to therapy.[2] Further trials of larger patient groups led to the current recommendation of an AHI between 15 and 65 per hour for optimal response to device therapy.[2,3,18] Further research is warranted as to whether this therapy could be effective in patients with an AHI >65.

Another sleep parameter of importance from the PSG study is the proportion of obstructive, central, and mixed events. The central and mixed index should be less than 25% of the overall AHI to include for implantation of upper airway stimulation. Central sleep apnea is a different pathophysiologic entity from OSA, and it is important to determine what proportion of an individual's sleep apnea is central versus obstructive in nature. Central sleep apnea is characterized by a cessation in respiratory drive during sleep, with

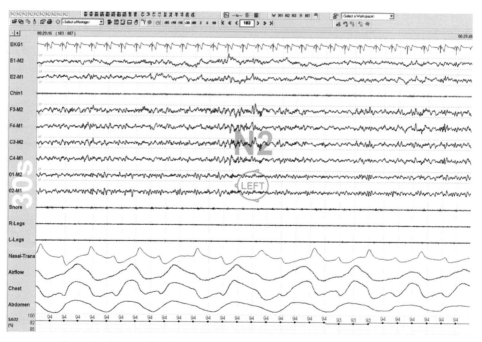

**FIGURE 5.1** Example of a typical polysomnogram (PSG) tracing. **(A)** Two-minute tracing of obstructive apneas, with thin arrows indicating no flow in nasal pressure transducer (NP), and associated oxygen desaturations (shown by wide arrows). Effort is seen in the chest and abdomen leads. **(B)** Two-minute tracing of episodes of central apneas (indicated by thin arrows) where no flow is seen in the CPAP signal, with no effort seen in chest and abdomen leads, and associated oxygen desaturations (shown by wide arrows).[34]

multiple causes, including a high hypercapnic responsiveness and an unstable ventilatory control system.[28-30] These are nonanatomic factors and are not likely to be altered or successfully treated by a hypoglossal nerve stimulator. Therefore, if greater than 25% of a patient's sleep apnea is central in nature, the patient is less likely to benefit from the device. The PSG also provides important patient information regarding sleep latency and number and length of awakenings, which may be indicative of emotional conditions or insomnia. It can also reveal additional comorbid sleep conditions such as periodic limb movements in sleep.

# 5.6. Drug-Induced Sleep Endoscopy

DISE is a procedure used to select appropriate patients for hypoglossal nerve stimulator implantation. Once patients have passed the initial screening in the clinic with a thorough history and physical exam, have undergone a PSG, and have been found to have OSA with an AHI within the inclusion criteria, the final step is a DISE. The details of this procedure and of anesthetic considerations will be discussed in Chapters 6 and 7. In brief, DISE is performed with patients sedated to mimic natural sleep and induce snoring, usually with midazolam and/or propofol.[31,32] Once an appropriate level of sedation is achieved, a flexible fiberoptic laryngoscope is inserted via the nose to examine the upper airway and determine the location and pattern of collapse. This is scored based on the site of collapse (Velum, Oropharyngeal walls, Tonsils, Epiglottis [VOTE] classification [Figure 5.2]), degree of collapse (partial or complete), and pattern of collapse

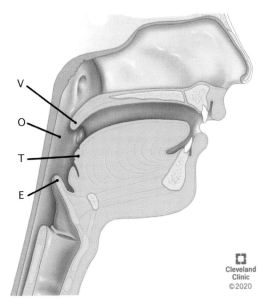

Cleveland
Clinic
©2020

**FIGURE 5.2** VOTE system of upper airway collapse with corresponding positions. V = velum (soft palate), O = oropharynx, T = tongue base, E = epiglottis. Image adapted from Mete and Akbudak.[35]

(anteroposterior, lateral, or concentric).[33] Collapse can be seen in one location, although many patients have collapse involving multiple levels.[31]

Studies have determined that some collapse patterns or anatomic observations are more favorable and predict response with the hypoglossal nerve stimulator, while some are considered contraindications. The main contraindication is the presence of complete concentric collapse at the level of the soft palate, as this was the only pattern of collapse on DISE that had a negative predictive value with therapy response.[19,31,32] While not contraindicated based on the manufacturer's recommendations, there is a growing expert opinion that significant lateral oropharyngeal wall collapse may also portend a poor clinical response.[36]

## 5.7. Conclusion

Appropriate patient selection prior to hypoglossal nerve stimulator implantation is paramount to therapy success. As outlined in this chapter, initial studies for the device were conducted to determine patient characteristics that were predictors of response to therapy.[2,3] Patients should be seen in the outpatient clinic for initial evaluation. Once a medical history has been obtained, physical examination and in-office flexible laryngoscopy should be performed. On exam, attention should be paid to patient's BMI, nasal airway, and upper airway anatomy. Although a BMI > 35 kg/m² is a relative contraindication for device implantation, the ADHERE database suggests that a lower BMI is associated with increased odds of success.[9] An up-to-date PSG should be reviewed to ensure that the patient meets AHI criteria (< 15 or ≥ 65) and apneic events do not consist of >25% central apneas. Patients who are deemed appropriate candidates must then undergo the final qualifying step, DISE, to evaluate for the pattern of collapse. On DISE, complete concentric collapse at the soft palate has been found to be a negative predictor for therapy success, so the presence of this pattern of airway collapse is a contraindication to device implantation. In a patient who has failed PAP therapy for OSA, motivation and the quantitative and qualitative considerations detailed in this chapter must be assessed and met before recommending a hypoglossal nerve stimulator device to ensure optimal results.

## References

1. Dioguardi A, Al-Halawani M. Oral appliances in obstructive sleep apnea. *Otolaryngol Clin North Am.* 2016;49(6):1343–1357. doi:10.1016/j.otc.2016.07.005
2. Van de Heyning PH, Badr MS, Baskin JZ, et al. Implanted upper airway stimulation device for obstructive sleep apnea. *Laryngoscope.* 2012;122(July):1626–1633. doi:10.1002/lary.23301
3. Strollo PJ, Soose RJ, Maurer JT, et al. Upper-airway stimulation for obstructive sleep apnea. *N Engl J Med.* 2014;370(2):139–149. doi:10.1056/NEJMoa1308659
4. Horner RL. Pathophysiology of obstructive sleep apnea. *J Cardiopulm Rehabil Prev.* 2008;28(5):289–298. doi:10.1097/01.HCR.0000336138.71569.a2

5. Davies RJ, Stradling JR. The relationship between neck circumference, radiographic pharyngeal anatomy, and the obstructive sleep apnoea syndrome. *Eur Resp J.* 1990;3(5):509–514.

6. Schwartz AR, Patil SP, Laffan AM, et al. Obesity and obstructive sleep apnea pathogenic mechanisms and therapeutic approaches. *Proc Am Thorac Soc.* 2008;5:185–192. doi:10.1513/pats.200708-137MG

7. Schwartz AR, Gold AR, Schubert N, et al. Effect of weight loss on upper airway collapsibility in obstructive sleep apnea. *Am Rev Respir Dis.* 1991;144(3 Pt 1):494–498. doi:10.1164/ajrccm/144.3_Pt_1.494

8. Isono S, Tanaka A, Tagaito Y, et al. Pharyngeal patency in response to advancement of the mandible in obese anesthetized persons. *Anesthesiology.* 1997;87(5):1055–1062. doi:10.1097/00000542-199711000-00008

9. Thaler E, Schwab R, Maurer J, et al. Results of the ADHERE upper airway stimulation registry and predictors of therapy efficacy. *Laryngoscope.* 2020;130(4):1333–1338. doi:10.1002/lary.28286

10. Ramar K, Dort LC, Katz SG, et al. Clinical practice guideline for the treatment of obstructive sleep apnea and snoring with oral appliance therapy : An update for 2015. *J Clin Sleep Med.* 2015;11(7):773–827.

11. Mahmoud AF, Thaler ER. Upper airway stimulation therapy and prior airway surgery for obstructive sleep apnea. *Laryngoscope.* 2018;128(6):1486–1489. doi:10.1002/lary.26956

12. Meleca JB, Kominsky AH. Reconfiguration of upper airway stimulation devices utilizing awake endoscopy. *Laryngoscope.* 2020 [E-pub before print, Feb. 25]. doi:10.1002/lary.28569

13. Camacho M, Certal V, Capasso R. Comprehensive review of surgeries for obstructive sleep apnea syndrome. *Braz J Otorhinolaryngol.* 2013;79(6):780–788. doi:10.5935/1808-8694.20130139

14. Awad MI, Kacker A. Nasal obstruction considerations in sleep apnea. *Otolaryngol Clin North Am.* 2018;51(5):1003–1009. doi:10.1016/j.otc.2018.05.012

15. Ambekar AA, Saksena SG, Bapat JS, Butani MT. Correlation of bedside airway screening tests with airway obstruction during drug-induced sleep endoscopy. *Asian J Anesthesiol.* 2019;57(4):117–124. doi:10.6859/aja.201912_57(4).0002

16. Amra B, Pirpiran M, Soltaninejad F, et al. The prediction of obstructive sleep apnea severity based on anthropometric and Mallampati indices. *J Res Med Sci.* 2019;24:66. doi:10.4103/jrms.JRMS_653_18

17. Eggerstedt M, Urban MJ, Chi E, et al. The anesthesia airway evaluation: Correlation with sleep endoscopy findings. *Am J Otolaryngol.* 2019;41(2):102362. doi:10.1016/j.amjoto.2019.102362

18. Vanderveken OM, Beyers J, Beeck S Op De, Dieltjens M. Development of a clinical pathway and technical aspects of upper airway stimulation therapy for obstructive sleep apnea. *Front Neurosci.* 2017;11(September):1–12. doi:10.3389/fnins.2017.00523

19. Ong AA, Murphey AW, Nguyen SA, et al. Efficacy of upper airway stimulation on collapse patterns observed during drug-induced sedation endoscopy. *Otolaryngol Head Neck Surg.* 2016;154(5):970–977. doi:10.1177/0194599816636835

20. Atkins JH, Mandel JE. Drug-induced sleep endoscopy: From obscure technique to diagnostic tool for assessment of obstructive sleep apnea for surgical interventions. *Curr Opin Anesth.* 2018;31(1):120–126. doi:10.1097/ACO.0000000000000543

21. Abramson Z, Susarla S, August M, et al. Three-dimensional computed tomographic analysis of airway anatomy in patients with obstructive sleep apnea. *J Oral Maxillofac Surg.* 2010;68(2):354–362. doi:10.1016/j.joms.2009.09.087

22. Barrera JE, Pau CY, Forest V–I, et al. Anatomic measures of upper airway structures in obstructive sleep apnea. *World J Otorhinolaryngol Head Neck Surg.* 2017;3(2):85–91. doi:10.1016/j.wjorl.2017.05.002

23. Neelapu BC, Kharbanda OP, Sardana HK, et al. Craniofacial and upper airway morphology in adult obstructive sleep apnea patients: A systematic review and meta-analysis of cephalometric studies. *Sleep Med Rev.* 2017;31:79–90. doi:10.1016/j.smrv.2016.01.007

24. Cosentini T, Le Donne R, Mancini D, Colavita N. Magnetic resonance imaging of the upper airway in obstructive sleep apnea. *Radiol Med.* 2004;108(4):404–416.

25. Uong EC, McDonough JM, Tayag-Kier CE, et al. Magnetic resonance imaging of the upper airway in children with Down syndrome. *Am J Respir Crit Care Med.* 2001;163(3 Pt 1):731–736. doi:10.1164/ajrccm.163.3.2004231

26. Finkelstein Y, Wolf L, Nachmani A, et al. Velopharyngeal anatomy in patients with obstructive sleep apnea versus normal subjects. *J Oral Maxillofac Surg.* 2014;72(7):1350–1372. doi:10.1016/j.joms.2013.12.006

27. Horner RL, Shea SA, McIvor J, Guz A. Pharyngeal size and shape during wakefulness and sleep in patients with obstructive sleep apnoea. *Q J Med.* 1989;72(268):719–735.

28. White DP. Pathogenesis of obstructive and central sleep apnea. *Am J Respir Crit Care Med.* 2005;172(11):1363–1370. doi:10.1164/rccm.200412-1631SO

29. Verbraecken JA, De Backer WA. Upper airway mechanics. *Respiration.* 2009;78(2):121–133. doi:10.1159/000222508

30. Eckert DJ, Jordan AS, Merchia P, Malhotra A. Central sleep apnea: Pathophysiology and treatment. *Chest.* 2007;131(2):595–607. doi:10.1378/chest.06.2287

31. Vroegop AV, Vanderveken OM, Boudewyns AN, et al. Drug-induced sleep endoscopy in sleep-disordered breathing: Report on 1,249 cases. *Laryngoscope.* 2014;124(3):797–802. doi:10.1002/lary.24479

32. Vanderveken OM, Maurer JT, Hohenhorst W, et al. Evaluation of drug-induced sleep endoscopy as a patient selection tool for implanted upper airway stimulation for obstructive sleep apnea. *J Clin Sleep Med.* 2013;9(5):433–438. doi:10.5664/jcsm.2658

33. Kezirian EJ, Hohenhorst W, de Vries N. Drug-induced sleep endoscopy: The VOTE classification. *Eur Arch Otorhinolaryngol.* 2011;268(8):1233–1236. doi:10.1007/s00405-011-1633-8

34. Rundo JV, Downey R. Polysomnography. *Handb Clin Neurol.* 2019;160:381–392. doi:10.1016/B978-0-444-64032-1.00025-4

35. Mete A, Akbudak İH. Functional anatomy and physiology of airway. In: Erbay RH, ed. *Tracheal Intubation.* Rijeka: IntechOpen; 2018:Ch. 1. doi:10.5772/intechopen.77037

36. Mulholland GB, Dedhia RC. Success of hypoglossal nerve stimulation using mandibular advancement during sleep endoscopy. *Laryngoscope.* 2020 [E-pub before print, Feb. 28]. doi: 10.1002/lary.28589

# Drug-Induced Sleep Endoscopy

Eric J. Kezirian, Madeline J. L. Ravesloot,
Winfried Hohenhorst, and Nico de Vries

## 6.1. Introduction

Because a substantial number of patients with obstructive sleep apnea (OSA) are unable to tolerate positive airway pressure therapy,[1,2] alternative treatments such as surgery, upper airway stimulation, or oral appliances may be required. Comprehensive patient evaluation is key to success for the latter group of treatments. The goal of evaluation is to determine the pattern of airway obstruction, with the ultimate aim of designing targeted, effective treatment.

The ideal evaluation technique would be an assessment of sleeping patients with spontaneous breathing, as this would provide a real-time, dynamic assessment. It would also be safe, noninvasive, and low in cost. The desire to visualize directly airway obstruction led some investigators to perform fiberoptic examination during natural sleep in the late 1970s and early 1980s.[3,4] However, these efforts were generally abandoned due to the discomfort experienced by patients, particularly caused by movement of the endoscope to view multiple areas of the pharyngeal airway.

Fiberoptic evaluation of the upper airway under conditions of sedation was developed in a number of centers in Europe in the late 1980s, and Croft and Pringle first described their technique of "sleep nasendoscopy" in 1991.[5] The nomenclature was changed to "drug-induced sleep endoscopy" (DISE) by Hohenhorst[6] to reflect the three key features of this method: (1) the potential use of various pharmacological agents to achieve sedation, (2) the target depth of sedation as approximating natural sleep as much as possible, and (3) the endoscopic evaluation of the upper airway. In contrast to other procedures that usually provide two-dimensional assessments during wakefulness in the upright sitting position, DISE may provide a three-dimensional evaluation of the airway during unconscious sedation, in a position similar to natural sleep.

This chapter presents recommendations regarding DISE technique and reviews the evidence concerning the role of DISE in the evaluation of OSA.

# 6.2. Technique

## 6.2.1. Indications and Contraindications

Any diagnostic evaluation will be useful if the benefits outweigh the risks. For DISE, the benefits include potential value in treatment selection and patient counseling, and the risks are related to the sedative agent used and the potential for significant airway compromise. Indications and contraindications are listed in Box 6.1.

## 6.2.2. Sedative Agent

Control of the depth of sedation is essential. The sedative agent is generally administered intravenously at the minimum dose to achieve the target depth of sedation: the loss of consciousness, defined as loss of response to verbal stimulation at a normal conversational volume, similar to a modified Ramsay score of 5.[7] Multiple sedative agents have been used as effective agents in the performance of DISE. The commonly used sedative agents included propofol, midazolam, propofol with midazolam, and dexmedetomidine. Pharmacological properties of these sedative agents are shown in Table 6.1.

---

**BOX 6.1. Indications and Contraindications for DISE**

Indications

OSA (or snoring, in some countries)

Unable to tolerate positive airway pressure (in countries where positive airway pressure is the first-line treatment modality for OSA)

Consideration of hypoglossal nerve stimulation, surgery, oral appliances, or combination approaches (including with positional therapy)

Contraindications

Allergy to sedative agents (or soy or certain types of egg allergy for propofol)

Pregnancy

Significant medical comorbidities

Optional contraindications used by some surgeons:

Markedly severe OSA (AHI >70 events per hour)

Obesity (body mass index >32/35 kg/m²)

The choice of sedative agent, to some extent, depends on its ability to reproduce some of the changes that occur in natural sleep. During sleep, upper airway patency relies on pharyngeal dilator muscle tone and changes in lung volume that counteract collapsing forces, principally intraluminal negative pressure generated during inspiration and anatomical narrowing of the airway.[8] OSA patients maintain pharyngeal patency with greater dilator (genioglossus) muscle tone during wakefulness, but sleep onset results in marked decreases in muscle tone due to the loss of the wakefulness stimulus and decreases in negative pressure reflex activity and lung volume.[9-15] Rapid-eye-movement (REM) sleep has greater reductions in muscle tone and lung volumes than non-REM sleep.[11-15] The continuum of sedation ranges from wakefulness to conscious sedation to unconscious sedation to general anesthesia, where arousability to all stimulation is lost. Deeper levels of sedation are associated with progressive decreases in upper airway dilator muscle tone and neuromuscular reflex activation that both increase airway collapsibility.[11,13-17]

Unconscious sedation represents a lesser degree of neural depression than anesthesia and may be a closer approximation to natural sleep. The interest in the transition from wakefulness to unconscious sedation is based on the concept of a thalamocortical switch determining consciousness or unconsciousness (no response to verbal stimulation) that may be common to natural sleep and sedation.[18,19]

Propofol can be administered with target-controlled infusion, with a continuous infusion, or using small boluses. The most detailed study of changes in upper airway physiology associated with propofol sedation had results consistent with the thalamocortical switch described in the previous paragraph, as changes in upper airway collapsibility (passive $P_{crit}$), Bispectral Index (BIS) score (based on frontal electroencephalographic activity), and muscle tone occurred at this transition from consciousness to unconsciousness disproportionate to changes in propofol concentration.[16] During propofol unconscious sedation, normals have decreases in genioglossus tone to 10% of maximum

**TABLE 6.1 Pharmacological Properties of Propofol, Midazolam, and Dexmedetomidine**

| Sedative Agent | Propofol | Midazolam | Dexmedetomidine |
|---|---|---|---|
| | 2-6-diisopropylphenol | Benzodiazepine | Alpha-2 adrenergic receptor agonist |
| Functional half-life | 4–6 minutes | 45 minutes | 6 minutes |
| Elimination half-life | 3 hours | 150 minutes | 2 hours |
| Accumulation | Inactive metabolite (no accumulation) | Active metabolite (alpha-hydroxymidazolam) | Inactive metabolite (no accumulation) |
| Therapeutic range | Small | Large | Small |
| Respiratory side effects (potential) | Respiratory depression and hypopharyngeal reflex depression | Respiratory depression | None |
| Cardiovascular side effects (potential) | Hypotension | Hypotension | Fluctuation of blood pressure and heart rate |

awake activity,[16,20] which is one-half to one-third of the level in NREM sleep in normals[10] but greater than during REM sleep in normals and patients with OSA.[21]

To achieve this depth of sedation, target-controlled infusion with the Diprifusor (Astra-Zeneca, Inc., United Kingdom) technology is available in many countries. It uses a proprietary algorithm to achieve effect site (brain) concentration using a three-compartment pharmacokinetic model.[20,22] This technology is not available in the United States and many other countries, so some surgeons use a protocol involving a continuous infusion (usually unconscious sedation requires 100 to 150 mcg/kg/min), with possible additional boluses (e.g., 20 to 50 mg). Other surgeons prefer using a continuous infusion without administration of boluses. It is important to remember that different individuals can require markedly different dosages of propofol to reach the target depth of sedation.[16,23]

Dexmedetomidine has been used extensively in anesthesia for a wide range of procedures and for prolonged periods of sedation, with comparable performance during general anesthesia.[24] As is true for midazolam, there has been no study evaluating the impact of dexmedetomidine on upper airway muscle tone and airway collapsibility.

Dexmedetomidine may achieve a depth of anesthesia comparable to propofol for general surgical procedures,[24] but in one study of DISE, half of the patients required supplemental propofol because they did not achieve adequate sedation despite a maximum dose of dexmedetomidine ($1.4$ microg/k$^{-1}$/h$^{-1}$).[25] We have seen a number of patients who underwent DISE using dexmedetomidine at other institutions in which no airway obstruction was visualized despite apparent loss of consciousness; this may reflect a lesser decrease in upper airway muscle tone with dexmedetomidine compared to propofol and midazolam, but there are no data evaluating this to date.

## 6.2.3. Preoperative Preparation

Preoperative anesthetics other than the sedative agent of choice should be avoided. To prevent regurgitation and aspiration, patients should remain nil per os (NPO) before the procedure. Anticholinergic agents such as atropine or glycopyrrolate can be administered intravenously 30 minutes prior to the procedure to reduce secretions, leading to better visualization and avoidance of coughing due to aspiration during the procedure; mild tachycardia is commonly observed with these anticholinergic agents.

A topical vasoconstrictor is generally applied to one or both nostrils, and a topical anesthetic can be applied to one nostril. The dose of topical anesthetic is minimized to avoid excessive pharyngeal anesthesia, which can lead to coughing during the procedure (again, due to aspiration of secretions) or blunting of muscular reflexes that promote upper airway patency.[26] Awake fiberoptic examination performed before initiating sedation can confirm adequate topical anesthesia. This awake examination also allows the anesthesia team the opportunity to visualize the patient's airway before administration of sedation, often providing some additional level of comfort.

Historically, DISE is performed in the supine position. Although it may be technically easier to perform the procedure in the supine position, various studies have found significantly different DISE findings in supine position versus nonsupine position.[27-30] Although it may be technically easier to perform DISE in the supine position, one must bear in mind that the majority of OSA patients are positional and have an increase in respiratory events specifically in the supine question, making examination of an individual's pattern of upper airway obstruction in both the lateral and supine position important.

Surgeons' preferences regarding patient positioning vary widely. Some prefer to use the supine position in all patients, as this body position is used by many patients for at least a portion of the night and may reflect the body position that is most problematic for OSA. Other surgeons prefer to use the patient's natural body position during sleep. Still others evaluate the patient in both the lateral and supine positions or turn the head to the side while the trunk is in the supine position.[31] Studies have questioned whether rotation of the head to the lateral position may suffice instead of positioning the head and trunk in the lateral position. In patients with positional sleep apnea (but not in those without positional changes), DISE findings differ between lateral head rotation and lateral head and trunk rotation.[32]

There is no single best approach, but if possible the surgeon should examine the body (or head) position that will provide the greatest amount of information to use in treatment selection. Based on our experience, we recommend starting the DISE procedure with the patient positioned on the right side, both head and trunk. After adequate observation in this position, tilt the patient into the supine position (both head and trunk).

## 6.2.4. Setting and Monitoring

DISE is usually performed in the operating room or procedure suite, but it is also possible to perform DISE in various outpatient settings, depending on the availability of personnel and appropriate equipment for administering sedation safely. The temperature of the room should be set as comfortable as possible. Lights should be dimmed, and the room noise should be minimized.

Oxygen saturation, cardiac rhythm, and blood pressure monitoring are required during the procedure. Supplemental oxygen may not be necessary, but it should be available for potential use. Some surgeons prefer routine administration of oxygen via nasal cannula or face mask placed on the upper chest in a "blow-by" fashion.

The most important evaluation of the depth of sedation is clinical, through the onset of snoring, disordered breathing events, and the loss of consciousness. The BIS score may provide additional monitoring of sedation.[16] The BIS score is associated with the depth of sedation, with a potential target BIS score of 55 to 70, based on changes in muscle tone and upper airway collapsibility.[16] Greater depth of sedation may produce greater loss of muscle tone and increased airway collapsibility. One study of DISE using propofol showed an increase in airway obstruction (both severity and contribution of the palate and tongue) at BIS scores of 50 to 60 versus 65 to 75.[33]

## 6.2.5. Risks and Disadvantages

No catastrophic events have been reported with DISE. Endotracheal intubation is extremely rare, and cricothyrotomy and tracheostomy also have not been reported. Oversedation that may lead to airway compromise or central apnea can be prevented by titrating the sedative agent to the lowest level that maintains the target of sedation. Supplemental oxygen or concurrent positive airway pressure administration may be an option to prevent complications in high-risk patients such as those with morbid obesity or greater medical comorbidity. Other DISE risks include local pain on intravenous infusion of propofol and allergic reaction to medications.

# 6.3. Diagnosis

## 6.3.1. Airway Evaluation: The VOTE Classification

DISE is principally an examination of the pharynx, and during the examination, the flexible fiberoptic laryngoscope is moved a number of times in order to evaluate the entire length of the pharynx across a number of cycles of airway obstruction and normal breathing. Surgeon must recognize that they are often visualizing only a portion of the pharynx at a single point in time, necessitating evaluation and reevaluation of different regions to understand, to the extent possible, the source(s) of airway obstruction over a period of time in different body positions, during various maneuvers, etc.

A variety of classification schemes have been described to characterize DISE findings. There are at least seven schemes reported in the literature, with a wide range of complexity.[5,34–39] The Velum, Oropharynx, Tongue, Epiglottis (VOTE) classification was proposed as a standard for DISE scoring because it incorporates the four major structures that contribute to airway obstruction in most patients: velum (palate), oropharyngeal lateral walls, tongue, and epiglottis. The hope is that widespread adoption of the VOTE classification would lead to the sharing of findings and results across centers, enhancing clinical and research communication and collaboration.

## 6.3.2. The Structures of VOTE

The VOTE classification allows the surgeon to characterize the structures that contribute to pharyngeal obstruction in a patient, incorporating the degree and configuration of airway narrowing related to these structures that are each composed of multiple components.

### 6.3.2.1. Velum

Velum-related obstruction is that related to the palate and occurs due to the soft palate, uvula, or lateral pharyngeal wall tissue at the level of the velopharynx. Airway closure related to the velum can occur with collapse in an anteroposterior (Figure 6.1), concentric, or, less commonly, lateral configuration. Because it is not always possible to distinguish between the soft palate, uvula, and lateral pharyngeal walls at the level of the velopharynx

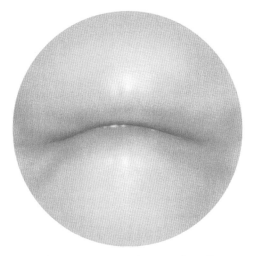

FIGURE 6.1. View of the velum demonstrating anterior posterior collapse.

on DISE, the VOTE classification groups them under the umbrella of the velum. The lateral pharyngeal walls at the level of the velopharynx have some interaction with the remainder of the lateral wall tissues, but in the VOTE classification there is an attempt to describe these separately.

## 6.3.2.2. Oropharyngeal Lateral Walls, Including Tonsils

The oropharyngeal lateral walls include the palatine tonsils and the lateral pharyngeal wall tissues that include muscles and the adjacent parapharyngeal fat pads, among other elements. In the VOTE classification, the oropharyngeal lateral walls collapse only in a lateral configuration (Figure 6.2), although there can be some collapse of

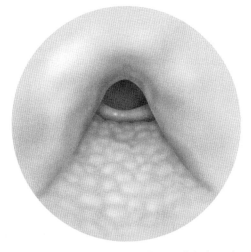

FIGURE 6.2. View of the oropharynx demonstrating collapse of the lateral walls.

tissues originating on the posterior pharyngeal walls that create the impression of a concentric pattern. In the presence of lateral wall collapse, it can be difficult (but certainly not impossible) to determine whether the tonsils alone are the source of airway obstruction or whether the other lateral pharyngeal tissues also contribute. The distinction can have important implications for treatment selection and outcomes. While the VOTE classification is largely based on DISE findings alone, the examination of tonsil size and lateral pharyngeal wall tissues during routine oral cavity examination can be invaluable in making a determination of potential contributions of each of these structural elements.

### 6.3.2.3. Tongue

Tongue-related obstruction is a common DISE finding, and it results in anteroposterior narrowing of the upper airway (Figure 6.3). In natural sleep, there is a reduction in upper airway muscle tone. Because the tongue is largely composed of muscle, fat, and lymphoid tissue (lingual tonsil), this muscle relaxation leads to tongue-related airway obstruction in many patients. Tongue-related obstruction occurs in an anteroposterior configuration only.

### 6.3.2.4. Epiglottis

Epiglottic collapse may occur in an anteroposterior (Figure 6.4) or lateral configuration. Anteroposterior collapse can result with folding of the epiglottis based on what appears to be decreased structural rigidity of the epiglottis or with a posterior displacement of the entire epiglottis against the posterior pharyngeal wall, with apparently normal epiglottic structural integrity. In the rarer lateral collapse, a lateral folding or involution is consistent with a central vertically oriented crease of decreased rigidity of the epiglottis. The

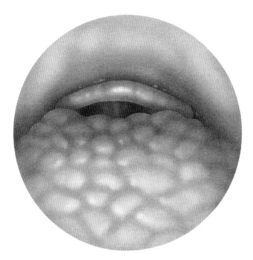

**FIGURE 6.3.** View of the base of tongue and epiglottis showing anterior posterior collapse.

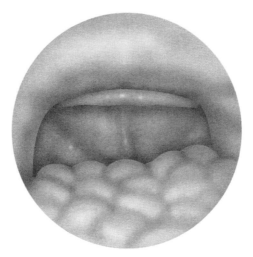

**FIGURE 6.4.** View of the base of tongue and epiglottis showing independent anterior posterior epi-glottic collapse.

epiglottis may be underrecognized as a factor in patients with sleep disordered breathing, and a substantial proportion of patients with OSA demonstrate a significant epiglottic contribution to airway obstruction during DISE.[23,40] Identification of an epiglottic contribution is unique to DISE, as its apparent role has not been demonstrated clearly with other evaluation techniques.[41,42]

## 6.3.3. Other Structures
Airway obstruction in sleep disordered breathing can be related to other structures. In rare cases, collapse superior to the VOTE structures (e.g., massive nasal polyps or naso-pharynx) or inferior to the VOTE structures (e.g., larynx) can be visualized, although at least the nasal airway is easily visualized with office fiberoptic examination. These are usually detected by awake examination prior to DISE and are noted separately. While these are important, the VOTE classification was developed to reflect the patterns of pharyngeal obstruction seen in the large majority of patients.

## 6.3.4. Degree of Airway Narrowing
The VOTE classification involves a qualitative assessment of the degree of airway narrowing for each structure, divided into the following:

- None (typically with no vibration or airflow limitation related to the involved structure),
- Partial (vibration, possible reduced airflow), or
- Complete (obstruction, markedly reduced or absent airflow).

Differentiating between the three categories is not always clear, although as outlined later in the chapter the evaluation of degree of obstruction has demonstrated moderate to substantial reliability.[23,43] Importantly, different structures can have different degrees (and configuration) of obstruction in the same patient.

The VOTE classification does not exclude additional assessments. DISE can be performed in various body positions, as described earlier in the chapter. If there are differential patterns of obstruction according to body position, this may require separate VOTE scoring for each body position.

DISE permits certain maneuvers, ranging from manual closure of the mouth only to the Esmarch maneuver (mandibular advancement). Open-mouth breathing is associated with reduction of the retropalatal and retroglossal areas and thus can worsen OSA.[44] One-third of patients with persistent OSA after previous palate surgery have moderate to severe mouth opening, with half demonstrating marked improvement in airway obstruction with manual mouth closure during DISE.[45] The Esmarch maneuver is performed by gently advancing the mandible by up to approximately 5 mm in an attempt to reproduce the effect of a mandibular repositioning appliance. Studies suggest that the use of a simulation bite (in maximal comfortable protrusion of the mandible) may be more effective in predicting the response of treatment with a mandibular advancement device.[46] As for differences according to body position, multiple separate VOTE assessments can be used during a single DISE to record changes in the pattern of collapse that occur after an assessment with these maneuvers.

# 6.4. Clinical Outcomes

## 6.4.1. Test Properties of DISE: Validity, Reliability, and Uniqueness of Information

Any useful diagnostic test must demonstrate key characteristics such as validity and reliability, and these have been examined for DISE.

DISE is not a perfect representation of natural sleep. Nevertheless, in one study light sedation with relatively low doses of propofol using target-controlled infusion did not produce marked changes in the apnea–hypopnea index (AHI) or oxygen saturations, compared to natural sleep.[47]

Administration of propofol at a wide range of doses (a relatively high dose at the maximum levels) did not cause any snoring or airway obstruction in 54 subjects without a history of snoring or witnessed apneas, whereas all 53 subjects with such a history demonstrated snoring and/or airway obstruction.[48] Another study showed greater airway collapsibility in those with OSA compared with those with primary snoring during sedation with propofol.[49]

Interrater reliability reflects the degree to which ratings from different reviewers are similar. Interrater reliability was moderate to substantial in one study of two experienced reviewers,[23] and another study showed greater interrater reliability for experienced versus nonexperienced reviewers.[50] Test–retest reliability, which evaluates the ratings on distinct

DISE examinations performed on the same patient, has also been shown to be moderate to substantial.[43] This is in sharp contrast to the marked variation seen among different patients undergoing DISE,[40] a reassuring finding that likely relates to the heterogeneity of anatomic factors contributing to OSA.

Information taken from DISE is different from other upper airway evaluation techniques. No association was seen between elevated modified Mallampati score (reflecting a tongue size that is large relative to space posterior to the mandible) and tongue-related obstruction during DISE performed with propofol.[41] Another study compared findings of DISE performed with propofol and the lateral cephalogram x-ray. Amid an extensive series of measurements, only the posterior airway space (anteroposterior dimension of the airway posterior to the tongue base) was associated with tongue-related obstruction.[42]

## 6.4.2. DISE and Airway Surgery

Because the purpose of DISE is guiding treatment selection, some have argued that DISE is helpful if it modifies the treatment plan. One study suggested that DISE may alter treatment recommendations in 78% of cases.[51]

Another approach is to consider whether there are associations between DISE findings and outcomes of various interventions. Multiple case series studies have examined this. Subjects with anteroposterior palate-related obstruction or obstruction related to the palatine tonsils on DISE performed with diazepam achieved better outcome after uvulopalatopharyngoplasty (UPPP), along with tonsillectomy in those without previous tonsillectomy, than those with concentric palate-related obstruction or obstruction related to structures other than the palate or tonsils (with or without palate- or tonsil-related obstruction).[38] Similarly, patients with nasal and palatal obstruction during DISE performed with propofol had better outcomes after UPPP than those with hypopharyngeal region obstruction.[52]

Preoperative findings of DISE performed with propofol have also been associated with surgical outcomes in cohort studies including single-level and multilevel surgery. Among a group of patients undergoing a range of procedures (including nasal surgery, UPPP, the pillar procedure, genioglossus advancement, tongue base resection, tongue stabilization, and hyoid suspension) that resulted in a 56% response rate ($\geq$50% reduction in the AHI to <20 events per hour), preoperative DISE findings of complete oropharyngeal lateral wall-related obstruction and complete epiglottis-related obstruction were associated with nonresponse to surgery.[53] Another study involving DISE performed with propofol included those undergoing one or more procedures from among UPPP, Z-palatoplasty, tongue base radiofrequency, and hyoid suspension; individuals with complete concentric collapse of the velum or complete tongue-related obstruction had poorer outcomes, after adjusting for age, gender, AHI, and body mass index.[54]

The largest study examining the association between DISE findings and surgery outcomes was a multicenter cohort study of individuals with OSA and without enlarged tonsils (0 to 2+ tonsils), incorporating review of preoperative DISE videos by four surgeon reviewers blinded to type of procedure and outcomes.[55] Among 275 study participants from 14 centers, partial or complete oropharyngeal lateral wall-related obstruction was associated with poorer surgical outcomes (adjusted odds ratio for surgical response 0.51; 95% confidence interval 0.27, 0.93). Complete tongue-related obstruction was associated with lower odds of surgical response (adjusted odds ratio 0.52; 95% confidence interval 0.28, 0.98). Surgical outcomes were not clearly associated with the degree and configuration of velum-related obstruction or the degree of epiglottis-related obstruction.

DISE has also been used to examine nonresponders to single-level or multilevel pharyngeal OSA surgery. DISE performed with propofol revealed a wide range of potential sources of residual airway obstruction, including that related to the velum or other VOTE structures and moderate to severe mouth opening that was associated with narrowing of upper airway dimensions.[45]

## 6.4.3. DISE and Hypoglossal Nerve Stimulation

In an early study of hypoglossal nerve stimulation using upper airway stimulation, complete concentric collapse related to the velum during DISE performed with propofol was associated with poorer outcomes; the response rate was 0% (0/5) versus 81% (13/16), based on a definition of response of ≥50% decrease in the AHI to <20 events/hour.[56] This study led to the use of DISE in patient selection for the Stimulation Therapy for Apnea Reduction (STAR) trial[57] and the requirement of DISE as a screening test prior to implantation, excluding those with complete concentric collapse related to the velum. A study performed at the completion of this trial revealed that during DISE performed with an individual in the supine body position, this technology produced an overall 180% enlargement of the cross-sectional area of the retropalatal airway and a 130% increase in the cross-sectional area of the hypopharyngeal region airway.[58] Interestingly, the increase in retropalatal airway cross-sectional area was limited to the anteroposterior dimension, whereas there was enlargement of the transverse and anteroposterior dimensions in the hypopharyngeal region airway.

Currently, DISE is required to confirm the absence of complete concentric collapse prior to proceeding with hypoglossal nerve stimulation. The impact of various sites and configurations of upper airway obstruction observed through DISE on hypoglossal nerve stimulation outcomes is under investigation.

## 6.4.4. Nonsurgical Approaches

Because positional OSA is so common, it is interesting to note the changes that have been demonstrated with changes in body position during DISE. Sleep position has been shown to alter the pattern of obstruction during DISE in individuals with positional (but not nonpositional) OSA.[28] The supine body position was associated with a greater presence and severity of obstruction related to the tongue and epiglottis in positional OSA. In another study, head turning to the side (with the body in the supine position) produced findings similar to those with the head and body both in the lateral position, with the exception of greater anteroposterior velum-related obstruction with the head and body both in the lateral position.[31] This suggests that head rotation may be a reasonable substitute, facilitating the assessment of positional therapy.

The Esmarch maneuver during DISE may indicate benefit of treatment with a mandibular repositioning appliance. Among OSA patients who showed a substantial improvement in airway dimensions with mandibular advancement during DISE performed with propofol, 97% achieved an improvement in subjective or objective measures (not defined clearly) with mandibular repositioning appliance treatment.[59] Another study from the same group showed that DISE performed with propofol with the patient wearing the mandibular repositioning device achieves similar changes in the airway as manual mandibular advancement.[60] Manual mandibular advancement may produce arousals and may not capture the degree of mouth opening that occurs with a mandibular repositioning appliance; it is possible to use a custom-fabricated mouthpiece to simulate the effect of mandibular advancement.[46]

# 6.5. Conclusion

Identifying the pattern of airway obstruction in OSA is critical. No single ideal method exists, although DISE is an attractive option. DISE is a structure-based surgical evaluation technique that may enable targeted, more effective, and less invasive treatment of snoring and OSA.

# References

1. Weaver TE, Grunstein RR. Adherence to continuous positive airway pressure therapy: The challenge to effective treatment. *Proc Am Thorac Soc.* 2008;5:173–178.
2. Cistulli PA, Armitstead J, Pepin JL, et al. Short-term CPAP adherence in obstructive sleep apnea: A big data analysis using real-world data. *Sleep Med.* 2019;59:114–116.
3. Borowiecki B, Pollak CP, Weitzman ED, et al. Fibro-optic study of pharyngeal airway during sleep in patients with hypersomnia obstructive sleep-apnea syndrome. *Laryngoscope.* 1978;88:1310–1313.
4. Rojewski TE, Schuller DE, Clark RW, et al. Synchronous video recording of the pharyngeal airway and polysomnograph in patients with obstructive sleep apnea. *Laryngoscope.* 1982;92:246–250.
5. Croft CB, Pringle M. Sleep nasendoscopy: A technique of assessment in snoring and obstructive sleep apnoea. *Clin Otolaryngol Allied Sci.* 1991;16:504–509.
6. Hohenhorst W. Personal communication; 2005.
7. Ramsay MA, Savege TM, Simpson BR, Goodwin R. Controlled sedation with alphaxalone-alphadolone. *Br Med J.* 1974;2:656–659.
8. White DP. Pathogenesis of obstructive and central sleep apnea. *Am J Respir Crit Care Med.* 2005;172:1363–1370.
9. Fogel RB, Trinder J, Malhotra A, et al. Within-breath control of genioglossal muscle activation in humans: Effect of sleep-wake state. *J Physiol.* 2003;550:899–910.
10. Fogel RB, Trinder J, White DP, et al. The effect of sleep onset on upper airway muscle activity in patients with sleep apnoea versus controls. *J Physiol.* 2005;564:549–562.
11. Horner RL, Innes JA, Morrell MJ, Shea SA, Guz A. The effect of sleep on reflex genioglossus muscle activation by stimuli of negative airway pressure in humans. *J Physiol.* 1994;476:141–151.

12. Malhotra A, Pillar G, Fogel RB, et al. Genioglossal but not palatal muscle activity relates closely to pharyngeal pressure. *Am J Respir Crit Care Med.* 2000;162:1058–1062.

13. Shea SA, Edwards JK, White DP. Effects of sleep-wake transitions and REM sleep on genioglossal response to upper airway negative pressure. *Am J Respir Crit Care Med.* 1998;157:A653.

14. Wheatley JR, Tangel DJ, Mezzanotte WS, White DP. Influence of sleep on response to negative airway pressure of tensor palatini muscle and retropalatal airway. *J Appl Physiol.* 1993;75:2117–2124.

15. Wheatley JR, White DP. The influence of sleep on pharyngeal reflexes. *Sleep.* 1993;16:S87–S89.

16. Hillman DR, Walsh JH, Maddison KJ, et al. Evolution of changes in upper airway collapsibility during slow induction of anesthesia with propofol. *Anesthesiology.* 2009;111:63–71.

17. Tangel DJ, Mezzanotte WS, White DP. Influence of sleep on tensor palatini EMG and upper airway resistance in normal men. *J Appl Physiol.* 1991;70:2574–2581.

18. Alkire MT, Haier RJ, Fallon JH. Toward a unified theory of narcosis: brain imaging evidence for a thalamocortical switch as the neurophysiologic basis of anesthetic-induced unconsciousness. *Conscious Cogn.* 2000;9:370–386.

19. Saper CB, Chou TC, Scammell TE. The sleep switch: Hypothalamic control of sleep and wakefulness. *Trends Neurosci.* 2001;24:726–731.

20. Eastwood PR, Platt PR, Shepherd K, et al. Collapsibility of the upper airway at different concentrations of propofol anesthesia. *Anesthesiology.* 2005;103:470–477.

21. Eckert DJ, Malhotra A, Lo YL, et al. The influence of obstructive sleep apnea and gender on genioglossus activity during rapid eye movement sleep. *Chest.* 2009;135:957–964.

22. Roblin G, Williams AR, Whittet H. Target-controlled infusion in sleep endoscopy. *Laryngoscope.* 2001;111:175–176.

23. Kezirian EJ, White DP, Malhotra A, et al. Interrater reliability of drug-induced sleep endoscopy. *Arch Otolaryngol Head Neck Surg.* 2010;136:393–397.

24. Chattopadhyay U, Mallik S, Ghosh S, et al. Comparison between propofol and dexmedetomidine on depth of anesthesia: A prospective randomized trial. *J Anaesthesiol Clin Pharmacol.* 2014;30:550–554.

25. Cho JS, Soh S, Kim EJ, et al. Comparison of three sedation regimens for drug-induced sleep endoscopy. *Sleep Breath.* 2015;19:711–717.

26. Fogel RB, Malhotra A, Shea SA, et al. Reduced genioglossal activity with upper airway anesthesia in awake patients with OSA. *J Appl Physiol.* 2000;88:1346–1354.

27. Lee CH, Kim DK, Kim SY, et al. Changes in site of obstruction in obstructive sleep apnea patients according to sleep position: A DISE study. *Laryngoscope.* 2015;125:248–254.

28. Victores AJ, Hamblin J, Gilbert J, et al. Usefulness of sleep endoscopy in predicting positional obstructive sleep apnea. *Otolaryngol Head Neck Surg.* 2014;150:487–493.

29. Vonk PE, Ravesloot MJL, Kasius KM, et al. Floppy epiglottis during drug-induced sleep endoscopy: An almost complete resolution by adopting the lateral posture. *Sleep Breath.* 2020;24(1):103–109.

30. Yalamanchili R, Mack WJ, Kezirian EJ. Drug-induced sleep endoscopy findings in supine vs. nonsupine body positions in positional and nonpositional obstructive sleep apnea. *JAMA Otolaryngology Head Neck Surg.* 2019;145:159–165.

31. Safiruddin F, Koutsourelakis I, de Vries N. Upper airway collapse during drug induced sleep endoscopy: Head rotation in supine position compared with lateral head and trunk position. *Eur Arch Otorhinolaryngol.* 2015;272:485–488.

32. Vonk PE, van de Beek MJ, Ravesloot MJL, de Vries N. Drug-induced sleep endoscopy: New insights in lateral head rotation compared to lateral head and trunk rotation in (non)positional obstructive sleep apnea patients. *Laryngoscope.* 2019;129:2430–2435.

33. Lo YL, Ni YL, Wang TY, et al. Bispectral Index in evaluating effects of sedation depth on drug-induced sleep endoscopy. *J Clin Sleep Med.* 2015;11(9):1011–1020.

34. Kezirian EJ, Hohenhorst W, de Vries N. Drug-induced sleep endoscopy: The VOTE classification. *Eur Arch Otorhinolaryngol.* 2011;268:1233–1236.

35. Abdullah VJ, Wing YK, van Hasselt CA. Video sleep nasendoscopy: The Hong Kong experience. *Otolaryngol Clin North Am.* 2003;36:461–471.

36. Friedman M, Ibrahim H, Bass L. Clinical staging for sleep-disordered breathing. *Otolaryngol Head Neck Surg.* 2002;127:13–21.

37. Fujita S, Conway W, Zorick F, Roth T. Surgical correction of anatomic abnormalities in obstructive sleep apnea syndrome: Uvulopalatopharyngoplasty. *Otolaryngol Head Neck Surg.* 1981;89:923–934.

38. Iwanaga K, Hasegawa K, Shibata N, et al. Endoscopic examination of obstructive sleep apnea syndrome patients during drug-induced sleep. *Acta Otolaryngol Suppl.* 2003;(550):36–40.

39. Vicini C, De Vito A, Benazzo M, et al. The nose oropharynx hypopharynx and larynx (NOHL) classification: A new system of diagnostic standardized examination for OSAHS patients. *Eur Arch Otorhinolaryngol.* 2012;269:1297–300.

40. Vroegop AV, Vanderveken OM, Boudewyns AN, et al. Drug-induced sleep endoscopy in sleep-disordered breathing: Report on 1,249 cases. *Laryngoscope.* 2014;124:797–802.

41. den Herder C, van Tinteren H, de Vries N. Sleep endoscopy versus modified Mallampati score in sleep apnea and snoring. *Laryngoscope.* 2005;115:735–739.

42. George JR, Chung S, Nielsen I, et al. Comparison of drug-induced sleep endoscopy and lateral cephalometry in obstructive sleep apnea. *Laryngoscope.* 2012;122:2600–2605.

43. Rodriguez-Bruno K, Goldberg AN, McCulloch CE, Kezirian EJ. Test-retest reliability of drug-induced sleep endoscopy. *Otolaryngol Head Neck Surg.* 2009;140:646–651.

44. Lee CH, Hong SL, Rhee CS, et al. Analysis of upper airway obstruction by sleep videofluoroscopy in obstructive sleep apnea: A large population-based study. *Laryngoscope.* 2012;122:237–241.

45. Kezirian EJ. Nonresponders to pharyngeal surgery for obstructive sleep apnea: Insights from drug-induced sleep endoscopy. *Laryngoscope.* 2011;121:1320–1326.

46. Vroegop AV, Vanderveken OM, Dieltjens M, et al. Sleep endoscopy with simulation bite for prediction of oral appliance treatment outcome. *J Sleep Res.* 2013;22:348–355.

47. Rabelo FA, Braga A, Kupper DS, et al. Propofol-induced sleep: Polysomnographic evaluation of patients with obstructive sleep apnea and controls. *Otolaryngol Head Neck Surg.* 2010;142:218–224.

48. Berry S, Roblin G, Williams A, et al. Validity of sleep nasendoscopy in the investigation of sleep related breathing disorders. *Laryngoscope.* 2005;115:538–540.

49. Steinhart H, Kuhn-Lohmann J, Gewalt K, et al. Upper airway collapsibility in habitual snorers and sleep apneics: Evaluation with drug-induced sleep endoscopy. *Acta Otolaryngol.* 2000;120:990–994.

50. Vroegop AV, Vanderveken OM, Wouters K, et al. Observer variation in drug-induced sleep endoscopy: Experienced versus nonexperienced ear, nose, and throat surgeons. *Sleep.* 2013;36:947–953.

51. Eichler C, Sommer JU, Stuck BA, et al. Does drug-induced sleep endoscopy change the treatment concept of patients with snoring and obstructive sleep apnea? *Sleep Breath.* 2013;17:63–68.

52. Hessel NS, Vries N. Increase of the apnoea-hypopnoea index after uvulopalatopharyngoplasty: Analysis of failure. *Clin Otolaryngol Allied Sci.* 2004;29:682–685.

53. Soares D, Sinawe H, Folbe AJ, et al. Lateral oropharyngeal wall and supraglottic airway collapse associated with failure in sleep apnea surgery. *Laryngoscope.* 2012;122:473–479.

54. Koutsourelakis I, Safiruddin F, Ravesloot M, et al. Surgery for obstructive sleep apnea: Sleep endoscopy determinants of outcome. *Laryngoscope.* 2012;122:2587–2591.

55. Green KK, Kent DT, D'Agostino MA, et al. Drug-induced sleep endoscopy and surgical outcomes: A multicenter cohort study. *Laryngoscope.* 2019;129(3):761–770.

56. Vanderveken OM, Maurer JT, Hohenhorst W, et al. Evaluation of drug-induced sleep endoscopy as a patient selection tool for implanted upper airway stimulation for obstructive sleep apnea. *J Clin Sleep Med.* 2013;9:433–438.

57. Strollo PJ Jr, Soose RJ, Maurer JT, et al. Upper-airway stimulation for obstructive sleep apnea. *N Engl J Med.* 2014;370:139–149.

58. Safiruddin F, Vanderveken OM, de Vries N, et al. Effect of upper-airway stimulation for obstructive sleep apnoea on airway dimensions. *Eur Respir J.* 2015;45:129–138.

59. Johal A, Battagel JM, Kotecha BT. Sleep nasendoscopy: A diagnostic tool for predicting treatment success with mandibular advancement splints in obstructive sleep apnoea. *Eur J Orthod.* 2005;27:607–614.

60. Johal A, Hector MP, Battagel JM, Kotecha BT. Impact of sleep nasendoscopy on the outcome of mandibular advancement splint therapy in subjects with sleep-related breathing disorders. *J Laryngol Otol.* 2007;121:668–675.

# Surgical Technique

## Device Implantation, Operative Device Programming, and Guidelines for Anesthesia

Clemens Heiser and J. Ulrich Sommer

## 7.1. Device Implantation

### 7.1.1. Materials

Beside basic surgical instruments for extended surgery in the head and neck region, a few specialties deserve mentioning:

- Two-channel neuromonitoring system (e.g., Medtronic NIM III)
- Bipolar "fork-like" probe for neuromonitoring system
- Microscope with attached monitor
- Small Overholt dissecting forceps
- Flexible brain ribbon retractor (~5 mm wide)

### 7.1.2. Introduction

Certain important points need to be considered when implanting a system for upper airway stimulation. The first and most important one is careful selection of the correct branches of the hypoglossal nerve. Therefore, using an intraoperative neuromonitoring device can be very helpful to provide a close look at the nerve's microanatomy and the functional effects of the stimulation. The second important step is the correct placement of the sensing lead because a bad respiratory sensing signal may make successful stimulation impossible.[1] The final point is the importance of maintaining sterile technique throughout surgery because an infection may necessitate removal of the whole system and will make it impossible to implant the system in a second attempt due to postinflammatory scarring.[2]

## 7.1.3. Preparation

Details regarding patient positioning and intubation are described in detail in the section on anesthesia later in this chapter. After finishing the positioning steps, the intraoral neuromonitoring electrodes are placed after exposure of the oral cavity.[3] Here, a compromise must be found between good exposure of the tongue and leaving enough space under the chin to perform surgery on the hypoglossal nerve.

For neuromonitoring, two Prass paired electrodes (18 mm long) are used (Figure 7.1). For monitoring of the genioglossus muscle, the first electrode is placed in the anterior floor of the mouth at the right side, directed in a vertical direction toward the inner side of the mandible. The styloglossus and hyoglossus muscles, necessary for the unwanted retraction of the tongue, may be monitored by placing an electrode along the ventrolateral aspect of the right tongue directed posteriorly, just underneath the mucosa.[4,5] After careful fixation of the neuromonitoring electrodes, leaving enough slack in the cables for the tongue to move, the surgical area is prepared, keeping all incisions in one sterile field. The mouth is covered with an incise sterile drape (e.g., transparent, adhesive polyurethane film) to allow visual control of the tongue movements during stimulation.

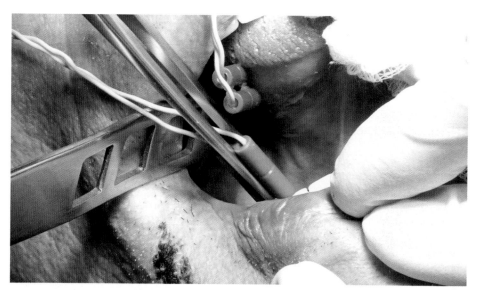

**FIGURE 7.1.** The blue electrode is placed in the anterior floor of the mouth (right side) to detect the electromyographic signals from the genioglossus muscle. The red electrode is placed along the corner of the right tongue underneath the mucosa to detect the electromyographic signals from the styloglossus and hyoglossus muscles.

## 7.1.4. Hypoglossal Nerve Dissection and Placement of the Cuff Electrode

Surgery begins by making a 3- to 5-cm-long incision starting ~1 cm from midline, 1.5 cm below the mandible (Figure 7.2). The platysma is dissected and the anterior belly of the digastric muscle is visualized. The next step is to identify the anterior edge of the submandibular gland as a posterior border of the surgical field. The posterior edge of the mylohyoid muscle is lifted carefully and the whole surgical field is exposed using three retractors. The first retractor holds back the submandibular gland, the second one lifts the mylohyoid muscle, and the third one draws the digastric muscle caudal. From there on, the hypoglossal nerve main trunk may be identified in the center of the resulting triangle, at the anterior edge of the submandibular gland. A large ranine vein (vena comitans of hypoglossal nerve) usually hinders further preparation of the anterior branching of the hypoglossal nerve and may be ligated at the very beginning of surgery (Figure 7.3). After that, the chances of uncontrolled bleeding during surgery are greatly reduced.

After that, the anterior branching of the hypoglossal nerve should be taken care of and the retractor branches need to be excluded; the protrusion branches need to be included. To accomplish this task, the microanatomy of the hypoglossal nerve should be carefully inspected. In many cases there is a clear and noticeable "breaking point" where the retracting fibers of the nerve leave the main trunk in a cranial direction (Figure 7.4).[6] Accompanying vasa nervorum that are running with the surrounding soft tissue of the nerve often make it easier to distinguish the different branches. After separating the branches, the nerve-integrity monitoring probe is used for further identification.

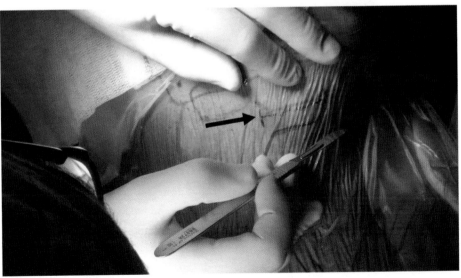

**FIGURE 7.2.** The black arrow marks the skin incision line. In most cases the incision line is 3 to 5 cm long, starting ~1 cm from midline, 1.0 cm below the mandible. The smallest incision, at 2 cm, was done by Mau Boon (world record, approved by Colin Huntley).

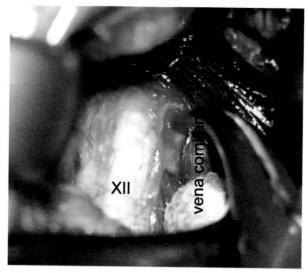

**FIGURE 7.3.** Separation of the vena comitans from the main trunk of hypoglossal nerve. MH = mylohoid muscle, XII = hypoglossal nerve.

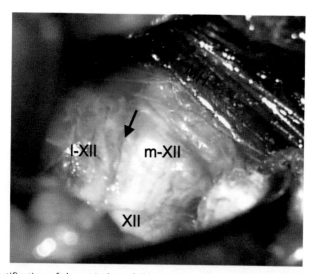

**FIGURE 7.4.** Identification of the main lateral (l-XII) and medial (m-XII) branches of the hypoglossal nerve. Arrow shows the first breakpoint of separation. MH = mylohoid muscle, XII = hypoglossal nerve.

A "fork-like" bipolar neuromonitoring probe is highly recommended for this task because it allows very selective stimulation of individual and closely coupled fibers compared to a monopolar stimulation probe.[3] The surgeon should have a close look at the neuromonitoring system to ensure that no unwanted retracting branches are included in the later-to-be-cuffed bundle (Figures 7.5 and 7.6). If differentiating the branches is unusually complicated, the tongue movement should be inspected to further distinguish

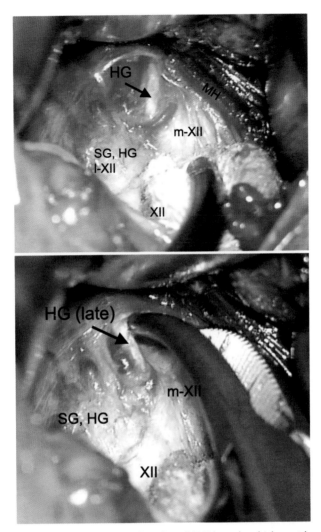

**FIGURES 7.5 AND 7.6.** Emergence of the last hyoglossal (HG) branch, which must be excluded in order to place selectively the stimulation lead. MH = mylohoid muscle, XII = hypoglossal nerve.

the branches. A contralateral or bilateral tongue movement serves as a good indicator for inclusion.

If possible the C1/C2 roots that travel with the hypoglossal nerve and also have a motor function should be included into the cuff electrode because it is known that stimulation of the geniohyoid muscle (to elevate the hyoid bone) and the thyrohyoid muscle (to depress the hyoid bone) contributes to successful airway opening.[3,7]

If the correct and final branches of the hypoglossal nerve have been identified, the silicone cuff is placed around the nerve with the wire end facing in the lateral direction (Figure 7.7). The easiest method usually is grabbing the uppermost right part of the rolled-out cuff electrode with a pair of tweezers, passing a small Overholt dissecting

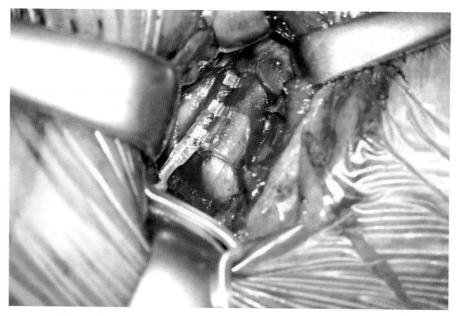

**FIGURE 7.7.** The stimulation lead has been placed around the medial branches of the hypoglossal nerve.

forceps under the nerve, and, after grabbing the corner of the silicone cuff, gently passing it under the nerve. It is important not to use instruments that may damage the silicone insulation when handling the stimulation and later on the sense lead during the placements. Depending on the anatomy, the wire is then passed under or over the digastric tendon to form a loop and the anchor is fixated with two braided permanent sutures to the muscle to create a strain relief from neck movement. The inner part of the cuff electrode is then flushed with saline to flush any air retained in the cuff and therefore decrease impedance for later testing. A gauze soaked in saline is placed in the surgical site and the most difficult part of the procedure is finished.[4]

## 7.1.5. Implantable Pulse Generator Pocket and Placement

The incision for the implantable pulse generator (IPG) pocket is created in a straight line at the right anterior chest wall, midway along the clavicle, ~3 to 4 cm inferior to it, and 4 to 5 cm in length. The dissection is continued to the fascia overlying the pectoralis major muscle, taking care not to damage it. The IPG pocket is then formed in this layer caudal to the incision line. The IPG should be a snug fit in the accommodating pocket and should be created by blunt dissection.

The stimulation leads are then tunneled with the provided disposable tunneling device. Some initial dissection with a Kelly clamp or a large scissor is useful to facilitate the tunneling procedure. The tunneling device is bent beforehand to match the curve of the neck so that the tunneling device passes over the clavicle by any means. Care must be taken to avoid the external jugular vein. Depending on the anatomy, tunneling may be done from the cranial incision toward the IPG pocket or in a reverse direction. After the tunneling device has been passed, the connector is fixed to it and the wire is pulled toward the IPG pocket. After careful cleaning, a short suction catheter should be placed over the connector to protect it during the following dissection of the respiratory sensor.

## 7.1.6. Respiratory Sensor

The incision for the respiratory sensor is made horizontally along the lateral chest, extending ~5 cm laterally to the midline of the axilla, medially to the inferolateral border of the pectoralis major. The height of the incision should be between the fifth and sixth rib, or ~5 cm below the mammilla. In women, the incision may be placed a little bit more posteriorly and caudally to prevent the scar from lying under the edge or the wire of the bra.

Dissection is continued down to the serratus anterior muscle, which is retracted cranially to expose the fifth/sixth intercostal space. After placing some self-holding retractors, the external intercostal muscle is exposed. When dissecting deeper and by watching the grain direction of the muscle, the internal intercostal is easily identified. Using the flexible brain ribbon retractor, a small tunnel is made between the internal and the external intercostal muscles. When the right plane of dissection is found, this should work out effortlessly (Figure 7.8).

The sensor is then passed underneath the ribbon retractor and advanced while the retractor is redrawn simultaneously. The orientation of the sensor, with the pressure-sensitive opening facing toward the pleura, is important to consider here. Afterward, the first anchor next to the sensor is sutured to the fascia using at least three of the four provided fixation points. The orientation of the anchor should be parallel to the chest wall, not tilted in any way, and should form a straight line with the sensor. An omega-shaped strain relief is formed now, and the second anchor is sutured to the fascia of the serratus muscle cranial to the first anchor.

Tunneling the sensing lead is done from the cranial side of the sensing incision and directed upward to the inferior aspect of the IPG pocket. For insertion in the IPG, one surgeon should keep pushing the connector into the IPG while the other surgeon tightens the locking screw with the provided torque-controlled screwdriver. This avoids the connector being pushed out by the so-called air-piston effect, which would result in a poor connection to the IPG.

After testing the system as a whole, the IPG is slid into the anterior chest wall pocket, with the manufacturer's etching facing outward, keeping the sense and stimulation wire under the generator, forming a loop. This prevents problems connecting the IPG with the telemetry unit and facilitates battery changes in the future.

The IPG is finally fixed to the fascia of the pectoralis muscle using a 2-0 braided permanent suture through the suturing hole in the upper left corner of the IPG (Figure 7.9).

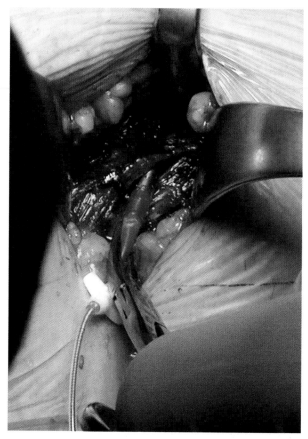

**FIGURE 7.8.** The respiratory sensor is placed between the external and internal intercostal muscles.

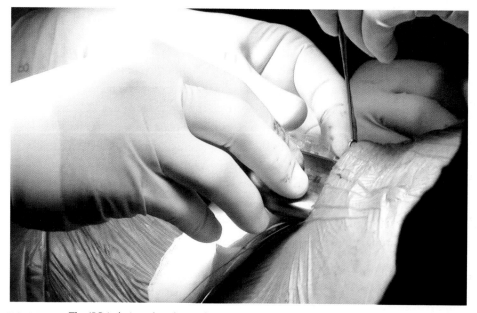

**FIGURE 7.9.** The IPG is being placed into the pocket, which is created in a straight line at the right anterior chest wall.

### 7.1.7. Final Steps

The incisions are sutured in a multilayer way, and a sterile dressing is applied. Inserting wound drainage is not recommended because it increases the risk of infection. On top of the sterile dressing a second dressing should be applied consisting of clouds of bulky gauze or fluff dressing with an elastic tape overlay.[4] The sterile dressing should be kept in place for ~48 hours before being changed for the first time.

## 7.2. Operative Device Programming

With the telemetry unit in a sterile sleeve, the unit is placed on top of the IPG with the grooves facing toward the IPG. The IPG rests on the patient's chest outside of the pre-formed pocket.

After establishing a successful connection, the first test should be to check the respiratory sensing waveform. After a few cycles of signal calibration, the surgeon should see a clear and synchronized breathing pattern free of major artifacts. The software performs an automatic zoom of the signal during the signal calibration phase, which makes interpreting the signal strength more complicated. A hint for assessing the amplitude of the sensing signal is to look for pressure changes resulting from the heartbeat. If the heartbeat amplitude is >30% of the respiratory amplitude, the signal-to-noise ratio is usually not adequate and the sensor should be repositioned. The signal should also be disapproved if the waveform looks edgy or pointy or differs from one breathing cycle to another by a considerable amount. A weak or faulty respiratory sensing signal complicates later successful titration to a significant amount or even may make it impossible.

The second test should be tongue movement. Starting from 0.5 V, the stimulation amplitude is raised until proper tongue movement has been visualized. If the tongue does not show a clear straight or right protrusion (which means a protrusion to the left side of the patient), an incorrect inclusion of the hypoglossal nerve branches and therefore a repositioning of the cuff electrode should be considered. A sign for correct inclusion of the C1/C2 fibers is a clear and strong lifting of the floor of the mouth.[7] It is also possible and, in some cases advisable, to let one person stick one finger into the mouth from underneath the drape and palpate the tongue base during stimulation. A very clear opening should be sought; a closing or no movement at all should also trigger a cuff repositioning.

All test results should be saved into the programming device for later evaluation and troubleshooting.

## 7.3. Anesthesia Guidelines

Anesthesiologic guidelines for implanting hypoglossal nerve stimulation systems differ from general head-and-neck–related procedures in some important ways that are necessary to understand. Induction and maintenance of general anesthesia should not interfere with the surgeon's ability to access the sites of implantation and identify the correct branches using a nerve integrity monitor system. Anesthesia devices should not obstruct the tongue's movement to determine the way of protrusion.

## 7.3.1. Preoperative Management

As nasotracheal intubation is usually preferred for implanting a hypoglossal nerve stimulator, the preoperative assessment should include an otolaryngologic exam with anterior rhinoscopy and/or fiberoptic evaluation of the upper airway to determine the wider nostril and scout for anatomic problems that could hinder successful insertion of the nasotracheal tube into the trachea. As sedating medication may trigger a collapse of the upper airway in patients with obstructive sleep apnea (OSA), these should be avoided in the preoperative management if possible, or patients should be monitored the whole time after administration of the sedating drugs.[8]

## 7.3.2. Preparation Before Induction

To facilitate visualization and reduce the secretion barrier to effective penetration of local anesthesia into the mucosa, atropine 0.5 to 1 mg or 100 mg succinylcholine should be administered prior to induction as an antisialagogue. To provide effective topical anesthesia and decongestion and to reduce bleeding of the nasal mucosa, 3 to 5 ml of a 1:1 mixture of oxymetazoline with xylocaine or another topical anesthetic jelly should be administered to both nostrils with a syringe. The jelly acts as a reservoir for the anesthetic and decongestion agent, producing a dense block. The tube should be prewarmed to soften it and facilitate its movement with minimal force into the nasal cavity.[9,10]

Finally, the standard American Society of Anesthesiologists (ASA) monitors are placed. Care should be taken not to place the electrocardiogram leads in the Mason-Likar configuration (i.e., both infraclavicular fossae, and the anterior axillary line midway between the iliac crest and the costal margin) as this will encroach on the surgical field. Instead, an alternative electrode placement, like placing electrodes on the left and right sides of the forehead and a third anywhere below the neck on the left side, seems like an viable option without creating abnormalities in R-wave amplitude.[11]

## 7.3.3. Intraoperative Management

### 7.3.3.1. Induction

Preoxygenation of the patient should be done with 100% oxygen for ≥3 minutes. Anesthesia then may be induced with intravenous 2 mg midazolam, 100 mcg fentanyl, and slow titration of 120 mg propofol with assurance of assisted ventilation. Succinylcholine may be used as a short-term muscle relaxant. After administration of the induction drugs, the tube is carefully inserted into the wider nostril.

There is a close relationship between OSA and difficult intubation because both are associated with upper airway abnormalities and morphologic changes. Thus, equipment for management of a difficult airway should be in place before induction of general anesthesia even though the airway has been evaluated in the awake condition. A laryngeal mask airway and fiberoptic devices may be useful. Two-person mask ventilation may be needed to attain adequate ventilation.[12]

When the tube has reached the oropharynx and while visualizing the glottis, using for example a C-MAC PM video laryngoscope, further manipulation of the tube is done with a Magill forceps to facilitate its movement into the trachea and to pass the glottis. Especially in OSA patients with hyperplasia of the tongue base, a Sellick maneuver facilitates tube passage into the glottis.

To avoid hypoglossal nerve palsy due to intubation, which may make proper implantation of the stimulation system impossible, all maneuvers involving manipulation of the upper airway should be conducted with the utmost diligence.[13]

A prophylactic antibiotic (e.g., 2 g cefazolin, or other coverage for skin flora if an allergy to cephalosporins is present) is given intravenously at the onset of anesthesia.[5]

### 7.3.3.2. Positioning

The neck is gently extended with a shoulder roll, and a positioning cushion is placed under the right half of the chest to better visualize the area where the respiration sensor is to be placed.[5] The arm should be placed in a loop of cloth, which is fixed by tunneling it under the patient, to remain as close to the body as possible.

The endotracheal tube is then secured to the left side of the mouth and a gauze packing is placed between the molar teeth of the left side, ensuring adequate space to visualize tongue movement during intraoperative assessment of tongue muscle activation. The endotracheal tube should be well secured as this is a shared airway and reintubation after an inadvertent extubation can be challenging intraoperatively. The operating room table is then positioned such that the patient's head is 180 degrees from the anesthesiologist and the anesthesia machine.[12]

### 7.3.3.3. Maintenance

Maintenance of anesthesia may be achieved using remifentanil with an infusion titrated to the rate of 0.05 to 0.2 mcg/kg/min and monitored anesthesia care (MAC) using desflurane with $FiO_2$ of 50%. No muscle relaxants are used after intubation to facilitate hypoglossal nerve integrity monitoring intraoperatively.[12]

While checking the correct pressure sensor placement with the telemetry unit, the positive end-expiratory pressure (PEEP) should be reduced to the minimal bearable value and ventilation of the patient should be done in pressure-controlled mode to achieve comparable and usable results while testing the sensing.

### 7.3.3.4. Emergence

Special emphasis should be placed on the fact that the cotton swab between the molars has been removed and the NIM electrodes have been removed from the tongue prior to emergence from anesthesia. As awake extubation is generally considered to be safer in OSA patients as the return of airway tone, reflexes, and respiratory drive allows the patient to maintain airway patency, extubation of the patient should be done "wide awake." All the anesthetic agents should be discontinued in advance and the oropharynx should be carefully suctioned. Extubation should then be conducted in a head-up position, and the patient should remain semi-upright during the early recovery period. As OSA patients tend to suffer from postoperative hypoxia, supplemental oxygen should be provided after extubation. The benefits of oxygen are supposed to excel the odds of the prolongation or masking of an apnea, atelectasis, or hypoventilation with $CO_2$ retention.

Dexamethasone and a 5HT3 antagonist may be administered for antiemetic prophylaxis.[12,14]

## 7.3.4. Postoperative Management

As patients with OSA are at high risk of developing postoperative complications, they should be closely monitored. The need for a postoperative intensive care unit is still debated, but a post-anesthesia care unit is recommended for OSA patients without any treatment.[14]

Because an upregulation of central opioid receptors and recurrent hypoxemia are pathognomonic to OSA, an increased analgesic sensitivity to subsequent morphine administration should be considered. Therefore, the analgesic requirement should be continuously evaluated and alternative medications such as acetaminophen, tramadol, ketorolac, ketamine, and dexmedetomidine should be used when appropriate to reduce narcotic use.[12,15] Due to the dissection next to the pleural area for placement of the respiratory sensor in the intercostal space, in the case of a sudden drop in oxygen saturation or dyspnea, a pneumothorax should be considered. If possible, an anteroposterior chest x-ray and lateral neck x-ray should be obtained to document the position of the IPG and the leads and to rule out pneumothorax.[4,16]

# References

1. Sommer JU, Heiser C, Hasselbacher K, Steffen A. Changes of respiratory cycle sensing affects therapy outcome in upper airway stimulation in obstructive sleep apnea. *Laryngo-Rhino-Otologie*. 2019;98(Suppl 02):11062.

2. Heiser C, Thaler E, Soose RJ, et al. Technical tips during implantation of selective upper airway stimulation. *Laryngoscope*. 2018;128(3):756–762. doi:10.1002/lary.26724

3. Heiser C, Hofauer B, Lozier L. Nerve monitoring-guided selective hypoglossal nerve stimulation in obstructive sleep apnea patients. *Laryngoscope*. 2016;126(12):2852–2858. doi:10.1002/lary.26026

4. Heiser C. Updates of operative techniques for upper airway stimulation. *Laryngoscope*. 2016;126(Suppl 7):S12–S16. doi:10.1002/lary.26158

5. Maurer JT. Operative technique of upper airway stimulation: An implantable treatment of obstructive sleep apnea. *Oper Techn Otolaryngol*. 2012;23(3):227–233.

6. Lewis R, Pételle B, Campbell MC, et al. Implantation of the Nyxoah bilateral hypoglossal nerve stimulator for obstructive sleep apnea. *Laryngoscope Invest Otolaryngol*. 2019;4(6):703–707. doi:10.1002/lio2.312

7. Zhu Z, Hofauer B, Heiser C. Improving surgical results in complex nerve anatomy during implantation of selective upper airway stimulation. *Auris Nasus Larynx.* 2018;45(3):653–656. doi:10.1016/j.anl.2017.10.005

8. Auckley D, Bolden N. Preoperative screening and perioperative care of the patient with sleep-disordered breathing. *Curr Opin Pulmon Med.* 2012;18:588–595.

9. Mahajan R, Gupta R, Sharma A. Another method to avoid trauma during nasotracheal intubation. *Anesth Analg.* 2005;101:928–929.

10. Prasanna D, Bhat S. Nasotracheal intubation: An overview. *J Maxillofac Oral Surg.* 2014;13(4):366–372.

11. Gupta S, Paliwal B, Kumar M, Bhatia P. Alternative electrocardiography electrode placement. *Anaesthesia.* 2018;73(4):525.

12. Sharma A, Scharoun J. Anesthesia for hypoglossal nerve stimulator: A case report and anesthesia implications. *J Anesth Intens Care Med.* 2018;4(5): 555650. doi:10.19080/JAICM.2018.04.555650

13. Aytuluk HG, Turk J. Unilateral hypoglossal nerve palsy after septoplasty under general anaesthesia. *Anaesthesiol Reanim.* 2018;46(3):241–244.

14. American Society of Anesthesiologists. Practice guidelines for the perioperative management of patients with obstructive sleep apnea: An updated report by the American Society of Anesthesiologists Task Force on Perioperative Management of Patients with Obstructive Sleep Apnea. *Anesthesiology.* 2014;120: 268–286.

15. Connolly LA. Anesthetic management of obstructive sleep apnea patients. *J Clin Anesth.* 1991;3(6):461–469.

16. Chung SA, Yuan H, Chung F. A systemic review of obstructive sleep apnea and its implications for anesthesiologists. *Anesth Analg.* 2008;107(5):1543–1563.

# Efficacy and Safety

Vaibhav H. Ramprasad and Ryan J. Soose

## 8.1. Preclinical Data

### 8.1.1. Animal Basic Science Studies

In the late 1980s, canine studies demonstrated incremental upper airway stability and reduced airway resistance with graded increases in stimulation of the genioglossus muscle.[1] Feline studies shortly afterward by Schwartz et al. showed that increasing bilateral hypoglossal nerve stimulation (HNS) frequencies were associated with increases in airflow and decreases in critical closing pressure ($P_{crit}$).[2] Improvements in upper airway stability with electrical stimulation were corroborated by Oliven et al. in anesthetized canines.[3] Additional animal studies have confirmed that the genioglossus muscle is the primary upper airway dilator and its stimulation advances the tongue anteriorly, whereas stimulation of the hyoglossus and styloglossus muscles retracts the tongue posteriorly and contributes to airway collapse.[4-7] Canine models were also used to study the effects of selective stimulation of different segments of the hypoglossal nerve versus nonselective HNS.[8]

### 8.1.2. Human Basic Science Studies

In the mid-1990s, multiple studies reported on the results of transoral or transcutaneous electrical stimulation of the human tongue.[9-13] Direct stimulation of the lingual musculature in patients with obstructive sleep apnea (OSA) was shown to decrease the frequency of obstructive respiratory events in a subset of the study participants without causing cortical arousal.[14] Oliven et al. demonstrated the airway effects of selective stimulation of tongue protrusor muscles versus tongue retractor muscles. Selective intramuscular stimulation of the genioglossus muscle, the primary tongue protrusor, improved airway stability (reduced $P_{crit}$) while selective stimulation of the styloglossus and hyoglossus muscles, the primary retractors, caused upper airway collapse (increased $P_{crit}$).[3] Co-activation of both sets of muscles (protrusors and retractors) resulted in a net improvement in airflow and reduction in $P_{crit}$. Flexible upper airway endoscopy was also used to confirm under direct visualization that genioglossus muscle stimulation can provide a multilevel effect, enlarging and stabilizing not only the tongue base portion of the airway but also the soft palate area. With the majority of OSA patients demonstrating *multilevel* upper airway collapse, this finding represented a key development in the therapy's potential to make the jump to a standalone OSA treatment and to further distinguish it from traditional tongue base surgeries.

## 8.1.3. Human Pilot and Feasibility Studies

Initial studies by Eisele et al. examined the effects of site-specific HNS.[15] A total of 20 patients were evaluated. Fifteen patients undergoing unrelated head and neck procedures resulting in exposure of the hypoglossal nerve underwent intraoperative site-specific stimulation. In these patients, stimulation of the distal medial branches to the genioglossus muscle produced exclusive tongue protrusion, whereas stimulation of the more proximal and lateral nerve (just distal to the ansa hypoglossi) resulted in tongue retraction. In this same study, five sleep-deprived patients with a clinical diagnosis of OSA underwent direct stimulation of the main trunk of the hypoglossal nerve, resulting in increased airflow by 176.1 ± 32.6 ml/s and direct stimulation of the specific genioglossus branches of the nerve showing further increase in airflow by a mean of 197.2 ± 112.0 ml/s. In addition, the arousal threshold for motor recruitment for tongue movement exceeded that of the cortical arousal threshold in this cohort, proving feasibility of UAS without sleep fragmentation due to the stimulation itself.

This study essentially established the foundation for upper airway stimulation (UAS) to provide safe and effective neuromodulation of the upper airway, and subsequently a capable therapeutic modality for OSA. No significant adverse events were reported in this pilot study except for one episode of bradycardia thought to be secondary to inadvertent stimulation of the vagal nerve. The same group implanted eight patients with a commercially made hypoglossal nerve pulse generator, electrode, and respiratory sensor with 1 year of follow-up.[16] UAS reduced the mean apnea–hypopnea index (AHI) during non-random eye movement sleep (NREM) from 52.0 ± 20.4 to 22.6 ± 12.1 events per hour and during REM sleep from 48.2 ± 30.5 to 16.6 ± 17.1 events per hour. Although no serious adverse events were reported, device-related malfunction (including electrode breakage, sensor malfunction, and pulse generator failure) precluded the ability to monitor long-term outcomes.

Following the first human pilot study in 2001, multiple investigators and medical device companies spent a decade improving the technology and studying their devices in larger trials. Eastwood et al. (n = 21) and Kezirian et al. (n = 31) studied the Hypoglossal Nerve Stimulation System (Apnex Medical, Inc., St. Paul, MN) and showed significantly reduced mean AHI at 6 and 12 months, respectively, with reported adverse events including a combined total of two infections requiring device removal and three cuff electrode dislodgements.[17,18] Mwenge et al. (n = 14) studied the aura6000 System (ImThera Medical, Inc., San Diego, CA), which consists of a cuff electrode that is continuously activated and therefore does not require a respiratory sensor. Results demonstrated a significant improvement in mean AHI at 12 months, with reported adverse events including two participants with transient tongue paresis.[19] Van de Heyning et al. studied the Inspire II system (Inspire Medical Systems, Inc., Maple Grove, MN) in an initial feasibility study that identified AHI <50 events per hour, body mass index (BMI) ≤32 kg/m$^2$, and absence of a complete concentric pattern of palatal collapse on drug-induced sleep endoscopy (DISE) as predictors of response to therapy.[20] These factors were implemented as inclusion criteria for a second cohort of eight patients. At the 6-month follow-up, the second feasibility cohort demonstrated a significant reduction in AHI from 38.9 ± 9.8 to 10.0 ± 11.0 events per hour. Serious adverse events in this study included postoperative pain and swelling at the incision site requiring inpatient admission and antibiotics in one patient and delayed infection requiring explantation in another patient.

# 8.2. Clinical Trials

## 8.2.1. Phase III Multicenter Trial

The pivotal Stimulation Therapy for Apnea Reduction (STAR) trial incorporated these findings from the feasibility study into the trial inclusion criteria. The STAR trial was a multicenter prospective observational cohort study with a randomized withdrawal arm at 12 months.[21] After clinical, polysomnographic (PSG), and anatomic screening, 126 patients who were intolerant of continuous positive airway pressure (CPAP)—with the feasibility study criteria of moderate to severe OSA (AHI 20 to 50 events per hour), BMI ≤32 kg/m$^2$, and absence of a complete concentric palatal collapse on DISE—underwent Inspire II device implantation. Both patient-reported and PSG outcome measures were assessed at regular intervals across a 5-year follow-up.

The 12-month primary (AHI, 4% oxygen desaturation index [ODI]) and secondary (Epworth Sleepiness Scale [ESS], Functional Outcomes of Sleep Questionnaire [FOSQ]) findings all demonstrated statistically significant improvement, and self-reported nightly adherence was 86%.[21] At 12 months, median AHI decreased by 68% from a baseline value of 29.3 to 9.0 events per hour. The median ODI score decreased by 70% from 25.4 to 7.4 events per hour. Median FOSQ scores increased from 14.6 to 18.2, and median ESS scores decreased from 11 to 6. At 12-month follow-up, serious adverse events were uncommon, with 2 of 126 participants requiring surgical repositioning of the generator (Table 8.1). There were no reports of hypoglossal nerve injury, no serious postoperative infections requiring explantation, and substantially less postoperative pain compared to traditional pharyngeal or skeletal surgery procedures. With therapy use, no changes in tongue function or morphology were identified. The most common non-serious adverse event, reported by 40% of participants at some point during the first year, was therapy-related tongue soreness due to either the stimulation itself or tongue abrasion from an adjacent

**TABLE 8.1. STAR Trial: Summary of Adverse Events**

| Adverse Events | No. of events | Number of Participants with Event (%) |
|---|---|---|
| **Serious adverse event** | **35** | **27 (21%)** |
| Device revision | 2 | 2 (2%) |
| Death, unrelated[‡] | 2 | 2 (2%) |
| Other unrelated* | 31 | 23 (18%) |
| **Procedure-related non-serious adverse event** | **169** | **72 (57%)** |
| Postoperative discomfort related to incisions | 46 | 33 (26%) |
| Postoperative discomfort not related to incision | 39 | 31 (25%) |
| Temporary tongue weakness | 35 | 23 (18%) |
| Intubation effects | 18 | 15 (12%) |
| Headache | 8 | 8 (6%) |
| Other postoperative symptoms | 22 | 14 (11%) |
| Mild infection | 1 | 1 (1%) |
| **Device-related non-serious adverse event** | **190** | **85 (67%)** |
| Discomfort due to electrical stimulation | 80 | 50 (40%) |
| Tongue abrasion | 33 | 26 (21%) |
| Dry mouth | 13 | 13 (10%) |
| Mechanical pain associated with device presence | 8 | 8 (6%) |
| Temporary internal device functionality complaint | 14 | 12 (10%) |
| Temporary external device usability or functionality complaint | 8 | 7 (6%) |
| Other acute symptoms | 25 | 19 (15%) |
| Mild or moderate infection** | 1 | 1 (1%) |

* Other unrelated serious adverse events included cardiac conditions: coronary artery disease, arrhythmias, and chest pain (n = 8), accidents or injuries (n = 11), and other surgeries (n = 12).
** Skin cellulitis
‡ One death occurred from a cardiac event thought to be unrelated to the device and one death was related to a homicide.
Reproduced with permission from Strollo PJ, Soose RJ, Maurer JT, et al. Upper-airway stimulation for obstructive sleep apnea. *N Engl J Med.* 2014;370(2):139–149. doi:10.1056/NEJMoa1308659

tooth. The majority of these local side effects resolved with adjustment of stimulation parameters or in some cases use of a protective dental guard. Two-thirds of the implanted participants (84 of 126) were considered therapy responders using previously published criteria for surgical success.

The STAR trial also examined a subset of 46 consecutive responders who underwent randomization for therapy withdrawal at the 12-month mark) (Figure 8.1).[22] AHI and ODI scores were similar in the two groups prior to randomization. Among the 23 participants in the therapy withdrawal group, AHI and ODI scores worsened, indicating recurrence of OSA. At the completion of 12 months, participants randomized to therapy withdrawal were reinitiated on UAS and showed normalization of pre-withdrawal primary and secondary outcomes after resumption of treatment—confirming the treatment effect of the nightly stimulation. Reported data at the 24-month mark showed continued significant improvement in ESS and FOSQ scores.[23] These scores remained stable from the 12-month follow-up evaluation. UAS also showed a large effect size (>0.8) at both 12 and 24 months for both FOSQ and ESS, which compares favorably to CPAP and other second-line therapies. Furthermore, patient- and bedpartner-reported snoring showed improvement, with the proportion of participants self-reporting "no" or "soft" snoring increasing from 22% to 88% at 12 months of follow-up and 91% at 24 months.

Data from 3 and 5 years after implantation further supported a durable treatment effect, with sustained long-term improvements in AHI as well as ESS and FOSQ scores.[24,25] At 5 years, 78% completed follow-up, and of the 97 patients, 71 underwent voluntary PSG. Primary outcome measures of AHI and ODI showed sustained improvement at the 60-month follow-up, with median AHI of 6.1 and median ODI of 4.6 in patients completing PSG. At the 60-month follow-up, median FOSQ improved from a baseline of 14.6 to 18.7, while median ESS improved from a baseline of 11 to 6. Serious adverse events remained uncommon at the 60-month follow-up. Eight participants had a total of nine device-related serious adverse events requiring hardware repositioning or replacement (one patient required two revision procedures). Discomfort due to electrical stimulation continued to be the most common non-serious adverse event, occurring 81 times in the first year. Again, stimulation-related discomfort was frequently resolved by adjusting the stimulation parameters and was reported only five times by the fifth year of follow-up. Similarly, tongue abrasion was reported 28 times in the first year and was reduced to 2 times during the fifth year.

## 8.2.2. U.S. and Europe Postmarket Studies

After approval of the Inspire II system in 2014 by the U.S. Food and Drug Administration, outcomes from routine clinical practice continued to show high therapy adherence rates measured by objective device adherence monitoring as well as objective improvements in OSA outcomes based on postoperative PSG that even exceeded STAR trial results, with an accompanying overall low rate of adverse events.[26] A meta-analysis in 2015 included results from six prospective studies with 200 total patients. At 12 months, the pooled fixed effects analysis demonstrated statistically significant reductions in AHI, ODI, and ESS.[27] Comparison of outcomes of consecutive patients between independent academic institutions demonstrated remarkably consistent outcomes and adherence, suggesting that the therapy could be broadly translated and applicable to routine clinical practices, outside of a clinical trial setting (Figure 8.2 and Table 8.2).[28]

Similarly, the German postmarket prospective single-arm study across three sites reported 60 implanted patients with a mean objective adherence of 5.6 hours per night,

(a) Apnea–Hupopnea Index

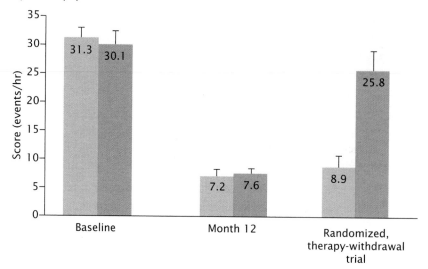

(b) Oxygen Desaturation Index

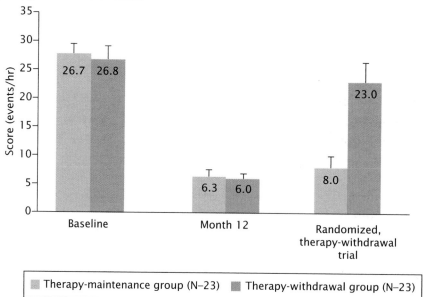

Therapy-maintenance group (N–23)      Therapy-withdrawal group (N–23)

**FIGURE 8.1.** STAR trial primary outcomes at 12 months after implantation and during the randomized therapy withdrawal trial. After 12 months, 46 consecutive participants who had a response to therapy were randomly assigned, in a 1:1 ratio, to the therapy maintenance group or the therapy withdrawal group. The therapy withdrawal group had the device turned off for ≥5 days during this phase, and it remained off until polysomnography was performed. The therapy maintenance group continued nightly use of the device. There was a significant difference between the groups with respect to the change in the AHI **(A)** and the ODI **(B)**, confirming the mechanism and effect of nightly stimulation. Results are expressed as the mean values, with T bars representing standard errors. Reproduced with permission from Strollo PJ, Soose RJ, Maurer JT, et al. Upper-airway stimulation for obstructive sleep apnea. *N Engl J Med.* 2014;370(2):139-149. doi:10.1056/NEJMoa1308659

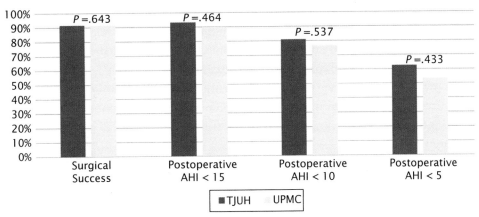

**FIGURE 8.2.** Comparison of preoperative and postoperative outcomes of consecutive UAS patients at two independent institutions, Thomas Jefferson University Hospital (TJUH) and University of Pittsburgh Medical Center (UPMC). Reproduced with permission from Huntley C, Kaffenberger T, Doghramji K, et al. Upper airway stimulation for treatment of obstructive sleep apnea: an evaluation and comparison of outcomes at two academic centers. *J Clin Sleep Med* 2017; 13(9):1075-9.

a median AHI reduction from 28.6 to 9.5 events per hour, and a responder rate of 73% at 12 months.[29,30] An additional study investigated UAS efficacy in patients with a BMI range higher than the traditional pivotal trial inclusion criteria.[31] Despite the published inverse correlation between outcomes and BMI, this multicenter retrospective review found no difference in postoperative AHI, oxygen desaturation nadir, subjective daytime sleepiness, or success rates in patients with a BMI greater than 32 kg/m² when compared to patients with a BMI below 32 kg/m², suggesting that select patients with an elevated BMI can still be successfully treated with HNS therapy.

## 8.2.3. Pediatric Down Syndrome Trial

While OSA is thought to affect 1% to 5% of the general pediatric population, the prevalence of OSA in children with Down syndrome (DS) is approximately 55%

**TABLE 8.2. Data from Consecutive UAS Patients at Two Independent Institutions**

|  | TJUH Preoperative | TJUH Postoperative | *p* | UPMC Preoperative | UPMC Postoperative | *p* |
|---|---|---|---|---|---|---|
| ESS | 11.09 ± 3.77 | 5.77 ± 3.35 | <.001 | 10.911 ± 4.89 | 6.60 ± 4.51 | <.001 |
| AHI | 35.98 ± 20.82 | 6.34 ± 11.50 | <.001 | 3529 ± 15.33 | 6.28 ± 6.10 | <.001 |
| O₂ nadir | 80.96 ± 7.90 | 88.04 ± 3.40 | <.001 | 79.58 ± 7.18 | 84.35 ± 4.74 | <.001 |

The table compares the percentage of patients meeting definitions of surgical success, postoperative AHI <15, postoperative AHI <10, and postoperative AHI <5.
Reproduced with permission from Huntley C, Kaffenberger T, Doghramji K, et al. Upper airway stimulation for treatment of obstructive sleep apnea: An evaluation and comparison of outcomes at two academic centers. *J Clin Sleep Med.* 2017;13(9):1075–1079.

to 90%, with severe OSA (AHI >10) affecting almost half of the DS population.[32] A number of pathophysiologic factors, including midface hypoplasia, mandibular deficiency, relative macroglossia, and hypotonia, all contribute to the increased prevalence. With high rates of congenital heart disease and early-onset dementia, DS children may be even more vulnerable to the neurocognitive and cardiovascular effects of untreated OSA. Furthermore, CPAP adherence rates remain poor in this population, and approximately 40% of DS children still have moderate to severe OSA after adenotonsillectomy.[33]

In 2015, the first pediatric HNS implant was performed in a 14-year-old with DS, asthma, congenital heart disease, chronic tracheostomy dependence, and severe refractory OSA despite prior adenotonsillectomy, lingual tonsillectomy, and CPAP trials. This therapy resulted in an AHI reduction from 48.5 preoperatively (with capped tracheostomy) to 3.4 postoperatively, leading to successful tracheostomy decannulation and long-term OSA management.[34] An additional five adolescents with DS were subsequently treated with similar successful OSA outcomes, good patient accommodation and adherence, and a low rate of adverse events—results that served as the genesis of the first multicenter pediatric DS trial of HNS therapy (Table 8.3).[35] Reports of the first 20 participants in the ongoing pediatric DS trial demonstrated 2-month PSG data with a median AHI reduction of 85% (interquartile range 75% to 92%).[36] The multicenter DS trial is ongoing at the time of writing, but early results are very promising that HNS may provide a safe and effective alternative for a pediatric DS population often in desperate need of effective OSA treatment. More studies are needed to assess long-term outcomes as these children grow and transition to adulthood, as well as to determine whether other neuromuscular, congenital, or syndromic subpopulations of OSA patients could similarly benefit from HNS therapy.

TABLE 8.3. Early Results from the UAS Pediatric Down Syndrome Trial

| Patient | Age (y) | BMI (kg/m²) | Preop. AHI | Postop. AHI | Use (avg. hr/night) |
|---------|---------|-------------|------------|-------------|---------------------|
| 1 | 14 | 24.6 | 48.5 | 5.0 | 9.6 |
| 2 | 15 | 26.1 | 17.1 | 2.7 | 10.0 |
| 3 | 13 | 19.2 | 30.7 | 4.6 | 9.3 |
| 4 | 12 | 20.3 | 22.7 | 4.7 | 5.6 |
| 5 | 17 | 28.8 | 13.9 | 5.4* | 9.0 |
| 6 | 18 | 25.8 | 25.6 | 1.5 | 9.4 |

The table shows patient characteristics, baseline findings, 12-month PSG results, and therapy adherence after UAS implantation.
*Only the 6-month postoperative AHI is available for patient 5.
Adapted and reproduced with permission from Diercks GR, Wentland C, Keamy D, et al. Hypoglossal nerve stimulation in adolescents with Down Syndrome and OSA. *JAMA Otolaryngol Head Neck Surg.* 2018;144(1):37–42.

# 8.3. Global Clinical Registry

The Adherence and Outcome of Upper Airway Stimulation for OSA International Registry (ADHERE registry) was established in 2016 to collect data on HNS therapy patients across multiple U.S. and European sites (Figure 8.3). Published outcomes from the first 300 registry patients demonstrated mean ± standard deviation AHI decreasing from 35.6 ± 15.3 preoperatively to 10.2 ± 12.9 events per hour postoperatively ($p < .001$), with an accompanying decrease in ESS and mean objective therapy utilization of 6.5 hours per

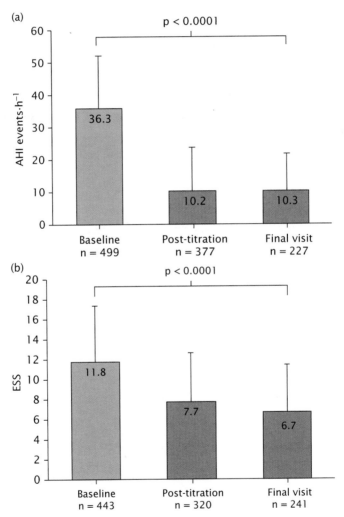

**FIGURE 8.3.** Outcomes data from the global clinical registry (ADHERE registry). Change in AHI **(A)** and ESS **(B)** measurements from baseline to post-titration and final 12-month visits. Results reported as mean and standard deviation. Reproduced from Heiser C, Steffen A, Boon M, et al. Post-approval upper airway stimulation predictors of treatment effectiveness in the ADHERE registry. *Eur Resp J.* 2019;53(1):1801405.

night.[37] At the time of writing, >1,600 patients at over 40 sites across the United States and Germany are included in the registry thus far, representing the largest cohort of patients studied with HNS therapy to date.

The safety profile of UAS continued to be favorable, with 98% of the 508 implanted participants with no reports of adverse events in the intraoperative and immediate post-operative period. Two cases of intraoperative bleeding with tunneling of the stimulation lead and two cases of postoperative seroma resolved without sequelae (Table 8.4). Other adverse events related to implantation included submandibular swelling, transient tongue weakness, transient dysarthria, and one dislodged stimulator cuff at activation at the 1-month post-implant visit. A total of 87 adverse events were reported in 23% of patients completing a post-titration visit and a total of 61 adverse events were reported in 23% of patients completing a final visit.[38]

With the number of UAS patients now in the thousands and growing rapidly, understanding predictors of therapy response and improving patient selection are critical to long-term success. One of the goals of the ADHERE registry is to identify predictors of therapy success by analyzing large cohorts of patients. Using traditional AHI definitions of treatment success, the currently available ADHERE registry data show that increasing age, decreasing BMI, and female gender are independent predictors of UAS therapy success.[39] Although both older (age ≥65) and younger (age <65) adult groups demonstrated significant AHI reduction at 12 months, the older group showed a greater degree of AHI

## TABLE 8.4. Adverse Events Data from the Global Clinical Registry (ADHERE Registry)

| Type | Post-Titration | | Final Visit | |
|---|---|---|---|---|
| | No. of Events | % of patients | No. of Events | % of patients |
| Tongue weakness | 3 | <1 | 0 | 0 |
| Swallowing or speech related | 4 | 1 | 1 | <1 |
| Discomfort, incision/scar | 14 | 4 | 8 | 2 |
| Discomfort, device | 10 | 3 | 5 | 1 |
| Infection | 2 | <1 | 0 | 0 |
| Postoperative other | 14 | 4 | 6 | 2 |
| Stimulation-related discomfort | 41 | 12 | 28 | 8 |
| Tongue abrasion | 12 | 3 | 14 | 4 |
| Insomnia/arousal | 10 | 3 | 17 | 5 |
| Revision interventions, including explantation | 1 | <1 | 2 | <1 |
| Other discomfort | 12 | 3 | 8 | 2 |
| Activation, other | 37 | 3 | 23 | 7 |
| *Total* | 161 | 46 | 113 | 32 |

Reproduced from Thaler E, Schwab R, Maurer J, et al. Results of the ADHERE upper airway stimulation registry and predictors of therapy efficacy. *Laryngoscope.* 2020;130(5):1333–1338. doi:10.1002/lary.28286 improvement.[40] Univariate regression analysis reported that every 1-year increase in age was associated with a 4% increase in the odds of OSA treatment success, whereas every 1-unit increase in BMI was associated with a 9% reduction in the odds of OSA treatment success.

# 8.4. Comparison of UAS to Other Treatments

## 8.4.1. Comparison to Traditional Medical Devices

Direct comparison studies or even randomized controlled trials evaluating the effectiveness of UAS versus CPAP are not currently available, particularly since UAS is only approved for use as *second-line* therapy in the setting of CPAP intolerance. Nevertheless, a recent study used mixed effect models to compare blood pressure and ESS outcomes between 201 UAS patients from the ADHERE registry and historical data from 201 matched CPAP patients.[41] The CPAP group showed greater improvement in diastolic blood pressure and mean arterial pressure compared to UAS; however, the UAS group showed greater improvements in ESS scores and objective therapy use.

Although head-to-head comparison data are limited, general comparisons of the device functionality and approach to patient care can be made. UAS has emerged as a hybrid *surgically implanted* yet *medically titratable* OSA treatment option, for at least a subset of the untreated OSA population. For clinicians familiar with CPAP, UAS may be thought of in similar terms as a medical device therapy that is adjustable across a longitudinal care model. The subcutaneous placement of UAS is unique, however, in that, unlike CPAP or oral appliance therapy (OAT), UAS does not require wearing an external apparatus (which is the root of many of the nonadherence concerns associated with CPAP and OAT therapies).

Based on data from the STAR trial, postmarket studies, and the ADHERE registry, objective adherence rates with UAS compare favorably to alternative forms of OSA treatment, including to CPAP adherence rates from the SAVE trial.[42] UAS therapy provides titratable parameters that can be modified in the clinic or sleep laboratory setting to optimize effectiveness as well as patient comfort and use. Furthermore, UAS therapy allows for device data download at follow-up, analogous to CPAP data download technology, and has an expected internal battery life of 10 to 12 years, facilitating longitudinal care in what is for the majority of OSA patients a chronic long-term condition.

Similar to troubleshooting with CPAP or even OAT, UAS therapy settings and programming (including electrode configuration, pulse width, amplitude, duration of stimulation, timing with respiration) can be systematically analyzed and modified in the outpatient setting, with or without concurrent upper airway endoscopy, to improve long-term outcomes. As clinically indicated, the addition of positional therapy, weight management, lowering of nasal resistance, mandibular repositioning, upper airway surgery, and other adjunctive measures may also provide an opportunity to further strengthen HNS outcomes. In summary, as with other OSA medical devices, for UAS patients with subop-timal response or inadequate adherence, implementation of best-practice approaches to device data analysis, patient education, therapy modifications, and close clinical follow-up will likely optimize long-term outcomes.

## 8.4.2. Comparison to Traditional Upper Airway Surgical Procedures

UAS differs from traditional OSA airway reconstructive surgery in several fundamental ways. It provides multilevel airway improvement with only one procedure, as evidenced by DISE and imaging studies demonstrating enlargement of the retropalatal space as well as the retrolingual space. Unlike pharyngeal or skeletal surgical procedures, again UAS can be titrated in the clinical or sleep laboratory setting and has been shown to provide an incremental multilevel response with increasing amplitude.[43] Furthermore, the im-plant procedure does not alter upper airway anatomy and is technically reversible. Unlike other tongue base or pharyngeal surgeries, the UAS surgical procedure is completely ex-ternal to the pharynx, thus substantially reducing postoperative discomfort and recovery time, and minimizing or even eliminating the traditional risks of throat hemorrhage, dysphagia, change in taste, or other untoward pharyngeal side effects of anatomy-altering procedures.

Early in the STAR trial, the question was raised whether prior uvulopalato-pharyngoplasty (UPPP) would improve outcomes with UAS therapy and perhaps even be a prerequisite to successful UAS outcomes. This hypothesis was nullified, as the 17% of STAR trial participants with prior UPPP had similar outcomes to the 83% of partici-pants without prior UPPP.[21] The ADHERE registry also examined whether prior pha-ryngeal surgery (e.g., palatoplasty, excisional tongue base surgery, hyoid suspension) was associated with UAS treatment efficacy: The authors similarly reported no differences in outcome measures in patients with or without prior pharyngeal sleep apnea surgery.[44] Prior surgery was not associated with likelihood of UAS response at both the 2-month to 6-month titration follow-up (0.69; 95% confidence interval [CI] 0.37, 1.27) and the final 12-month follow-up (0.55; 95% CI 0.22, 1.34). Further, smaller retrospective cohort studies of patients undergoing UAS also corroborate the lack of association between prior OSA surgery and postoperative outcomes.[45,46]

A retrospective analysis of patients undergoing transoral robotic tongue base sur-gery (TORS) versus UAS implantation at one institution reported significant differences in outcomes between the two, with OSA-related outcome measures, length of hospital stay, and readmission rates all favoring UAS therapy. The authors reported "surgical success" rates of 86% for UAS versus 54% for TORS, and "cure" rates of 59% for UAS versus 21% for TORS.[47] Another retrospective study compared PSG outcomes of a cohort undergoing TORS base of tongue resection to a cohort undergoing UAS. This study spe-cifically included patients undergoing TORS base of tongue resection who met inclusion criteria for UAS. Average AHI reduction in the UAS cohort was 33.3 compared to 12.7 in the TORS, with a cure rate (defined as AHI <5) of 10% in the TORS cohort and 70.3% in the UAS cohort.[48]

Similarly, a single-center retrospective review comparing outcomes of expansion sphincter pharyngoplasty to UAS therapy reported overall comparable outcomes between the two, trending toward improved AHI reduction and higher success rates with UAS.[49] UAS was also compared to UPPP outcomes in another retrospective review. In this study, 20 patients undergoing modified UPPP (defined as either the uvulopalatal flap technique or expansion sphincter pharyngoplasty technique) were compared to 20 patients undergoing UAS. Mean AHI in the UAS cohort decreased from 38.9 ± 12.5 to 4.5 ± 4.8 events per hour, and all patients achieved AHI <20, with 65% achieving AHI <5. In comparison, mean AHI in the UPPP cohort only decreased from 40.3 ± 12.4 to 28.8 ± 25.4 events per hour, with only 20% achieving AHI <5.[50] These studies suggest that UAS therapy may be appropriately employed as an effective alternative to pharyngeal surgery rather than just a salvage option after failed pharyngeal surgery. A need exists to develop treatment algorithms and clinical care pathways to assist clinicians in treatment decision making when faced with CPAP-intolerant patients in need of an effective alternative.

## 8.5. Conclusions

Electrical stimulation of the hypoglossal nerve through implantable UAS has evolved from a basic science concept to a widely available second-line treatment for CPAP-intolerant OSA patients over the last decade. Initially corroborated by animal studies and subsequent human feasibility studies, UAS now has consistent safety and efficacy data across multiple observational cohort studies, including the landmark phase III multicenter STAR trial. These studies have demonstrated improvement in both objective PSG measures and subjective patient-reported outcome measures in patients meeting specific anatomic and clinical inclusion criteria. Furthermore, follow-up from thousands of patients in the multicenter global ADHERE registry confirms positive outcomes in routine clinical practice, including a favorable safety profile and good patient adherence. Early studies comparing UAS with traditional OSA surgical treatments, including UPPP and tongue base reduction, currently favor UAS with improved outcomes and reduced postoperative morbidity, although multimodality therapy likely represents the future, with UAS being implemented in combination with other medical and surgical OSA treatments. More studies are needed to (1) evaluate long-term cardiovascular and general health outcomes and (2) define the role of UAS in the OSA treatment armamentarium to better guide medical decision making for clinicians. Opportunities also abound for improved patient selection, clinical phenotyping, technology developments, and advanced therapy titration to further improve efficacy.

# References

1. Miki H, Hida W, Shindoh C, et al. Effects of electrical stimulation of the genioglossus on upper airway resistance in anesthetized dogs. *Am Rev Respir Dis.* 1989;140:1279–1284.
2. Schwartz AR, Thut DC, Russ B, et al. Effect of electrical stimulation of the hypoglossal nerve on airflow mechanics in the isolated upper airway. *Am Rev Respir Dis.* 1993;147:1144–1150.
3. Oliven A, Odeh M, Schnall RP. Improved upper airway patency elicited by electrical stimulation of the hypoglossus nerves. *Respiration.* 1996;63:213–216.
4. Eisele DW, Schwartz AR, Hari A, et al. The effects of selective nerve stimulation on upper airway airflow mechanics. *Arch Otolaryngol Head Neck Surg.* 1995;121:1361–1364.
5. Bishara H, Odeh M, Schnall RP, et al. Electrically-activated dilator muscles reduce pharyngeal resistance in anaesthetized dogs with upper airway obstruction. *Eur Respir J.* 1995;8:1537–1542.
6. Fregosi RF. Influence of tongue muscle contraction and dynamic airway pressure on velopharyngeal volume in the rat. *J Appl Physiol.* 2008;104:682–693.
7. Bailey EF, Fregosi RF. Pressure-volume behaviour of the rat upper airway: Effects of tongue muscle activation. *J Physiol.* 2003;548:563–568.
8. Yoo PB, Durand DM. Effects of selective hypoglossal nerve stimulation on canine upper airway mechanics. *J Appl Physiol.* 2005;99:937–943.
9. Miki H, Hida W, Chonan T, et al. Effects of submental electrical stimulation during sleep on upper airway patency in patients with obstructive sleep apnea. *Am Rev Respir Dis.* 1989;140:1285–1289.
10. Guilleminault C, Powell N, Bowman B, Stoohs R. The effect of electrical stimulation on obstructive sleep apnea syndrome. *Chest.* 1995;107:67–73.
11. Decker MJ, Haaga J, Arnold JL, et al. Functional electrical stimulation and respiration during sleep. *J Appl Physiol.* 1993;75:1053–1061.
12. Edmonds LC, Daniels BK, Stanson AW, et al. The effects of transcutaneous electrical stimulation during wakefulness and sleep in patients with obstructive sleep apnea. *Am Rev Respir Dis.* 1992;146:1030–1036.
13. Smith PL, Eisele DW, Podszus T, et al. Electrical stimulation of upper airway musculature. *Sleep.* 1996;19:S284–S287.
14. Schwartz AR, Eisele DW, Hari A, et al. Electrical stimulation of the lingual musculature in obstructive sleep apnea. *J Appl Physiol.* 1996;81:643–652.
15. Eisele DW, Smith PL, Alam DS, Schwartz AR. Direct hypoglossal nerve stimulation in obstructive sleep apnea. *Arch Otolaryngol Head Neck Surg.* 1997;123(1):57–61.
16. Schwartz AR, Bennett ML, Smith PL, et al. Therapeutic electrical stimulation of the hypoglossal nerve in obstructive sleep apnea. *Arch Otolaryngol Head Neck Surg.* 2001;127:1216–1223.
17. Eastwood PR, Barnes M, Walsh JH, et al. Treating obstructive sleep apnea with hypoglossal nerve stimulation. *Sleep.* 2011;34:1479–1486.
18. Kezirian EJ, Goding GS, Malhotra A, et al. Hypoglossal nerve stimulation improves obstructive sleep apnea: 12-month outcomes. *J Sleep Res.* 2014;23:77–83.
19. Mwenge GB, Rombaux P, Dury M, et al. Targeted hypoglossal neurostimulation for obstructive sleep apnoea: A 1-year pilot study. *Eur Resp J.* 2013;41:360–367.
20. Van de Heyning PH, Badr MS, Baskin JZ, et al. Implanted upper airway stimulation device for obstructive sleep apnea. *Laryngoscope.* 2012;122:1626–1633.
21. Strollo PJ, Soose RJ, Maurer JT, et al. Upper-airway stimulation for obstructive sleep apnea. *N Engl J Med.* 2014;370(2):139–149. doi:10.1056/NEJMoa1308659
22. Woodson BT, Soose RJ, Maurer JT, et al. Randomized controlled withdrawal study of upper airway stimulation on OSA: Short- and long-term effect. *Otolaryngol Head Neck Surg.* 2014;151(5):880–887.
23. Soose RJ, Woodson BT, Gillespie MB, et al. Upper airway stimulation for obstructive sleep apnea: Self-reported outcomes at 24 months. *J Clin Sleep Med.* 2016;12:43–48.
24. Woodson BT, Soose RJ, Gillespie MB, et al. Three-year outcomes of cranial nerve stimulation for obstructive sleep apnea. *Otolaryngol Neck Surg.* 2016;154(1):181–188. doi:10.1177/0194599815616618

25. Woodson BT, Strohl KP, Soose RJ, et al. Upper airway stimulation for obstructive sleep apnea: 5-year outcomes. *Otolaryngol Neck Surg.* 2018;159(1):194–202. doi:10.1177/0194599818762383

26. Kent DT, Lee JJ, Strollo PJ Jr, Soose RJ. Upper airway stimulation for OSA: Early adherence and outcome results of one center. *Otolaryngol Head Neck Surg.* 2016;155(1):188–193. doi:10.1177/0194599816636619

27. Certal VF, Zaghi S, Riaz M, et al. Hypoglossal nerve stimulation in the treatment of obstructive sleep apnea: A systematic review and meta-analysis. *Laryngoscope.* 2015;125(5):1254–1264. doi:10.1002/lary.25032

28. Huntley C, Kaffenberger T, Doghramji K, et al. Upper airway stimulation for treatment of obstructive sleep apnea: An evaluation and comparison of outcomes at two academic centers. *J Clin Sleep Med.* 2017;13(9):1075–1079.

29. Heiser C, Maurer JT, Hofauer B, et al. Outcomes of upper airway stimulation for obstructive sleep apnea in a multicenter German postmarket study. *Otolaryngol Neck Surg.* 2017;156(2):378–384.

30. Steffen A, Sommer JU, Hofauer B, et al. Outcome after one year of upper airway stimulation for obstructive sleep apnea in a multicenter German post-market study. *Laryngoscope.* 2018;128(2):509–515.

31. Huntley C, Steffen A, Doghramji K, et al. Upper airway stimulation in patients with obstructive sleep apnea and an elevated body mass index: a multi-institutional review. *Laryngoscope.* 2018;128(10):2425–2428.

32. Chamseddin BH, Johnson RF, Mitchell RB. OSA in children with Down syndrome: Demographic, clinical, and polysomnographic features. *Otolaryngol Head Neck Surg.* 2019; 160:150–157.

33. Farhood Z, Isley JW, Ong AA. Adenotonsillectomy outcomes in patients with Down syndrome and OSA. *Laryngoscope.* 2017;127:1465–1470.

34. Diercks GR, Keamy D, Kinane TB, et al. Hypoglossal nerve stimulator implantation in an adolescent with Down syndrome and sleep apnea. *Pediatrics.* 2016;137(5):e20153663. doi:10.1542/peds.2-15-3663

35. Diercks GR, Wentland C, Keamy D, et al. Hypoglossal nerve stimulation in adolescents with Down Syndrome and OSA. *JAMA Otolaryngol Head Neck Surg.* 2018;144(1):37–42.

36. Caloway CL, Diercks GR, Keamy D, et al. Update on hypoglossal nerve stimulation in children with down syndrome and obstructive sleep apnea. *Laryngoscope.* 2020;130(4):E263–E267. doi:10:1002/lary.28138

37. Boon M, Huntley C, Steffen A, et al. Upper airway stimulation for obstructive sleep apnea: Results from the ADHERE registry. *Otolaryngol Neck Surg.* 2018;159(2):379–385. doi:10.1177/0194599818764896

38. Thaler E, Schwab R, Maurer J, et al. Results of the ADHERE upper airway stimulation registry and predictors of therapy efficacy. *Laryngoscope.* 2020;130(5):1333–1338. doi:10.1002/lary.28286

39. Heiser C, Steffen A, Boon M, et al. Post-approval upper airway stimulation predictors of treatment effectiveness in the ADHERE registry. *Eur Resp J.* 2019;53:1801405.

40. Withrow K, Evans S, Harwick J, et al. Upper airway stimulation response in older adults with moderate to severe obstructive sleep apnea. *Otolaryngol Head Neck Surg.* 2019;161(4):714–719.

41. Walia HK, Thompson NR, Strohl KP, et al. Upper airway stimulation vs. positive airway pressure impact on BP and sleepiness symptoms in OSA. *Chest.* 2020;157(1):173–183.

42. McEvoy RD, Antic NA, Heeley E, et al. CPAP for prevention of cardiovascular events in OSA. *N Engl J Med.* 2016; 375:919-31. doi:10.1056/NEJMoa1606599

43. Strohl M, Strohl K, Palomo M, Ponsky D. Hypoglossal nerve stimulation rescue surgery after multiple multilevel procedures for obstructive sleep apnea. *Am J Otolaryngol.* 2016;37(1):51–53.

44. Kezirian EJ, Heiser C, Steffen A, et al. Previous surgery and hypoglossal nerve stimulation for obstructive sleep apnea. *Otolaryngol Head Neck Surg.* 2019;161(5):897–903.

45. Mahmoud AF, Thaler ER. Upper airway stimulation therapy and prior airway surgery for obstructive sleep apnea. *Laryngoscope.* 2018;128:1486–1489.

46. Huntley C, Vasconcellos A, Doghramji K, et al. Upper airway stimulation in patients who have undergone unsuccessful prior palate surgery: An initial evaluation. *Otolaryngol Head Neck Surg.* 2018;159(5):938–940.

47. Huntley C, Topf MC, Christopher V, et al. Comparing upper airway stimulation to transoral robotic base of tongue resection for treatment of obstructive sleep apnea. *Laryngoscope.* 2019;129(4):1010–1013.
48. Yu JL, Mahmoud A, Thaler ER. Transoral robotic surgery versus upper airway stimulation in select obstructive sleep apnea patients. *Laryngoscope.* 2019;129(1):256–258.
49. Huntley C, Chou DW, Doghramji K, et al. Comparing upper airway stimulation to expansion sphincter pharyngoplasty: A single university experience. *Ann Otol Rhinol Laryngol.* 2018;127(6):379–383.
50. Shah J, Russell JO, Waters T, et al. Uvulopalatopharyngoplasty vs. CN XII stimulation for treatment of obstructive sleep apnea: A single institution experience. *Am J Otolaryngol.* 2018;39(3):266–270.

# Special Considerations in the Acute Post-Implantation Period

Maria V. Suurna and Jolie L. Chang

## 9.1. Adverse Events and Complications and Their Management

All patients undergoing implantation of an upper airway stimulator (UAS) should be appropriately counseled on the risks of surgery and expectations for postsurgical care. Many centers in the United States are performing UAS as outpatient surgery, with patients returning home the day of surgery. Due to travel considerations, certain medical conditions, and management of postoperative anesthesia-related issues, patients can be kept overnight (23-hour stay). If patients are amenable to using positive airway pressure (PAP) perioperatively, they should continue nightly PAP use and bring their equipment to the hospital.[1]

### 9.1.1. Expected Postoperative Course

After surgery and prior to discharge, an upright chest x-ray should be obtained in all patients in the post-anesthesia care unit to document implant and lead location and to screen for pneumothorax. Expected changes after surgery include lower lip depressor weakness or asymmetric smile due to an incision of the unilateral platysma muscle (common) or neurapraxia of the marginal mandibular nerve (uncommon). In rare cases of marginal mandibular nerve injury, lip depressor weakness usually resolves over time with no intervention. Some surgeons elect to use a neuro-integrity monitoring (NIM) electrode pair in the lip depressor muscle to prevent inadvertent injury to the marginal mandibular nerve.

Temporary weakness of the tongue on protrusion in the postoperative period can be observed and has been reported in <1% of cases[2] due to probable neurapraxia from hypoglossal nerve dissection, and most patients can be managed with observation. Dysphagia, voice changes, or globus sensation after surgery can be related to intubation and muscle dissection and resolve within several days after surgery. Studies looking at the long-term voice and swallowing problems after UAS implantation showed no changes in voice handicap and swallowing function.[3,4]

Currently, there are no reports of permanent tongue paralysis after UAS surgery. When acute neurapraxia and tongue mobility abnormalities are noted, it is recommended to wait for resolution prior to UAS therapy activation. In most cases the tongue weakness resolves within 6 to 8 weeks without any intervention. There are anecdotal reports that early activation may prolong neurapraxia and may lead to higher stimulation settings to achieve functional tongue motion. Once neurapraxia resolves, the higher stimulation level may be uncomfortable, requiring repeat titration and setting adjustments. Neurapraxia of the marginal mandibular nerve does not require a delay in therapy activation.

Significant swelling of the submandibular incision area is expected for several weeks postoperatively. Patients and physicians should be alerted regarding the anticipated tissue swelling and expected gradual complete resolution over 2 to 4 weeks. Bruising of the skin around the incisions and tunneled wire sites can also be notable in many patients.

Postoperative management of pain requires limited opiate use, if any.[5] Most incisional pain can be managed with activity restriction, ice, acetaminophen, and ibuprofen, if not contraindicated. Patients should expect significant pain in the submandibular space, in the jaw, and over the chest incisions in the immediate postoperative period and at times lasting for several weeks after surgery. Significant sore throat and odynophagia in the immediate postoperative period are commonly reported and resolve within a few weeks. Pain in the lower intercostal space can contribute to atelectasis and splinting, so early mobility and full lung expansion with deep breathing are encouraged. Pressure dressings on the chest and neck incisions remain in place for a few days after surgery. Patients are advised to keep the incisions dry for 48 hours. Local incisional care includes moisturization and keeping wounds out of sunlight for best cosmetic results. For women, a supportive sports bra can help with healing and reduce tension on the upper chest incision.

Activity limitation includes no over-the-head lifting of the operated-side arm or strenuous activity for at least 2 weeks. Repeated arm and shoulder motions should be restricted to include avoiding swimming, golf, yoga, tennis, and weightlifting during the recovery period. For patients who do repeated lifting for work, activity modification should be limited for 4 weeks to avoid excessive motion of the implant site. An arm immobilizer can be a good reminder for the patient to limit lifting and arm motion. Routine neck stretching in the first month can help with tension/tethering of the tunneled stimulation lead in the neck, which in some patients is visible when the neck is extended. This

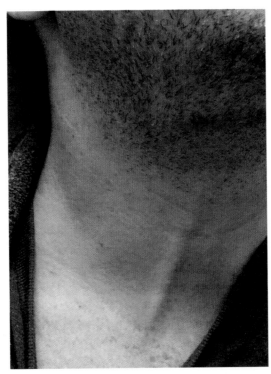

**FIGURE 9.1.** A patient with visible neck lead during neck extension managed with early neck stretching and massage of the region.

complication is rare if the tunneling was subplatysmal. Early stretching can prevent development of fibrous banding around the neck wire site (Figure 9.1).

## 9.1.2. Pneumothorax

Placing the sensor lead between the external and internal intercostal muscles is associated with the risk for injury to the pleura and subsequent pneumothorax. Intraoperative measures to reduce the risk for pneumothorax include proper visualization of the muscle layers in the intercostal space and following the curvature of the ribcage when creating the small tunnel for sensor lead placement. Intraoperative signs of pneumothorax include air rushing or leaking sounds during sensor lead manipulation or a positive air leak when the wound is filled with fluid and positive pressure ventilation is applied (leak test). Immediate management of a suspected pleural injury includes communication with the anesthesiologist regarding the patient's stability in terms of ventilation and vital signs. A small pneumothorax can occur as a result of parietal pleural injury. If a minor pleural injury is recognized, the sensor lead should be removed and the muscular layers of the dissected intercostal space should be closed. If the patient is stable, the sensor lead can be placed in the more superior intercostal space and possibly reoriented in the posterior lateral direction. More severe symptoms of iatrogenic pneumothorax can occur when both the parietal and visceral layers of pleura are inadvertently injured. If this occurs, cardiothoracic surgery consultation is recommended, and management may require chest tube placement. If the chest tube is placed, clinical judgment should be used to decide whether to proceed with completing the implant placement. If the patient is stable, the sensor lead can be placed with care to spatially separate the sensor lead from the chest tube site to minimize the possibility of infection. Alternatively, the patient can be allowed to heal and return for the completion of implantation at a later date, once the pneumothorax has resolved.

Tension pneumothorax in the setting of UAS surgery has not been reported, although this is a potential adverse event. The signs of tension pneumothorax include hypotension and hypoxia. Tension pneumothorax requires immediate decompression with a chest tube into the pleural space and an intraoperative cardiothoracic surgery consult.

In the majority of cases, pneumothoraces are recognized intraoperatively, but they can present postoperatively. A postoperative chest x-ray in the recovery area in the upright position is obtained on all patients to screen for ipsilateral pneumothorax. If the pneumothorax is diagnosed after surgery and the air collection is small, the patient can be observed over 12 to 24 hours to ensure there is no progression. Most small pneumothoraces resolve slowly with supportive care.

## 9.1.3. Bleeding

Superficial bleeding from the incision sites can occur in the immediate postoperative period. Most of the time it can be managed by application of pressure and observation. Patients who are taking anticoagulant medications are more prone to postoperative bleeding. These patients, especially the ones who require immediate anticoagulation, should be carefully monitored for bleeding complications or hematoma formation.

## 9.1.4. Hematoma

Hematoma, or collection of blood under the skin, is a rare complication after UAS implant surgery, although patients on chronic anticoagulation or with a bleeding disorder are at higher risk (Figure 9.2). In most cases, patients with hematoma or seroma can be observed for a few weeks. Due to the presence of an implant and concern for infection, aspiration of the fluid or blood collection should be avoided unless necessary. Needle aspiration carries a risk for lead damage and could introduce skin pathogens (e.g., *Cutibacterium acnes*) that can lead to severe infections. Progression of the hematoma may require evacuation, exploration for the source of bleeding, and wound reclosure in the operating room under sterile conditions. If aspiration or evacuation is required, it is critical to perform adequate preparation of the wound and maintain sterile technique. Delayed progressive skin swelling, pain, and drainage are suggestive of developing infection at the implant site, which requires further treatment.

Management of perioperative anticoagulation is done in collaboration with the patient's surgeon, primary care physician, cardiologist, and anesthesia team. For elective

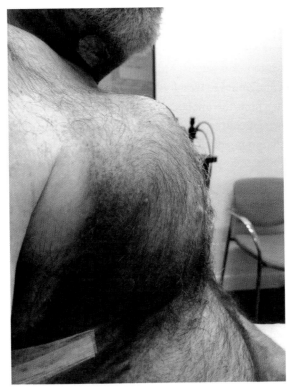

**FIGURE 9.2.** Postoperative hematoma at the IPG site after restarting warfarin 24 hours after surgery.

surgery, current guidelines advise continuing acetylsalicylic acid (ASA) therapy whenever possible.[6] UAS implant placement falls into the category of an elective surgery with low risk for significant blood loss and if indicated can be performed with concurrent anticoagulation on board. Decisions regarding anticoagulation should be made based on cardiopulmonary risk and should be guided by the patient's cardiologist and primary care team. In most cases surgery can proceed with 81 mg or 325 mg ASA on board. If a patient is taking warfarin, the medication should be stopped 5 days prior to surgery, with low-molecular-weight heparin or enoxaparin bridging, and warfarin can be restarted 12 to 24 hours postoperatively. Apixaban, dabigatran, and rivaroxaban are newer oral anticoagulants that should be discontinued ~48 hours prior to surgery and can be restarted 24 hours postoperatively. Perioperative anticoagulation is associated with an increased risk for hematoma and associated potential for infection of the implant site postoperatively.

## 9.1.5. Infection

Postsurgical complications related to infection are uncommon, and most occur within the first year and are associated with contamination at the time of surgery. Early infections occur in the first 30 days, late infections 30 days to 1 year, and delayed infections

>1 year after surgery. Minimal erythema at the surgical sites during the immediate post-operative period is common and usually resolves within 7 to 10 days without intervention. However, progressive erythema and swelling at the incision sites can be a sign of superficial skin infection or cellulitis. Most early superficial infections can be managed with 7 to 10 days of antibiotics to treat local skin flora–related infections. Deeper surgical site infections can occur at the implantable pulse generator (IPG) insertion site and are best described in the neurosurgery and cardiology literature for similar implants.[7] If deep infection is suspected, immediate antibiotic therapy should be initiated. Deep or persistent surgical site infections will most likely require removal of hardware and possible treatment with intravenous antibiotics in severe cases.

The most effective prevention of surgical site infections involves meticulous skin preparation and disinfection, adherence to universal sterile techniques and precautions, improved glycemic control, and good surgical technique. The guidelines for cardiac implantable electrical device placement recommend a single dose of pre-incision prophylactic antibiotics based on controlled trials showing reduction of postoperative device-related infections.[8] All patients undergoing implantation should receive appropriately dosed prophylactic antibiotics 1 hour prior to incision. Cefazolin is most commonly used, followed by clindamycin or vancomycin in those with beta-lactam allergies. Although there is no clear evidence in the literature, most surgeons use bacitracin or gentamicin irrigation of the surgical sites during the implantation. Postoperative antibiotics are not routinely recommended. Based on the literature for cardiac permanent pacemakers and defibrillators, data on postoperative antibiotic use and duration are mixed and there is some evidence that they can cause harm.[9] Antibacterial absorbable envelopes have been used for cardiac pacemakers and implantable cardioverter-defibrillators (ICDs) in high-risk patients, demonstrating reduction of postoperative infections,[7] but this area merits further investigation to identify the best candidates.

## 9.1.6. Persistent Long-Term Pain

Pain around the surgical sites is expected for up to 1 month after surgery. Conservative use of electrocautery and careful tissue dissection can prevent significant discomfort after surgery. Persistent pain in the IPG or intercostal space sites has been described. IPG-related pain should be assessed for infection and motion of the implant. Intercostal pain can be a sign of nerve irritation, most commonly of perforating intercostal nerve fibers as a result of superior or medial placement of the respiratory sensing lead tip. Placing the lead in the inferior portion of the intercostal space helps to prevent irritation of the neurovascular bundle that travels underneath each rib. If pain is significant and persistent, revision of the sensory lead might be required. During revision, the sensor lead should be removed from the original intercostal space and repositioned to another intercostal space, preferably in the posterior lateral direction. Referred pain secondary to scar formation should improve and eventually resolve over time. Evaluation of persistent pain may require further imaging, non-opiate pain control, local injections, or physical therapy for management.

Patients may additionally report persistent neck, jaw, or occipital pain triggered by UAS stimulation. Pain can occur due to stimulation of cervical nerve branches that are adjacent to the hypoglossal nerve with associated referred pain to the supraclavicular, postauricular, and occipital regions of the head and neck. Most pain of the head or neck will improve over time with supportive care and analgesic use as needed. When pain is triggered by UAS therapy, stimulation can be adjusted to allow for more comfortable settings.

## 9.1.7. Lead Visibility and Exposure of the Implant

Cosmetic concerns include local scarring at incision sites or visibility of the tunneled stimulation lead wire under the skin of the neck (Figure 9.1). Wire visibility, tension, or pain can be associated with tethering of the stimulation wire when the neck is fully extended or with contraction of the platysma. Care on tunneling beneath the platysma muscle and allowing for appropriate laxity of the wire is important. Immediate and routine postoperative stretching of the neck in all directions has also been helpful in the healing phase. For notable wire tension, gentle massage and stretching can help alleviate the tension of the skin around the wire. In rare cases when patients have persistent tethering and pain with neck movement, lead revision might need to be performed.

Eruption of the leads or the IPG implant can also occur (Figure 9.3). Attention to closure and tunneling in the proper layer to avoid superficial wire placement will prevent this complication. In the event of lead eruption, the entire UAS implant is removed followed by antibiotic therapy if infection is present, and subsequent reimplantation once the infection has cleared.

## 9.1.8. IPG Migration and Twiddler's Syndrome

IPG device migration has been reported for UAS implantation[10] and has also been described in the cardiology and neurosurgery literature. Motion of the IPG can present months after surgery and can cause tension on the stimulation or sensing leads. X-ray examination and comparison with immediate postoperative IPG and lead locations can assist with migration diagnosis, and the device may need to be resecured in a new pocket with dual anchoring on the anterior chest wall. Twiddler's syndrome has been described for cardiac and deep brain stimulation implants due to spontaneous rotation or intentional manipulation of the IPG by the patient and associated with lead dislodgement/ fracture and malfunction of the device[11,12] (Figure 9.4). Migration of the IPG is associated with tissue laxity, obesity, older age, large pocket creation, and inadequate fixation at IPG implantation. The IPG should be secured with a suture through both anchoring holes in accordance with most recent manufacturer recommendations.

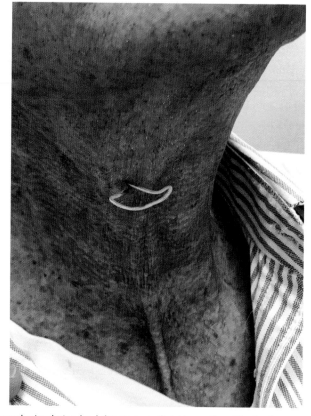

**FIGURE 9.3.** Exposed stimulation lead due to superficial tunneling. The lead was surgically replaced.

## 9.1.9. Absence of Tongue Movement with Stimulation and Improper Cuff Placement

Identification of the hypoglossal nerve and proper cuff placement around the medial branches of the nerve is essential for optimal therapy outcomes. Even though the tongue movement and therapy testing is thoroughly performed intraoperatively, no tongue motion with stimulation can sometimes be observed postoperatively during activation. In these cases, cuff dislodgement or improper placement of the cuff should be suspected. Patients can be evaluated with anteroposterior and lateral neck x-rays or preferably computed tomography of the neck to assess the electrode location. If cuff dislodgement or improper placement is confirmed, stimulation lead revision will be required.

## 9.1.10. Device Lead Damage

Inadvertent lead damage during dissection, due to cautery, improper lead handling, or damage from scissors or needles during suturing, may cause insulation breach, lead fractures, and postoperative current leaks with associated device malfunction. Prevention requires proper and careful handling of all portions of the implant by the surgeons and

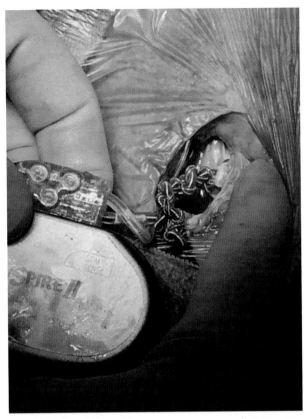

**FIGURE 9.4.** IPG migration and twiddler's syndrome due to excessive mobility of the IPG in the pocket. Properly securing the IPG to the pectoralis fascia helps prevent motion during healing.

operating room staff. Troubleshooting during system validation, when unexpected findings occur, may identify damaged system components, allowing for immediate replacement to avoid a future revision surgery.

## 9.2. Postoperative Considerations for Patients with Preexisting Medical Conditions

Prior neck procedures, such as neck dissection, submandibular gland excision, spinal surgery, Port-A-Cath placement in the neck or infraclavicular area, and cosmetic surgery, can contribute to difficulties not only during implant placement but also during the recovery period. Scarring and tissue devascularization can contribute to poor healing and increased risk for infection. Prior neck radiation treatment is not a contraindication for placement of the implant, but risks of delayed healing and device infection are higher in this patient group. Patients with a history of immunosuppressive disorders and organ transplant are also at an increased risk of postoperative device infection, and they should be closely monitored.

Insomnia screening and discussion of its implications are important during the evaluation of UAS implant candidacy. Comorbid OSA and insomnia is common and seen in up to 42% to 55% of patients.[13] Patients should be screened for insomnia with history of proper sleep habits, typical nightly hours, and ability to maintain sleep. Validated instruments such as the Insomnia Severity Index (ISI) can also be helpful for patient assessment.[14] Treatment of OSA can improve sleep and insomnia symptoms, but primary insomnia can persist and limit the ability to comfortably use the UAS therapy during sleep hours. Patient expectations regarding the efficacy of UAS therapy for sleep apnea versus symptoms of insomnia should be discussed thoroughly. Cognitive-behavioral therapy for insomnia is a preferred treatment. However, sleep aids may still be necessary in some patients. Limited hours of UAS therapy use and poor compliance with other OSA treatment devices may be exacerbated by insomnia, and patients should be aware of this relationship and potential associated challenges. Expectations for UAS therapy use and the importance of proper sleep habits and adequate hours of sleep should be discussed with all patients considering surgery.

## 9.3. Special Considerations in Women

Based on published experience with implantable devices in female patients, women may be more concerned about how incisions and scarring will make them feel about their body, clothing fit, and swimsuit wear.[15] With that in mind, care should be taken to place incisions within neck and chest skin creases, and attention should be given to meticulous cosmetic closure. Figure 9.5 demonstrates incision placement in the neck crease for the stimulation lead, a modified lateral anterior axillary crease for the IPG, and inframammary crease for the respiratory sensor lead.

Potential limitations regarding breast cancer surveillance should be discussed with all female patients. There are no contraindications for mammographic exams in patients with the UAS implant. Mammography should be completed with the same protocol used with other devices (e.g., pacemakers) implanted in the chest. Proper positioning under the breast tissue and more superior placement of the IPG will minimize interference of the device with mammograms. The current hypoglossal nerve simulation (HGNS) implant is not approved for chest, abdomen, or body magnetic resonance imaging (MRI). With current limitations, women who anticipate MR surveillance for breast cancer should not undergo HGNS implant placement.

Special considerations during surgical planning and counseling should be addressed in female patients with a history of radical mastectomy, breast reduction, reconstruction surgery, or breast augmentation implants. The surgeon should know the consistency of the breast augmentation implant (silicone vs. saline) and whether placement was done in the subglandular/submammary or subpectoral/submuscular plane. Prior placement of the incisions will help navigate and avoid areas of fibrosis. Chest x-ray or ultrasound

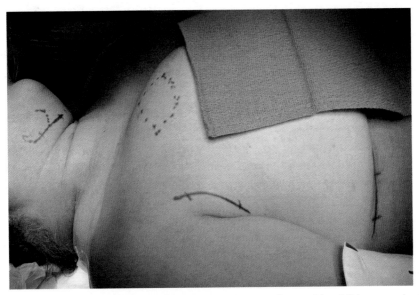

**FIGURE 9.5.** Implant incision planning for a woman who wanted to avoid a visible upper chest incision: one incision in the neck crease for the stimulation lead, a modified lateral anterior axillary crease for the IPG pocket, and inframammary crease for the sensor lead.

could be performed preoperatively to assess the location of the breast implants, and the IPG should not be placed in their direct proximity. Damage or rupture of the breast implant during tunneling is a potential risk. Lateral IPG incision placement and tunneling laterally and away from the implant can help avoid damage. Rupture or leak of the silicone gel implants is often asymptomatic and can go undetected. MRI is a widely accepted and effective radiographic method to detect silicone breast implant rupture. The U.S. Food and Drug Administration (FDA) currently recommends that women with silicone breast implants undergo screening for implant rupture 3 years after implantation and then every 2 years thereafter to detect silent leak.[16] However, current MRI restrictions for patients with a UAS implant will preclude women with suspected silicone breast implant leak from getting recommended MR imaging with the UAS implant, and candidates should be aware of this issue.

# 9.4. Considerations in Patients with Occupational Requirements for a Left-Sided Implant and Other Implanted Medical Devices

Incision and placement of IPG can be modified based on certain individual factors, such as routine use of straps or equipment that may sit near or on the anterior chest wall. Patients who report right-handed recreational or occupational rifle use or use equipment that crosses the deltopectoral groove and anterior chest may require more attention to the IPG incision planning and placement. Figure 9.6 demonstrates more a medial IPG incision planned for a patient with routine right-sided rifle use. In addition, cosmetic concerns regarding the implant location and visibility should be discussed and reasonable expectations reviewed preoperatively.

The existence of implanted devices on the right side (i.e., pacemaker, ICD, Port-A-Cath) or occupational needs may require HGNS system implantation on the left side. Left-sided implantation is performed with similar anatomic landmark identification and minor alteration in the placement of the stimulation lead electrode that requires the outer portion of the electrode cuff to be placed from the inferior to the superior direction, for the wire edge of the electrode will be directed laterally. This is opposite of the conventional right-sided nerve electrode placement. Respiratory sensor placement on the left chest will pick up more cardiac artifact due to the proximity of the heart ventricle. The respiratory sensor distal lead should be placed more laterally to position it farther away from the ventricle; this can be ensured by tunneling in the posterior lateral direction toward the axilla. During implant programming and testing, care should be taken to investigate the amount of cardiac artifact. If there is a concern for significant interference, the sensor lead may need to be

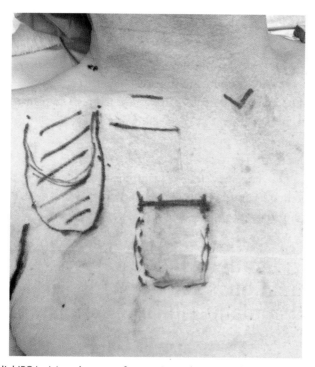

**FIGURE 9.6.** Medial IPG incision placement for a patient who required right-sided rifle use. Avoidance of wire and IPG placement in the deltopectoral groove region was achieved with more medial IPG incision planning.

repositioned farther away from the body of the left ventricle, typically positioning it posterior-laterally toward the axilla. Patients should be informed about the alternative implant location and should ensure the left-sided HGNS implants are not mistaken for cardiac devices.[17]

Various implantable devices are used for treatment of medical disorders, such as cardiac devices (pacemakers and defibrillators), spinal cord stimulators, deep brain stimulators, and bladder stimulators. Simultaneous use of the HGNS implant therapy and other implantable devices, including pacemakers, ICDs, and cardiac resynchronization therapy devices, was found to be safe and effective; there were no device–device interactions. There were no inappropriate ICD shocks, inappropriate pacemaker inhibitions, inappropriate mode switches, or noise reversion noted during intraoperative implant testing and during a 1-year follow-up period.[18] During surgery, both devices should be interrogated with multiple settings to ensure appropriate function. Multiple electrode configurations and supratherapeutic levels of HGNS therapy should be tested to demonstrate that HGNS signals are not identified inappropriately by the ICD as a cardiac event requiring defibrillation.[17]

## 9.5. Conclusions

Successful UAS implantation requires certain preoperative considerations and proper patient counseling and surgical planning. Thorough review of prior surgical and medical history, specifically of head and neck radiation, medical device implants, breast surgery (including augmentation implants), and individual occupational and recreational needs, is essential for planning the UAS implant procedure. Recognizing insomnia during preoperative patient evaluation is important for proper counseling and post-implant therapy management. Each patient should be advised on the expected postoperative course, pain management, and incisional care. Adherence to proper surgical techniques and postoperative care can minimize potential adverse events such as infection, hematoma, pneumothorax, cosmetic issues, and need for implant removal or replacement.

## References

1. Chung F, Nagappa M, Singh M, Mokhlesi B. CPAP in the perioperative setting: Evidence of support. *Chest.* 2016;149(2):586–597.
2. Thaler E, Schwab R, Maurer J, et al. Results of the ADHERE upper airway stimulation registry and predictors of therapy efficacy. *Laryngoscope.* 2020;130(5):1333–1338.
3. Bowen AJ, Nowacki AS, Kominsky AH, et al. Voice and swallowing outcomes following hypoglossal nerve stimulation for obstructive sleep apnea. *Am J Otolaryngol.* 2018;39(2):122–126.
4. Huntley C, Vasconcellos A, Mullen M, et al. The impact of upper airway stimulation on swallowing function. *Ear Nose Throat J.* 2019;98(8):496–499.

5. Strollo PJ Jr, Soose RJ, Maurer JT, et al. Upper-airway stimulation for obstructive sleep apnea. *N Engl J Med.* 2014;370(2):139–149.

6. Darvish-Kazem S, Gandhi M, Marcucci M, Douketis JD. Perioperative management of antiplatelet therapy in patients with a coronary stent who need noncardiac surgery: A systematic review of clinical practice guidelines. *Chest.* 2013;144(6):1848–1856.

7. Mittal S, Shaw RE, Michel K, et al. Cardiac implantable electronic device infections: Incidence, risk factors, and the effect of the AigisRx antibacterial envelope. *Heart Rhythm.* 2014;11:595–601.

8. Padfield GJ, Steinberg C, Bennett MT, et al. Preventing cardiac implantable electronic device infections. *Heart Rhythm.* 2015;12(11):2344–2356.

9. Korantzopoulos P, Sideris S, Dilaveris P, et al. Infection control in implantation of cardiac implantable electronic device: Current evidence, controversial points, and unresolved issues. *Europace.* 2016;18:473–478.

10. Tabatabai GM, Karepelis P, Hsia JC. Hypoglossal nerve stimulator generator migration: INSPIRE device reimplantation with parallels to cardiac implantable electronic devices. *Am J Otolaryngol.* 2018;29:639–641.

11. Bayliss CE, Beanlands DS, Baird RJ. The pacemaker-twiddler's syndrome: A new complication of implantable transvenous pacemakers. *Can Med Assoc J.* 1968;99:371–373.

12. Geissinger G, Neal JH. Spontaneous twiddler's syndrome in a patient with a deep brain stimulator. *Surg Neurol.* 2007;68:454–456.

13. Benetó A, Gomez-Siurana E, Rubio-Sanchez P. Comorbidity between sleep apnea and insomnia. *Sleep Med Rev.* 2009;13(4):287–293.

14. Bastien CH, Vallières A, Morin CM. Validation of the Insomnia Severity Index as an outcome measure for insomnia research. *Sleep Med.* 2001;2:297–307.

15. Davis LL, Vitale KA, Irmiere CA, et al. Body image changes associated with dual-chamber pacemaker insertion in women. *Heart Lung.* 2004;33(5):273–280.

16. U.S Food and Drug Administration. Update on the Safety of Silicone Gel-Filled Breast Implants (2011)—Executive Summary. https://www.fda.gov/medical-devices/breast-implants/update-safety-silicone-gel-filled-breast-implants-2011-executive-summary

17. Heiser C, Thaler E, Soose RJ, et al. Technical tips during implantation of selective upper airway stimulation. *Laryngoscope.* 2018;128(3):756–762.

18. Parikh V, Thaler E, Kato M, et al. Early feasibility of hypoglossal nerve upper airway stimulator in patients with cardiac implantable electronic devices and continuous positive airway pressure-intolerant severe obstructive sleep apnea. *Heart Rhythm.* 2018;15(8):1165–1170.

# Technical Considerations Following Implantation

Armin Steffen and Katrin Hasselbacher

## 10.1. Postoperative Stimulator Programming

The surgical implantation of upper airway stimulation (UAS) is beyond the scope of this chapter and is discussed in Chapter 7. After the UAS device has been implanted, patients are seen 7 to 10 days postoperatively for assessment of their wounds and removal of sutures. They are then seen again 4 to 6 weeks postoperatively for activation of the device.

The aim of implant activation and programming is to check for proper technical function and to adapt the implant settings to the patient's individual needs. The physician or experienced sleep technologist needs to instruct patients and familiarize them with the setup so they understand how to control the stimulation system with the remote and get acclimated to stimulation. Follow-up calls and/or appointments are arranged to review usage, assess tolerance to therapy, and assess symptomatic benefit. Communication between the implanting center and the sleep physician should be established for upcoming home sleep testing or polysomnographic (PSG) titration.

One must be familiar with several technical aspects of the implanted neurostimulation system (Table 10.1). The voltage or stimulation amplitude is highly variable between subjects and strongly dependent on electrode configuration. Published data on the impact of the voltage or electrode configuration on upper airway opening and treatment outcome are available.[1–4]

For better comparability over time for individuals, documentation of amplitude thresholds is recommended. The three recommended thresholds to be tested are (1) sensation level, (2) functional level, and (3) sub-discomfort level. The sensation level is the

**TABLE 10.1. Important Stimulation Parameter and Comfort Settings with Standard Value and Clinically Relevant Alternatives**

| Stimulation Parameter | Standard Setting | Alternative Setting (examples) |
|---|---|---|
| Electrode configuration | Bipolar + - + | Unipolar - - - or o - o |
| Impulse configuration | 90 μs 33 Hz | 120 μs 40 Hz |
| Start delay | 20–30 min | Longer for patients with insomnia |
| Pause function | 15 min | Longer for patients with insomnia |
| Therapy duration | 8 hours | Longer for late risers at weekends |

voltage level at which the patient first feels the stimulation. Sensation level is qualitative, such as impedance measurements for phenomena of nerve recovery or that of altering scar/connective tissue between cuff electrodes and hypoglossal nerve branches. The functional level is the voltage level at which the patient's tongue motion is observed to reach the level of the lower incisors. Functional level is relevant as it is usually close to the therapeutic level. The sub-discomfort level is the voltage level at which the patient declines further increase of voltage. The sub-discomfort level limits further increases of voltage, but during sleep patients often tolerate higher voltages than when they are awake.

Therapy activation usually takes about 30 to 45 minutes, depending on technical observation and the patient's preexisting knowledge about the therapy. It is strongly recommended to invite the bedpartner so that he or she is equally informed. Before the activation, the clinician should determine whether there are any swallowing or speech problems and healing difficulties. In cases of abnormal tongue motion indicating neurapraxia, wound dehiscence at incisions, incisional discomfort, or other signs of implant infection, the activation should be postponed and the implanting sleep surgeon should be contacted (see Chapter 9). The patient is seated in an upright position with the ability to recline. For evaluation of respiratory sensing in non-supine positions, the patient should lie down. The clinician should be aware of any electrical interferences in the vicinity (e.g., old-fashioned video monitors), which may interfere with the telemetry signal and make therapy activation problematic.

The sleep physician should be aware of the patient's previous sleep endoscopy and intraoperative findings, as well as challenges encountered during implantation. Patients with isolated retropalatal collapse have similar therapy outcomes compared to other types of collapse pattern, and this preoperative finding on drug-induced sleep endoscopy (DISE) should not have any negative impact on outcomes.[5] This can be explained as an effect of palatoglossus coupling.[6] Palatal obstructions require a sufficient tongue protrusion and not only submental activation. There are signs that the tongue protrusion patterns impact therapy outcomes,[3,7] so the patterns under several electrode configurations should be tested at implantation as well as during activation and follow-up (Table 10.2). In more than half of patients, the tongue motion patterns changed between activation and the 1-year follow-up.[3] Intraoperative factors that might have an impact on tongue motion with

**TABLE 10.2. Classification of Tongue Motion Patterns**

| Tongue Protrusion | Description | Prognostic |
|---|---|---|
| Right protrusion | Ipsilateral extension of the tongue | Good |
| Bilateral protrusion | Bilateral tongue elongation and anterior displacement | Good |
| Left protrusion | Contralateral extension of the tongue | Uncertain as retracting nerve fibers are co-stimulated |
| Mixed activation including retraction | Every other kind of tongue motion, such as shortening or curling of the tongue | High risk of unfavorable results |

Note that future efforts might include other aspects of tongue motion for outcome analysis.

neurapraxia include repeated cuff repositioning, cauterization close to the nerve, intense neuromonitoring stimulation with higher voltage, and repeated and longer activation for unnecessary demonstration to others (see Chapter 7).

Prior to the activation, the process of activation should be explained to the patient. This helps the patient to relax so that the observation of tongue motions is easier and respiratory signals have fewer artifacts. Tests for correct technical function should start with respiration in an upright or preferably supine position. If the patient prefers a lateral position during sleep, this should be tested as well (Figure 10.1). A pattern of smooth curves without sharp spikes reveals good sensing lead function. Talking or limb movements disturb the signal. The patient should not hold the telemetry header as this provokes artifacts.

As reflections within the intercostal space could interfere with the piezo-sensing head of the lead, sometimes the patient's respiration cycle and the stimulation appear to be off-phase and stimulation could start during expiration. Patients sometimes report this off-phase sensation or have an "awkward" feeling related to this. By selecting the "Invert Signal" box on the telemetry page of the programmer, patients become on-phase again (Figure 10.2). Proper respiratory sensing is needed for a good therapy outcome. Inverting the sensing might harm control of obstructive sleep apnea (OSA) with this therapy.[8] As off- and on-phase might differ between supine and nonsupine position in

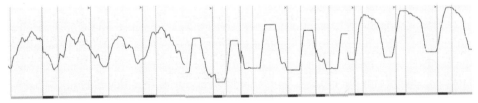

**FIGURE 10.1.** Respiratory sensing in the same patient: supine position (left), left-side position (middle), and right-side position (right).

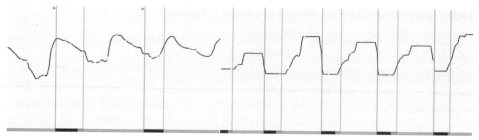

**FIGURE 10.2.** Respiratory sensing in the same patient: off-phase with "Inverting Signal Off" incorrect (left) and again on-phase with "Inverting Signal On" correct (right).

some cases, the settings should be made for the preferred sleep body position. Later, PSG controls are needed to evaluate the situation asleep.

After respiratory sensing, it is appropriate to check the impedance at 1.5 and 2.0 volts, which are automatically done at bipolar and unipolar (o - o, - o -) electrode configurations. Thus, baseline measurements are done for comparing with later analysis and the impedance can be used for the threshold-level voltages.[9] Higher impedance values correlate with higher voltages for sensing and functional thresholds. Finally, all three thresholds are measured for not only bipolar but also unipolar (- - - and o - o) electrode configurations. The type of tongue motion patterns is noted (see Table 10.2) and might change between functional and sub-discomfort level (mainly from bilateral to right protrusion) or electrode configuration. Stable tongue motion patterns between bipolar and unipolar settings are a good prognostic sign, whereas changes from right/bilateral in a bipolar setting to left protrusion in a unipolar setting indicate more retractor activation. Those cases should be followed closely for optimal outcome.[3]

After activation, therapy is adjusted to the patient's individual settings. It is recommended to start with the standard bipolar electrode configuration (see Table 10.1) as the increase from one voltage step to the next is much smoother compared to the unipolar configurations. Thus, increases in voltage are better tolerated by the patient. If a more sufficient tongue protrusion in unipolar settings appears, alternative configurations should be used, especially when complete palatal obstruction was seen in DISE. As the threshold-tested voltage might differ from the voltage with therapy switched on, it is recommend to assess whether the installed voltage has similar effects as in testing the thresholds. Usually, the voltage range covers 11 steps, starting with a step that is 0.1 volt below the functional threshold.

After testing the technical function and adjusting parameters to individual settings, patients are taught to control the implant with the remote. Patients should know about the acoustic confirmation tone and light status ring indicating voltage changes, pause function, and therapy duration. Patients should demonstrate that they can initiate, pause, and stop the therapy and implement voltage changes on their own. Typical start delay is set at 20 to 30 minutes (see Table 10.2). However, this can be shorter if the patient has a short sleep latency. The start delay should be made longer in patients who have co-morbid insomnia. The patient's bedpartner should also be taught, as many patients are anxious and might not take in all the information. Patients should be encouraged to use the stimulation with slow incremental increases in voltage to allow adequate acclimation to therapy. In contrast to positive airway pressure (PAP) therapy, the therapy allows the patient the flexibility to lower the voltage on less susceptible nights or to increase it after an evening of alcohol intake, which may be of great benefit for the patient and the bedpartner, who might be disturbed by snoring. In addition to the accompanying remote manual, there is a short brochure that serves as a quick reference for the patient with straightforward questions.

Finally, it is necessary to arrange follow-up calls and appointments. The first recommended contact with the patient is after 1 or 2 weeks of activation. This interaction focuses on therapy handling and comfort with the therapy. Most problems can be managed just by re-explaining the training. A common question is about the impulse perception in morning hours: When the therapy starts, patients feel a strong impulse but get used to it during the night and often do not feel the impulse in the morning. This phenomenon has to be differentiated from therapy ending with a short therapy duration of 6 to 7 hours, especially on weekends. Approximately 4 to 6 weeks after activation and prior to the post-activation titration, patient contact focuses on initial experiences: Is the device used regularly? What voltage was used on the previous nights? Can the patient can tolerate the impulse? Does the bedpartner notice any differences in snoring volume or breathing stops? By requesting the patient's feedback, therapy adherence can be enhanced. As many sleep physicians have a wait time for their sleep lab, or even home sleep testing, it should be confirmed that the appointments are made. Any abnormal findings at therapy activation should be communicated to the entire team involved in the patient's care, when the implanting surgeon is not involved in the activation process or following therapy adjustments.

At therapy activation, several situations maybe encountered. As mentioned, in cases with neurapraxia or wound healing problems, activation should be postponed. If a protrusion pattern other than right, bilateral, or a shifting of the tongue protrusion pattern is seen under different electrode configurations, the patient should be followed up closely. When the impedance is similar at different voltages, in two or even all three electrode configurations, the implanting sleep surgeon and/or manufacturer should be contacted. This could be an early sign of damage to the sensing lead. The same should be done in abnormal sensing patterns with low amplitudes or repeated spikes (Figure 10.3). If in doubt, it is helpful to contact the manufacturer for additional guidance.

A PSG therapy adjustment is helpful in analyzing whether these sensing findings impact the therapy effect and can be solved by adjusting the sensing setting. This involves

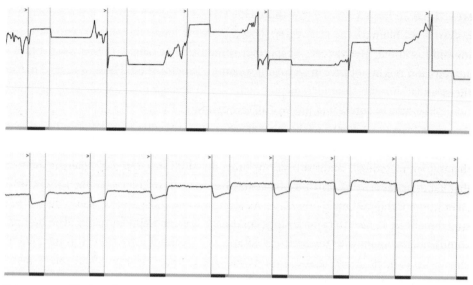

**FIGURE 10.3.** Tracings from two patients with broken isolation of the respiratory sensing lead.

an advanced titration in most cases (see Chapter 10). When therapy can be started with telemetry but not with the remote, there are often simple solutions like new batteries or the implant is not set to telemetry mode. In the rare cases in which there is no tongue motion with either telemetry or the remote, despite highest voltages in several electrode configurations and proper sensing signals and impedance values, it is possible that the cuff of the stimulation lead was not properly secured or has detached from the nerve branches. In such situations, a postoperative x-ray should be obtained to evaluate for abnormal position to dictate if there is a need for revision surgery. In the event of no tongue motion in isolated electrode configurations and abnormal impedances in the corresponding setting, but adequate response in other electrode configurations, the implanting sleep surgeon and/or manufacturer should be contacted, as there could be a problem with one of the three cuff contacts. For example, no tongue motion at bipolar + - + and unipolar o - o, but proper reaction with unipolar - - -/- o -, implies an issue with the middle contact. As most of these situations can be adjusted with use of alternative electrode configurations, no revision surgery is needed.

# 10.2. Protocol and Time Course for Postoperative Sleep Studies

Compared to the past, where therapy adjustment was performed in a shorter and stricter time period, current protocols focus on a more relaxed acclimatization. This allows more feedback calls to ensure regular usage and proper voltage increase (see Section 10.1 earlier in the chapter). A rushed and brisk increase in voltage makes it problematic to incorporate hypoglossal nerve stimulation into daily life for the patient. If patients have not appropriately acclimated to therapy, the post-activation titration study often produces unreliable information to dictate further therapy.

This can be seen in the key publication from 2014, the Stimulation Therapy for Apnea Reduction (STAR) trial,[10] and in the later prospective multicenter German postmarket study.[11,12] Both of these studies had a relatively strict time schedule for PSG therapy optimization 2 months after implantation. With this approach, there is the risk that some patients are prematurely scheduled for post-activation titration with insufficient initial usage or voltage increase. As a result, they wake up frequently during the study, even at smaller voltage changes. So if patients still feel uncomfortable using the stimulation at night, it is preferable to do an interim visit. In this case, it is possible to change the patient's comfort settings (see Chapter 11) or voltage ranges and postpone the PSG titration. Many problems can be simply solved with only an additional explanation of the therapy handling in a phone call.

In some cases the stimulation is too strong or too weak, even at the extreme voltage levels, after several weeks. In both situations, the patient should be scheduled for assessment. The same technical checkups should be done as during the initial activation (see Section 10.1). The threshold settings at several electrode configurations and the impedances at a minimum of two voltages can be compared with the previous values.

If the stimulation at the highest installed voltage is too weak, increased thresholds and impedances can be observed. If the voltage range is adapted to the actual thresholds and the tongue protrusion is the same at activation as at the functional threshold, the problem is solved. The reason for these threshold changes in such a short time span is unclear and may relate to changes in cuff electrode position relative to the nerve branches as a result of scar tissue.

Some patients are very cautious during activation and get more comfortable at home. Here, impedances help as an objective measurement. In the case of excessive sensitivity to stimulation, the technical checkup may show similar impedances but lower thresholds. Minimal nerve damage during the implantation with acute recovery might explain this. Both situations could impact the post-activation titration, depending on the voltage changes and the time left to get accustomed to the new installed settings. It is rare but has been observed by the author that both can occur in the same patient: The same settings that are too weak initially can become too intense within a relatively short time span. Under these circumstances, the implanting surgeon and/or the manufacturer should be informed whether the implanted components, especially the sensing lead, are working properly.

# 10.3. PSG Device Voltage Titration to Achieve Optimal Therapeutic Amplitude, including Controversies in This Area

For most patients, it is appropriate to offer a post-activation PSG titration. This allows the therapy to be adjusted during an in-laboratory PSG to optimize OSA control. The goals of the PSG device titration are as follows:

- Ensure proper technical function of the implant
- Adjust therapy for optimal OSA reduction, including synchronizing respiratory sensing
- Find the most suitable setting that will enable nightly usage for the patient, which reduces therapy-related sleep disturbances and improves sleep architecture[13,14]
- Exclude over-titration during the self-adjusting time period after therapy activation
- Control OSA reduction with so-called titrated sleep parameters
- Direct the next steps of therapy.

Some patients can achieve a good outcome without the formal post-activation titration, but under most circumstances a PSG is strongly recommended (Box 10.1). In all cases, however, a postoperative non-titration PSG is necessary to document treatment efficacy.

Patients with claustrophobia or those who have difficulty sleeping under laboratory conditions may be best served without formal in-laboratory post-activation titration. In these situations, subjective assessment of the patient and bedpartner's sleep should be made and home sleep testing may be used for objective measurement of apnea reduction. This approach has been validated for therapy outcomes even at 2 years after implantation.[15] The advantage of this home testing approach is that it reduces the loss of working

---

**BOX 10.1 Situations with a Strong Indication for PSG Therapy Titration**

- Centers starting a hypoglossal nerve stimulation program
- Higher percentage of non-obstructive events in baseline testing
- Positional or REM-sleep-dependent sleep apnea potentially requiring different voltages
- Improper respiratory sensing at therapy activation
- Low number of voltage steps between functional and sub-discomfort thresholds
- Comorbidities and cognitive impairments that risk proper quality of bio-signals in home sleep tests

days for the patient and increases sleep lab capacity. It is also easier to accommodate patient volume and patients who live far from the implanting center. However, home sleep testing tends to underestimate OSA severity.

In contrast to PSG titration nights with major adjustments, today the recommendation is to ensure proper OSA reduction with as few interventions as possible for the sleep technicians. If this cannot be achieved using standard therapy settings, more and more commonly a second PSG for advanced titration is initiated. Alternatively, other tools such as awake endoscopy or DISE with activated therapy should be considered (see Chapter 11).

Before starting the PSG, the patient is interviewed about his or her experiences during the first weeks of usage (see Section 10.2). Via telemetry, objective data from the weekly usage can be obtained. If the cloud-based readout is available at the center, this tool will allow further detailed night-to-night variability. With information about repeated start and pause function, handling problems could be identified as well.

It is very useful to repeat the steps of therapy activation, including the checkups for correct respiratory sensing. Special care should be taken to actualize the functional and sub-discomfort thresholds at several electrode configurations, mainly bipolar + - + and unipolar o - o and - - - . A voltage beyond sub-discomfort level is less likely to promote regular use and may lead to repeated restarts and therapy-related awakenings in the future.

The PSG recording should be done using the sleep laboratory's typical settings for the diagnostic approach. In all cases, it is necessary to use an oronasal thermal airflow sensor to monitor airflow to define apneas, and a nasal pressure transducer to monitor airflow to define hypopneas. The telemetry header should be placed using the double-sided adhesive rings supplied by the manufacturer. If the patient reports frequent body position changes during sleep, the proper telemetry signal quality should be evaluated not only in the supine position but also in lateral position. It is common for patients with more loose subcutaneous tissue or more fat to show telemetry contact problems while lying on the right side with a shifted impulse generator. The room environment should be checked for potential electric interferences with telemetry. Inductive respiratory effort bands may interfere with the telemetry signal, so piezoelectric or pneumatic bands for thoracic and abdominal breathing detection are preferable. As the sleep technician will have to make changes with the patient programmer, the room should be as close as possible to the programmer or accessible without disturbing the patient's sleep. Ideally, the telemetry wire can be routed through a cable conduit.

Patients should be informed of potential changes in therapy settings at night and should know that the PSG is not a noninterventional procedure. They should be warned that some settings may stimulate them to wake up. Therapy should be initiated when the patient falls asleep and the first obstructive events occur. It is recommended that initial therapy settings should start two steps (0.2 volts) below the functional threshold in order to avoid awakenings and to establish the lowest possible effective voltage. The same electrode and impulse configuration settings to which the patient is accustomed should be used. More recent recommendation direct apply the incoming voltage. This carries the risk of underestimating the role of overstimulation, but in real life, the functional threshold and the incoming voltage rarely differ that much. The synchronization of the patient's breathing cycle should be checked once again. Here, adjustments should be made only if there is an obvious mismatch, which can be handled by inverting the respiratory signal.

It is very likely that obstructive events will occur at a voltage level below the functional threshold. The voltage is increased gradually, in a stepwise fashion, at intervals of ≥10 minutes, to observe if hypopnea or apnea still occurs. Further increases are necessary in this case or when loud snoring is present. Isolated events without snoring are watched closely to avoid awakenings and over-titration. If the patient wakes up, the therapy is stopped and reinitiated like at the beginning of the night. A voltage level two steps (0.2 volts) below the level that led to awakening (see Figure 10.3) is then recommended. The therapeutic level is determined when OSA is controlled for ~30 minutes in the patient's preferred body position. It is preferable that rapid-eye-movement (REM) sleep is achieved during a portion of the total sleep time at a specific level to assess effectiveness.

In general, positional OSA is not an exclusion criterion anymore as it was in the STAR trial.[10,16] For preferred body position, the patient's view should be considered, as well as the data from the initial sleep recordings. These documents show how much time was spent in the lateral or the supine position. Nonetheless, a compromise is required if the therapeutic level differs significantly between body positions. It is not easy to determine optimal levels if the therapeutic level for the supine position leads to awakenings in the lateral position. The recommendation is to install a broader range of voltage levels and suggest gradual acclimatization at home. This should be followed up with clinical evaluation and home sleep testing for effectiveness. Some sleep physicians advise positional therapy during the use of upper airway stimulation in such circumstances. A patient with REM-dependent OSA might also need different therapeutic levels, but this phenomenon is far less common in the care of neurostimulation patients.

In the morning, the patient should be interviewed to assess his or her experiences with the PSG changes. With sufficient OSA control and normal cases, the installed voltage range can be narrowed to three to five steps. Especially in cases where much higher therapeutic voltages are determined by PSG titration, the programmed voltage range should never exceed the maximum stimulation level achieved before the study. This prevents complaints, interim visits for readjusting the remote, and/or low usage following the study. If the therapeutic voltage could not be determined and is either close to or even beyond sub-discomfort levels, further advanced therapy adjustment steps should be initiated (see Section 10.4). If OSA control is sufficient, the next follow-up appointment should be scheduled (see Chapter 11). It is helpful to agree on a feedback call or email within the next months. Functional thresholds can differ at PSG and the 1-year follow-up. This is mainly due to different tissue changes around the nerve branches and the cuff, resulting in different tongue motion patterns.[3] At our center, we maintain the protocol used in the German postmarket study,[11,12] which includes a clinical visit and home sleep test 6 months after implantation.

## 10.4. Complex Titration to Address Suboptimal Therapeutic Results

The main indication for complex or advanced titrations (see Chapter 11) is when OSA control could not be established during therapy acclimatization and titration (see Section 10.3). Other treatment problems, such as insufficient clinical benefit despite proper OSA control (see Chapter 11) or low therapy use, will not be reliably addressed by this. These situations need other approaches, such as:

- Patient retraining and motivation
- Reevaluation of comorbidities such as insomnia, alcohol abuse, and depression (see Chapter 11)
- Changes in impulse configuration[9] and patient comfort settings (see Chapter 11)
- Awake endoscopy[2] or DISE[1] (see Chapter 11)
- Possible additional soft palate surgery.[17]

Therefore, the main aspects evaluated at advanced titration are the effects of other electrode configurations and the sufficient synchronization between the respiratory sensing and the breathing cycle. In most and preferably all cases, office-based treatment adjustments for patient comfort settings and obvious mismatch of respiratory synchronization have already been implemented. This means the optimization of respiratory sensing by simply inverting the signal is not helpful. Instead, changes in the duty cycle, maximum stimulation time, or the sensitivity of the breathing cycle detection may be needed. Insufficient respiratory sensing may harm OSA control.[8] Therefore, it pays to seek optimal sensing quality at the time of implantation (see Chapter 7). It is strongly recommended to contact the manufacturer for titration consultancy. With a very low-quality signal, reducing the maximum stimulation time increases the chances that coincidentally the breathing cycle and stimulation will be phased better. If everything other than respiratory sensing problems has been excluded, revision of the sensing lead can be considered. This is particularly relevant if signs of technical failure from broken isolation occur (see Figure 10.3 and Section 10.1).

Another major advantage of advanced titration is the ability to change the electrode configuration, as this may lead to a more profound stabilization of the upper airway. The altered electric field activates the hypoglossal nerve branches and surrounding muscle differently, which can be identified in changed tongue motion patterns,[3] awake endoscopy,[2] and/or DISE.[18] The PSG is initiated similar to the previous titration attempt with regard to the increase in voltage steps. The choice of electrode configuration depends on tongue motion patterns and thresholds for these settings. It can be helpful to conduct an awake endoscopy or even a DISE to identify the most promising settings. One has to consider that in contrast to bipolar + - + configurations, the unipolar o - o or even - - - configurations have less tolerable voltage increments between functional and sub-discomfort thresholds.[9] When using unipolar electrode configurations, increasing the voltage should be done with care in order to avoid awakenings. It is important after an advanced titration that a feedback call or ideally a clinical visit including home sleep testing occurs. This is done to evaluate therapy and, if required, to conduct further steps in the case of insufficient OSA control. Examples of this would be DISE with activated stimulation (see Chapter 11) or even additional soft palate surgery.[17] The idea of additional soft palate surgery is that often the tongue base obstruction is addressed by the therapy but the palate obstruction remains, or the voltage needed to improve palatal collapse is intolerable for the patient.

# References

1. Safiruddin F, Vanderveken OM, de Vries N, et al. Effect of upper-airway stimulation for obstructive sleep apnoea on airway dimensions. *Eur Respir J.* 2015;45:129–138.
2. Meleca J, Kominsky A. Reconfiguration of upper airway stimulation devices utilizing awake endoscopy. *Laryngoscope.* 2020 [E-pub before publication, February 25].
3. Steffen A, Kilic A, König IR, et al. Tongue motion variability with changes of upper airway stimulation electrode configuration and effects on treatment outcomes. *Laryngoscope.* 2018;128:1970–1976.
4. Johnson MD, Dweiri Y, Durand D, et al. Model-based analysis of implanted hypoglossal nerve stimulation for the treatment of obstructive sleep apnea [submitted].
5. Mahmoud AF, Thaler ER. Outcomes of hypoglossal nerve upper airway stimulation among patients with isolated retropalatal collapse. *Otolaryngol Head Neck Surg.* 2019;160:1124–1129.
6. Heiser C, Edenharter G, Bas M, et al. Palatoglossus coupling in selective upper airway stimulation. *Laryngoscope.* 2017;127:E378–E383.
7. Heiser C, Maurer JT, Steffen A. Functional outcome of tongue motions with selective hypoglossal nerve stimulation in patients with obstructive sleep apnea. *Sleep Breath.* 2016;20:553–560.
8. Steffen A, Sommer JU, Strohl K, et al. Changes in breath cycle sensing affect outcomes in upper airway stimulation in sleep apnea. *Laryngoscope Invest Otolaryngol.* 2020;5(2):326–329.
9. Steffen A, Jeschke, S, Soose RJ, et al. Impulse configuration in upper airway stimulation in obstructive sleep apnea: The effect of modifying electrical comfort settings [submitted].
10. Strollo PJ Jr, Soose RJ, Maurer JT, et al.; STAR Trial Group. Upper-airway stimulation for obstructive sleep apnea. *N Engl Med J.* 2014;370:139–149.
11. Heiser C, Maurer JT, Hofauer B, et al. Outcomes of upper airway stimulation for obstructive sleep apnea in a multicenter German postmarket study. *Otolaryngol Head Neck Surg.* 2017;156:378–384.
12. Steffen A, Sommer JU, Hofauer B, et al. Outcome after one year of upper airway stimulation for obstructive sleep apnea in a multicenter German post-market study. *Laryngoscope.* 2018;128:509–515.
13. Hofauer B, Philip P, Wirth M, et al. Effects of upper-airway stimulation on sleep architecture in patients with obstructive sleep apnea. *Sleep Breath.* 2017;21:901–908.
14. Bohorquez D, Mahmoud AF, Yu JL, Thaler ER. Upper airway stimulation therapy and sleep architecture in patients with obstructive sleep apnea. *Laryngoscope.* 2020;130(4):1085–1089. doi:10.1002/lary.28057

15. Steffen A, König IR, Baptista PM, et al. Benefits of initial home sleep testing to direct upper airway stimulation therapy optimization for obstructive sleep apnoea [submitted].

16. Steffen A, Hartmann JT, König IR, et al. Evaluation of body position in upper airway stimulation for obstructive sleep apnea-is continuous voltage sufficient enough? *Sleep Breath.* 2018;22:1207–1212.

17. Steffen A, Abrams N, Suurna MV, et al. Upper-airway stimulation before, after, or without uvulopalatopharyngoplasty: A two-year perspective. *Laryngoscope.* 2019;129:514–518.

18. Heiser C. Advanced titration to treat a floppy epiglottis in selective upper airway stimulation. *Laryngoscope.* 2016;126(Suppl 7):S22–S24.

# Long-Term Follow-Up Considerations

B. Tucker Woodson and Abhay Varun Sharma

## 11.1. Introduction

Hypoglossal nerve stimulator therapy for obstructive sleep apnea (OSA), approved by the U.S. Food and Drug Administration in 2014, has provided a huge addition to the field of surgical therapies for the disease. The Stimulation Therapy for Apnea Reduction (STAR) trial cohort included patients intolerant of continuous positive airway pressure (CPAP) with moderate to severe OSA. The initial exclusion criteria consisted of a body mass index (BMI) >32 kg/m$^2$ and excluded patients with an apnea–hypopnea index (AHI) <20 or >50 events per hour, severe cardiopulmonary disorders, active psychiatric disease, neuromuscular disease, and comorbid nonrespiratory sleep disorders that could interfere with assessment of sleep. Those who qualified after this initial exclusion process were set up for in-lab polysomnography (PSG), consultation with the surgeon, and a drug-induced sleep endoscopy (DISE). The core requirements then were an AHI between 20 and 50, central or mixed apnea consisting of <25% of total AHI, nonsupine AHI > 10, and no concentric collapse of the velopharynx on DISE.[1,2] In total, there were 126 participants in the trial.

Now years out from the original trial, long-term follow-up for patients implanted with the therapy is available. As a result, data on a variety of factors can be obtained that allow continued adjustment and improvement in therapy. These factors can be separated into routine follow-up considerations and managing the medical complexities found in the long-term setting. Both objective and subjective data on patients need to be considered. In addition, factors such as device-related maintenance issues must be taken into account. This chapter will explore these questions to provide a guideline on how to manage upper airway stimulation (UAS) therapy in the long term.

# 11.2. Routine Follow-Up

There are a variety of important long-term factors to consider after UAS implantation. Success after device implantation is generally determined by the Sher criteria, which require an AHI <20 and a 50% reduction in AHI.[3] Exploring the frequency of visits, device checks, criteria for repeat sleep studies, monitoring of patient subjective and objective parameters, monitoring of adverse events, and long-term device maintenance are all important in the context of the overall long-term follow-up after device placement. Following patients regularly after therapy ensures continued effectiveness of the device and the ability to make adjustments if necessary.

## 11.2.1. Frequency of Visits

After the 1-month activation, continued evaluation is important to ensure the UAS therapy is working appropriately. The second visit typically occurs 2 to 3 months postoperatively with a sleep titration study to maximize therapy effectiveness. This time period may be flexible for patients who are having difficulty acclimating to therapy. A home sleep test (HST) at ~4 to 6 months after the titration study verifies adequate patient adherence and AHI reduction. Thereafter it is reasonable to follow the patient every 6 to 12 months to ensure continued device effectiveness and patient satisfaction. Figure 11.1 demonstrates the time course from initial evaluation to regular follow-up.

## 11.2.2. Device Checks

The UAS device needs to be monitored to ensure continued functionality. At each follow-up visit, a device check entails connecting to the generator using the physician's programmer tablet. Through this, the battery status, adherence to therapy, current settings, and stimulation thresholds are tested. In the currently approved Inspire device, the generator lasts approximately 11 years and therefore needs to be replaced at that time.[4] Approximately, six months before the device battery dies, the remote will indicate that the battery is low. This should prompt the patient to call to set up a generator replacement. Information on patient usage of the device can clue clinicians in to the need for any changes in parameters.[5]

The current generation of UAS device allows for download of patient data from the patient remote to obtain more granular detail related to patient adherence. It is recommended that this be performed and reviewed at each follow up visit to identify adequate compliance and opportunities to improve usage of the device.

Another important step during the device check involves visually verifying that the programmed stimulation results in adequate and appropriate movement of the tongue. The functional threshold refers to the stimulation required to move the tongue just past the incisors. Though rare, some patients experience changes in their functional threshold, and an alteration of the functional threshold could signal a need for a corresponding alteration of the therapeutic voltage. Overall, the ability to access all of this information at

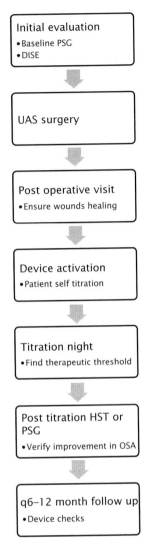

**FIGURE 11.1.** Sequence of steps from initial evaluation to regular follow-up.

device checks can be invaluable for determining the need for repeat sleep studies, device adjustments, and overall effectiveness of the UAS therapy on a regular basis.

## 11.2.3. Repeat Sleep Studies

As shown in Figure 11.1, repeat sleep studies are built into the regular follow-up. Patients initially self-titrate the device by increasing the voltage nightly to allow them to improve tolerance to the device and prepare them for the titration study. An in-lab monitored PSG is normally performed at the 2- to 3-month postoperative period in order to titrate to the therapeutic voltage, the level that eliminates the maximum number of obstructive events while maintaining patient comfort and ability to sleep. Afterward, patients can adjust the amplitude on their own within a 0.2-V range to achieve maximum comfort during sleep while still being therapeutic.[4,5] At some institutions, an HST rather than a titration PSG is done at the 2- to 3-month postoperative period after the patient acclimates to the initial device settings.

After the titration study, repeat sleep studies can still be indicated. Though much of this is at the discretion of the provider, an HST 4 to 6 months after the initial titration study is reasonable to monitor the continued effectiveness of UAS therapy. There have been cases where various changes have been necessary after a longer period of stimulation. In addition, further sleep studies can be scheduled based on either subjective changes relative to sleep or changes noted during device checks.

In the future, much of the information garnered by repeat sleep studies may be instead be obtained by the device itself, similar to how current-generation CPAP systems work. This will simplify the process of monitoring patients receiving UAS therapy.

## 11.2.4. Clinical Parameters

Clinicians should follow specific clinical parameters to ensure device effectiveness. Objective parameters include AHI, oxygen desaturation index (ODI), and BMI, while subjective parameters include a comprehensive sleepiness assessment and partner-reported snoring.

In general, objective measures like AHI, ODI, and BMI have been shown to remain stable over time. Evidence from the 5-year follow-up of the original Stimulation Therapy for Apnea Reduction (STAR) trial patients indicates that improvements in AHI remain stable. These patients received PSGs at 12 months, 18 months, 3 years, and 5 years after implantation, providing an excellent method to screen for changes that could occur with persistent stimulation. Administering a validated sleepiness scoring system such as the Epworth Sleepiness Scale (ESS) or Functional Outcome of Sleep Questionnaire (FOSQ) provides another tool for ensuring that UAS therapy is still effective. Based on the 1-year follow-up in the Adherence and Outcome of Upper Airway Stimulation for OSA International Registry (ADHERE registry), which currently has >1,000 patients enrolled, as well as the 5-year follow-up from the original STAR trial patients, ESS and FOSQ remain significantly improved (Figure 11.2).[1,6]

Other clinical parameters to follow are subjective complaints such as snoring, morning headaches, and sleep architecture. The improvement in bedpartner-reported snoring noted after UAS therapy implantation remains stable after 5 years (Figure 11.3). Worsening headaches or snoring could indicate that a therapy adjustment is necessary. Sleep architecture improvement remains stable after UAS, with an increase in N3 sleep and no change in rapid-eye-movement (REM) sleep noted up to 5 years after surgery.[1,2,7]

Various parameters have been shown to be statistically significant in affecting UAS therapy. Based on information from the ADHERE registry, the only parameters that affect the response to UAS therapy based on current data are gender and BMI. Women had a 90% increased odds of success based on the Sher criteria. In addition, each unit decrease

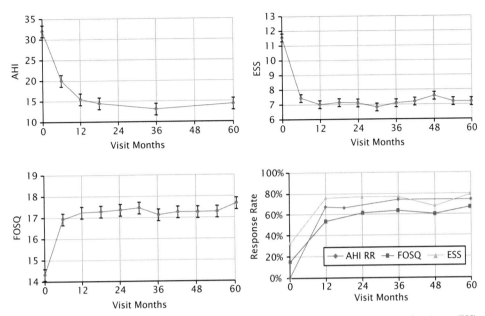

**FIGURE 11.2.** Sixty-month outcome of AHI, sleep quality of life (FOSQ), and daytime sleepiness (ESS). Values are presented as mean ± SD. Response rates (in percentages) are based on the following parameters: AHI >50% reduction to <20 events per hour, ESS score <10, and FOSQ score >17.9. From Figure 2 of Woodson BT, et al. Upper airway stimulation for obstructive sleep apnea: 5-year outcomes. *Otolaryngol Head Neck Surg.* 2018;159(1):194–202.

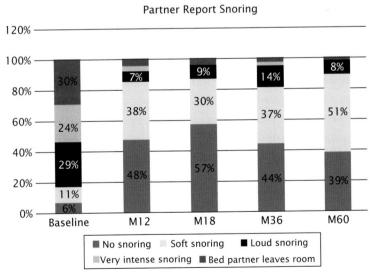

**FIGURE 11.3.** Bedpartner-reported snoring intensity over time. From Figure 3 of Woodson BT, et al. Upper airway stimulation for obstructive sleep apnea: 5-year outcomes. *Otolaryngol Head Neck Surg.* 2018;159(1):194–202.

in BMI increased the effectiveness of UAS by 8.5%.[6] However, in another study based on multiple cohorts, BMI, younger age, and lower preoperative AHI were negatively correlated with success with UAS therapy. These results held true at both 6 and 12 months after surgery.[8] Based on the STAR trial data alone, the only factor that was statistically significant in determining responders versus nonresponders to UAS therapy was the ODI, with a lower ODI predictive of 5-year responders.[1] This demonstrates the continued need to evaluate which patients benefit most from this therapy.

## 11.2.5. Monitoring for Adverse Events

Adverse events are separated into procedure-related events and device-related events. Serious adverse events are defined as any events that led to death, life-threatening illness, permanent impairment, or new or prolonged hospitalization with serious health impairment. In the STAR trial at 5 years, a total of nine serious device-related adverse events occurred to eight patients. One patient required repositioning of the sensing lead twice in order to resolve discomfort, four patients required replacement of the sensing lead, and one patient required replacement of the stimulation lead after it was inadvertently cut.[1]

The most common non-serious adverse events that were procedure-related include discomfort from stimulation and tongue abrasion. The discomfort from electrical stimulation was high in the first 12 months (81 total events), but reprogramming the stimulus levels reduced this significantly at 5 years to 5 total events. Of the original 126 participants in the STAR trial, 60.3% had this event at some point during their 5-year follow-up. Similarly, tongue abrasion occurred at a higher rate within the first 12 months (28 times) but was reduced to a total of 2 events at 5 years.[1] A meta-analysis of UAS therapy found similar complication rates in other patient cohorts, including a 6.1% rate of serious adverse events (Table 11.1).[9]

Resolving patient discomfort from stimulation is paramount as it can be a huge deterrent to using therapy. There are two types of thresholds for stimulation: sensation and functional. Sensation threshold is the first point where the patient subjectively feels the stimulation. Changing the threshold to make the device comfortable during sleep is an important step in the initial titration study and the follow-up 2- to 3-month study. This plays an even bigger role in patients with insomnia, as will be discussed later in the chapter. Patients have the ability to adjust the voltage within 0.2 V of their therapeutic threshold. However, if there are still adherence issues, further adjustments may be necessary to find the appropriate settings for optimal comfort. This will be discussed later as part of the complex titration portion of the chapter.

To resolve tongue abrasion issues, one of two methods can be used. First, the phenotype of the stimulation can be changed to allow for the tongue to sit well within the mouth while the UAS therapy is active. This involves changing the settings and having the patient comment on the comfort level with the new stimulation. The other approach is to use a tongue guide, which functions as a bite guard that allows the tongue to remain off the teeth during therapy (Figure 11.4).

## TABLE 11.1. Non-serious Adverse Events

| Adverse Event | No. of Events | | | | | Total | Participants with Event, % (n of 126) |
|---|---|---|---|---|---|---|---|
| | 0–12 months | 12–24 months | 24–36 months | 36–48 months | >48 months | | |
| Procedure-related | | | | | | | |
| Postoperative discomfort related to incisions | 47 | 1 | 2 | 1 | 1 | 52 | 30.2 (38) |
| Postoperative discomfort independent of incisions | 41 | 0 | 1 | 0 | 0 | 42 | 27.0 (34) |
| Temporary tongue weakness | 34 | 0 | 0 | 0 | 0 | 34 | 18.3 (23) |
| Intubation effects | 18 | 0 | 0 | 0 | 0 | 18 | 11.9 (15) |
| Headache | 8 | 0 | 0 | 0 | 0 | 8 | 6.3 (8) |
| Other postoperative symptoms | 22 | 0 | 0 | 0 | 0 | 22 | 11.1 (14) |
| Mild infection | 1 | 0 | 0 | 0 | 0 | 1 | 0.8 (1) |
| Device-related | | | | | | | |
| Discomfort due to electrical stimulation | 81 | 23 | 26 | 7 | 5 | 142 | 60.3 (76) |
| Tongue abrasion | 28 | 12 | 4 | 3 | 2 | 49 | 27.0 (34) |
| Dry mouth | 10 | 5 | 2 | 0 | 3 | 20 | 15.1 (19) |
| Mechanical pain associated with presence of the device | 7 | 2 | 3 | 1 | 1 | 14 | 11.1 (14) |
| Temporary internal device usability or functionality complaint | 7 | 2 | 3 | 1 | 1 | 14 | 16.7 (21) |
| Temporary external device usability or functionality complaint | 11 | 11 | 8 | 9 | 6 | 45 | 26.2 (33) |
| Other acute symptoms | 21 | 14 | 1 | 2 | 1 | 39 | 24.6 (31) |
| Mild infection | 1 | 0 | 0 | 0 | 0 | 1 | 0.8 (1) |

From Table 5 in Woodson BT, et al. Upper airway stimulation for obstructive sleep apnea: 5-year outcomes. *Otolaryngol Head Neck Surg.* 2018;159(1):194–202.

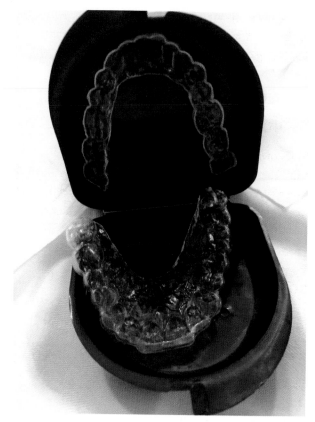

**FIGURE 11.4.** Example of a tongue guide to help avoid abrasions caused by teeth during stimulation.

Procedure-related non-serious adverse events include discomfort from the incisions, discomfort independent of the incisions, tongue weakness, intubation effects, headache, and infection. These symptoms, other than one patient with continued discomfort from the incision, all resolved at 5 years.[1]

## 11.2.6. Long-Term Device Maintenance

Device maintenance issues arise at various times. Most commonly patients will present with problems that are usually the result of user error that can be fixed in the clinic. Scheduling a 6- to 12-month follow-up visit will allow clinicians to keep track of the battery life of the implantable pulse generator (IPG) as well as to pick up on any device-related issues. In addition, the sleep remote battery needs to be changed every 2 to 4 months.

## 11.2.7. Long-Term Routine Device Replacement

The battery for the UAS made by Inspire lasts 11 years.[4] Replacing the old device is a relatively simple procedure involving general anesthesia. An incision is made over the same area in the upper chest and carried down to the IPG device, which normally lies over the pectoralis major muscle. The leads are removed, the new device is inserted, and the incision is then closed. A few patients have already reached this point and have successfully undergone IPG replacement. Device replacement is described in further detail in Chapter 12.

# 11.3. Complexities in Long-Term Care

As we continue to follow patients after UAS implantation, new problems arise that require diligence to fix. These issues highlight the importance of regular follow-up. In this portion of the chapter we will discuss suboptimal clinical response to UAS, weight gain, comorbid medical conditions, surgical complications in the long-term setting, device malfunction, complex device programming, complex PSG titration, awake versus sleep endoscopy for titration, and complex clinical profiles.

## 11.3.1. Suboptimal Clinical Response

In a recent update on the ADHERE UAS registry as well as the STAR trial patients, UAS continues to have excellent responses in patients 1 to 5 years after surgery. The ESS scores and AHI remain significantly improved, and therapy usage remained high at 5.7 hours per night.[6] In the STAR trial participants, there was an increase in AHI at the 12-month follow-up, but levels remained stable at 5 years. There was a 75% success rate of UAS therapy at 5 years as well.[1] Given that a certain number of patients remain inadequately responsive to therapy, there are some situations in which patients require optimization. A stepwise approach is necessary for dealing with these patients. As will be discussed later in the chapter, obtaining data on patient adherence and making in-office adjustments represents the first step in this process. Threshold settings are checked to ensure that the functional and sensation thresholds are the same. Changes in these could signal a corresponding need to change the therapeutic amplitude. A variety of more nuanced changes can be made in the clinic setting as well, and this can be aided with an awake endoscopy if the initial adjustments are unsuccessful. If this fails to relieve the issues, a repeat titration sleep endoscopy is indicated. Occasionally, a DISE titration is necessary if there continues to be persistent obstruction despite these attempts to alleviate them.

## 11.3.2. Weight Gain

The criteria for UAS therapy include BMI <32. Based on the ADHERE registry results, each unit decrease in BMI increases the effectiveness of UAS therapy by 8.5% in terms of the effect on AHI reduction.[6] However, some evidence shows that BMI does not play a role in its effectiveness.[6,10] As a result, there continues to be controversy over the upper limit of BMI for considering UAS therapy. After UAS implantation, weight tends to remain stable, though drastic increases in weight would certainly diminish the effectiveness of the therapy.

## 11.3.3. Medical Conditions

Following medical conditions after UAS is an important consideration due to the connection between untreated OSA and other medical comorbidities. Untreated OSA, causing nocturnal intermittent hypoxemia, is known to be a significant contributor to neurocognitive, behavioral, and cardiovascular disease, along with all-cause mortality.[11] The ODI has been found to be the most important indicator for cardiovascular disease, specifically a desaturation of 4% for >10 seconds. In addition, there is a correlation between hypopneas that are associated with a 4% desaturation and increased cardiovascular disease risk.[12] CPAP improves both cardiovascular and cerebrovascular health by reducing mortality from ischemic heart disease by 4% to 5% and stroke mortality by 6% to 8%, and the hope is that future studies will show UAS to provide a similar improvement in health.[13]

OSA is by far the most common secondary cause of hypertension, with a hypertension prevalence of 30% to 70% in OSA patients. Various studies have observed the effect of different OSA therapies on hypertension, with CPAP having a small benefit in improving hypertension on its own.[13] There is currently a double-blinded, sham-controlled, randomized crossover trial, CARDIOSA-12, exploring the effect of the UAS therapy primarily on ambulatory systolic blood pressure. This will help elucidate prospectively some of the expected effects that improvement in OSA from UAS should have on hypertension and heart disease.[14]

Atrial fibrillation (Afib) is also known to be accentuated by untreated OSA, leading to worsened cardiovascular outcomes. Specifically, studies have shown that OSA is an independent risk factor for developing Afib, increases recurrence of Afib after ablation, and results in a higher incidence of Afib in patients after coronary artery bypass graft surgery.[15] Though not proven, CPAP does seem to improve atrial and ventricular ectopy after long-term use.[15] As a result, following the status of Afib in patients implanted with the UAS is an important aspect of postoperative care.

Though patients with congestive heart failure (CHF) can sometimes have more prevalent central sleep apnea with Cheyne-Stokes respirations, OSA has also been shown to worsen CHF by causing ventricular remodeling. Studies show that for patients with OSA and CHF, CPAP is valuable in improving systolic function.[16] Again, this highlights another medical condition that can be improved by treating OSA. Evaluating the effects of UAS on these cardiac conditions will be important in future research.

## 11.3.4. Surgical Complications

Surgical complications in the long-term setting differ from those found in the immediate postoperative period. Some of these complications are more theoretical, and none are very common. However, it is important to keep some of these in mind and to have a treatment plan to resolve them if they occur.

One reasonable complication to consider is dysphagia. Due to continued stimulation, muscle fatigue or tongue hypertrophy could cause issues with swallowing. Though there are some reports of tongue weakness at the post-titration visit, long-term data from the ADHERE registry report showed no residual tongue weakness at 12 months.[6] One case report by Stevens et al. described a woman who developed cricopharyngeus muscle dysfunction after activation of UAS. Stopping therapy resolved the dysphagia, and the dysphagia returned after attempting to restart it again. A videofluoroscopic study showed posterior pharyngeal wall protrusion with narrowing at the level of the cricopharyngeus, which resolved after stopping therapy. The device was eventually explanted in this patient.[17] However, this represents an isolated case that does not appear to be the norm. A study of 27 patients by Huntley et al. showed no change in swallowing function based on a subjective dysphagia assessment, the EAT-10 survey, at 3 months after UAS activation.[18] Though more long-term data on dysphagia are necessary, it does not appear to be a common complication in implanted patients.

Device migration is another complication that, though rare, has been reported in the literature. Tabatabai el al. describes a patient who required surgery to relocate an IPG that had migrated in the chest. This is a known complication in cardiac implantables as well. In this case, the IPG migrated inferiorly, causing the stimulating wire to be pulled taut. As a result, the stimulating wire also became visible in the neck. The problem was eventually solved when the pocket was placed more superiorly. This patient was an obese female with a large amount of breast tissue, possibly leading to the issues with migration. In addition, the stimulating lead had to be tunneled to the IPG after it had become taut and visible in the neck. Smaller device pockets, secure suturing to the fascia, and appropriate placement more superiorly in female patients with a large amount of breast tissue appear to help most with avoiding this complication.[19] Stimulator electrode dislodgement has been reported, as well as a need to reposition the stimulator electrode.[6] The first step in managing a device issue such as this is to obtain an x-ray of the chest and neck to view the position of the IPG and stimulating electrode.

Twiddler syndrome represents another complication seen with implantable cardiac devices that can also cross over to UAS therapy. In this syndrome, patients have a tendency to manipulate the implanted device, leading to damage to the leads or device migration. Though this is a rare complication seen in a quoted range of 0.7% to 7% of patients with implanted cardiac devices, this can certainly occur with the IPG of the UAS therapy, as it is in an easy location to manipulate.[20]

## 11.3.5. Device Malfunction

A variety of complications can lead to device malfunction and can require anything from a simple reset in clinic to revision surgery. Some of these problems are related to device placement issues or patient factors, as noted in the previous section. Cardioversion is another adverse event that has been encountered, leading to deactivation of the UAS therapy. An estimated 40% to 50% of patients with Afib have concurrent OSA, and effective treatment of OSA can help prevent recurrences of Afib. Vasconcellos et al. describe the experience of the two senior authors with a four-patient case series of people requiring revision surgery after electrical cardioversion for Afib. When this occurs, there is a stepwise approach to resolving the issue, which will be explored further in Chapter 12. To avoid this complication, the manufacturer's guidelines for the UAS therapy state that, if possible, pharmaceutical cardioversion is preferred. In addition, a biphasic waveform is preferred over a monophasic one, and total energy given should be minimized if possible.[21] However, electrical cardioversion will continue to be given for these patients when necessary, leading to the possibility of revision surgery.

## 11.3.6. Complex Device Programming

One of the methods used to improve on suboptimal UAS therapy is advanced device programming. The three settings that can be changed are stimulation amplitude, electrode configuration, and pulse width and rate. There is a stepwise approach to improving UAS effectiveness after the 2- to 3-month titration study that has been elucidated with increasing experience with the device (Figure 11.5).

If a patient with the device continues to have issues, they can be categorized into three main sections: poor adherence, poor effectiveness, and a combination of both. Any of these will lead to a need for more complex device programing. In the ADHERE registry's most recent report, device discomfort occurred in 12% of patients at 6 months and 8% of patients at 12 months. Stimulator discomfort can be a large problem for adherence purposes. The sensation threshold is the point at which the patient feels stimulation, while the sub-discomfort threshold is the amplitude at which the patient feels discomfort or feels that the intensity of the stimulation might cause them to wake up. Occasionally

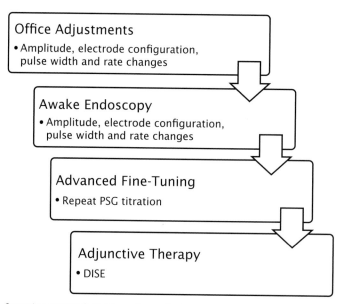

**FIGURE 11.5.** Stepwise approach to improving patient response to upper airway stimulation.

patients can have changes in these thresholds that result in a need to adjust the amplitude, though most will remain at the amplitude set after the initial titration study.[5]

For patients with comfort issues, the first step involves changing settings in the office. It is often possible for some patients to become over-titrated if they come in with continued sleepiness despite being at a therapeutic level based on the PSG titration study. Amplitude is the simplest setting to change and allows real-time evaluation of the effect on the tongue. One of the important points about this kind of change, however, is that there can be a tendency to increase the amplitude too extensively if a patient continues to come in with persistent sleepiness. Over-titration will cause decreased adherence and failure of the device to work effectively. After amplitude has been adjusted or determined to not be the problem, the start delay can be changed to ensure patients actually have time to fall asleep before the therapy starts. Other comorbid sleep conditions, especially insomnia, need to be considered to obtain optimal comfort during UAS therapy. Finally, changing the pulse width and rate can provide a more subtle adjustment. With a change in these settings, the amplitude will need to be decreased as well to maintain the same therapeutic effect. Changing the pulse width and rate can improve the sensation of the impulse, allowing for more comfortable sleep during stimulation.

If instead a patient is having issues with continued sleepiness despite adherence, the problem could be persistent suboptimal AHI. In this case an HST or PSG is warranted to evaluate the AHI. One of the advantages of a PSG in this situation is that it is possible to determine if positional therapy could be helpful. If AHI is still elevated despite adherence to UAS and positional therapy provides no benefit, changing the electrode setting can drastically improve results. It is important to start at an amplitude 50% lower than the original setting in order to find the new appropriate amplitude after the change. The default electrode setting for the UAS device is bipolar, meaning the stimulation current loop is completely within the stimulating electrode. This allows the device to fire a more local current loop to ideally avoid stimulating the retrusor portion of the hypoglossal nerve. However, this setting can be changed to a monopolar configuration, which provides a larger area of stimulation.[5] A case report by Heiser demonstrated an improvement in a patient's device function with a change to the monopolar setting. He hypothesized that the broader current loop allowed stimulation of C1, which innervates the geniohyoid, for improved tongue protrusion. This kind of a simple change can make a large difference in results, with the aforementioned patient going from an AHI of 20.7 events per hour with a bipolar setting to 4.8 events per hour with a monopolar setting.[5,22,23]

## 11.3.7. Complex PSG Titration

The first titration study, which takes place 2 to 3 months after the 1-month activation appointment, allows for adjustment of the device parameters to eliminate obstructive events. This often involves mostly changes in amplitude to ensure a therapeutic effect without exceeding the arousal threshold. If the patient fails to have a subjective improvement in symptoms or shows inadequate improvement on an HST, then a repeat PSG titration may be necessary if in-office adjustments do not resolve the situation.[5] Repeat PSG titration allows for more subtle adjustments than the original titration study, with the sleep technician changing the pulse width and rate, making electrode configuration adjustments, and attempting supplemental therapies such as positional therapy, chin-straps, cervical pillows, or oral appliances.

## 11.3.8. Awake Versus Sleep Endoscopy for Titration

Awake endoscopy can initially be used in the office setting to make changes based on how the airway appears subjectively to the physician. Patients reach this step in advanced titration when they have failed to respond to the standard adjustments in amplitude, pulse width and rate, and electrodes that are attempted looking just at external tongue motion. During awake endoscopy, the patient is placed as flat as possible and a flexible endoscope is inserted transnasally. The UAS is turned on, and different settings are tried in an attempt to find the optimal configuration that improves the airway opening.

In addition, supplemental techniques can be used to optimize the airway. Nasal breathing stabilizes the upper airway during sleep, and its benefits have been shown in its ability to improve CPAP compliance.[24,25] Though not objectively shown to actually lower obstructive events, a chinstrap to promote nasal breathing can selectively improve the effectives of UAS. A case report by Ramaswamy et al. describes a patient who underwent UAS implantation and failed to have complete response, improving from a supine AHI of 43 to 27 events per hour. However, with the addition of a chinstrap applied during DISE, he had significant improvement in airway opening and his supine AHI improved to 3 events per hour (Figure 11.6).[26] Other cases have shown improvement in AHI after placement of an oral appliance or use of a cervical pillow if moving the chin to the sternum improves the airway.

Repeat DISE after implantation may be necessary if advanced finetuning during a PSG does not improve the AHI. The case reports by Heiser and Ramaswamy mentioned previously show how DISE can provide a vast improvement in UAS effectiveness

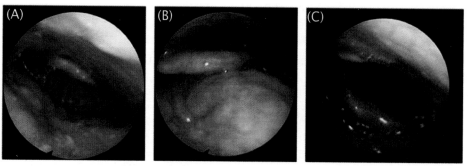

**FIGURE 11.6.** DISE images from advanced titration. (A) Total collapse with no hypoglossal nerve stimulation or mouth closure. (B) With new unipolar settings. (C) Unipolar settings with mouth closure. From figure 1 of Ramaswamy et al. A case of hypoglossal nerve stimulator-resistant obstructive sleep apnea cured with the addition of a chin strap. *Laryngoscope.* 2017;128(7):1727–1729.

by changing the setting from bipolar to monopolar or adding a supplemental device like a chinstrap.[22,26] This step is generally the last recourse used to find the optimal way to improve the results of UAS.

## 11.3.9. Complex Clinical Profiles

Comorbid sleep conditions can cause a variety of issues with UAS. Insomnia can be a particularly difficult problem to deal with for those implanted with the UAS. This specifically becomes an issue when the stimulation from the UAS prevents patients from falling asleep or wakes them up, as insomniacs will then have difficulties using the device consistently. As a result, in these patients it is especially important to find the appropriate level of therapeutic stimulation that prevents awakenings. In addition, the start delay and pause time need to be long enough to allow the patient to initially fall asleep and fall back asleep, respectively. Treating restless leg syndrome and periodic limb movement disorder will also help eliminate non-OSA-related causes for failure of the UAS therapy.

Depression, bipolar disorder, and schizophrenia all represent comorbidities that can present with OSA. They are not absolute contraindications to UAS therapy, but clinicians must exercise judgment when recommending the procedure for these patients. One case report by Mingo et al. details a patient with the stimulator implanted who underwent electroconvulsive therapy for bipolar depression without disruption of the function of the therapy.[27] Uncontrolled manic episodes could lead patients to not use the device, resulting in failed therapy. Schizophrenic patients may also be unsuitable for UAS therapy due to an inability to handle the device. Overall, the most important factors in these patients is their ability to tolerate an implanted device as well as to reliably turn the device on and off.

# 11.4. Conclusions

UAS represents the newest and one of the most effective advancements in sleep surgery. As we have gathered more data on the long-term effects of this therapy, we have gained knowledge on how to improve its efficacy. The future includes new devices from different companies, continued advancements in technology that allow for recording of objective parameters such as AHI by the implant itself, and research that provides more information on the effects of UAS on cardiac health.

# References

1. Woodson BT, et al. Upper airway stimulation for obstructive sleep apnea: 5-year outcomes. *Otolaryngol Head Neck Surg.* 2018;159(1):194–202.
2. Woodson BT, et al. Three-year outcomes of cranial nerve stimulation for obstructive sleep apnea: The STAR trial. *Otolaryngol Head Neck Surg.* 2016;154(1):181–188.
3. Sher AE, Schechtman KB, Piccirillo JF. The efficacy of surgical modifications of the upper airway in adults with obstructive sleep apnea syndrome. *Sleep.* 1996;19(2):156–177.

4. Doghramji K, Boon M. The role of upper airway stimulation therapy in the multidisciplinary management approach of obstructive sleep apnea in the adult patient. *Laryngoscope*. 2016;126(Suppl 7):S9–S11.

5. Vanderveken OM, et al. Development of a clinical pathway and technical aspects of upper airway stimulation therapy for obstructive sleep apnea. *Front Neurosci*. 2017;11:523.

6. Thaler E, et al. Results of the ADHERE upper airway stimulation registry and predictors of therapy efficacy. *Laryngoscope*. 2020;130(5):1333–1338.

7. Bohorquez D, et al. Upper airway stimulation therapy and sleep architecture in patients with obstructive sleep apnea. *Laryngoscope*. 2020;139(4):1085–1089.

8. Kent DT, et al. Evaluation of hypoglossal nerve stimulation treatment in obstructive sleep apnea. *JAMA Otolaryngol Head Neck Surg*. 2019;145(11):1044–1052.

9. Costantino A, et al. Hypoglossal nerve stimulation long-term clinical outcomes: A systematic review and meta-analysis. *Sleep Breath*. 2020;24(2):399–411.

10. Huntley C, et al. Upper airway stimulation in patients with obstructive sleep apnea and an elevated body mass index: A multi-institutional review. *Laryngoscope*. 2018;128(10):2425–2428.

11. Dempsey JA, et al. Pathophysiology of sleep apnea. *Physiol Rev*. 2010;90(1):47–112.

12. Punjabi NM, et al. Sleep-disordered breathing and cardiovascular disease: An outcome-based definition of hypopneas. *Am J Respir Crit Care Med*. 2008;177(10):1150–1155.

13. Patel AR, et al. The association of obstructive sleep apnea and hypertension. *Cureus*. 2019;11(6):e4858.

14. Dedhia RC, et al. Cardiovascular endpoints for obstructive sleep apnea with twelfth cranial nerve stimulation (CARDIOSA-12): Rationale and methods. *Laryngoscope*. 2018;128(11):2635–2643.

15. Abumuamar AM, et al. Cardiac effects of CPAP treatment in patients with obstructive sleep apnea and atrial fibrillation. *J Interv Card Electrophysiol*. 2019;54(3):289–297.

16. Kourouklis SP, et al. Effective sleep apnoea treatment improves cardiac function in patients with chronic heart failure. *Int J Cardiol*. 2013;168(1):157–62.

17. Stevens BJ, et al. Cricopharyngeal muscle dysfunction following hypoglossal nerve stimulator placement. *JAMA Otolaryngol Head Neck Surg*. 2018;144(10):948–949.

18. Huntley C, et al. The impact of upper airway stimulation on swallowing function. *Ear Nose Throat J*. 2019;98(8):496–499.

19. Tabatabai GM, Karempelis P, Hsia JC. Hypoglossal nerve stimulator generator migration: INSPIRE device reimplantation with parallels to cardiac implantable electronic devices. *Am J Otolaryngol*. 2018;39(5):639–641.

20. Tahirovic E, Haxhibeqiri-Karabdic I. Twiddler's syndrome: Case report and literature review. *Heart Views*. 2018;19(1):27–31.

21. Vasconcellos AP, et al. Dysfunctional hypoglossal nerve stimulator after electrical cardioversion: A case series. *Laryngoscope*. 2019;129(8):1949–1953.

22. Heiser C. Advanced titration to treat a floppy epiglottis in selective upper airway stimulation. *Laryngoscope*. 2016;126(Suppl 7):S22–S24.

23. Heiser C, et al. Technical tips during implantation of selective upper airway stimulation. *Laryngoscope*. 2018;128(3):756–762.

24. Kempfle JS, et al. A cost-effectiveness analysis of nasal surgery to increase continuous positive airway pressure adherence in sleep apnea patients with nasal obstruction. *Laryngoscope*. 2017;127(4):977–983.

25. Camacho M, et al. The effect of nasal surgery on continuous positive airway pressure device use and therapeutic treatment pressures: A systematic review and meta-analysis. *Sleep*. 2015;38(2):279–286.

26. Ramaswamy AT, Li C, Suurna MV. A case of hypoglossal nerve stimulator-resistant obstructive sleep apnea cured with the addition of a chin strap. *Laryngoscope*. 2018;128(7):1727–1729.

27. Mingo K, Kominsky A. Electroconvulsive therapy for depression in a patient with an Inspire hypoglossal nerve stimulator device for obstructive sleep apnea: A case report. *Am J Otolaryngol*. 2018;39(4):462–463.

# 12

# Special Circumstances

## Maurits S. Boon and Colin T. Huntley

## 12.1. Introduction

There are emerging unique circumstances that may impact the deployment and clinical approaches of upper airway stimulation (UAS) in regard to patient populations not well represented in the U.S. Food and Drug Administration (FDA) trials and early postmarket reports. This chapter details some of these considerations.

## 12.2. Implants and Gender

The experience of assessment and implant for men is numerically greater than for women. While indications, assessments, and implant devices for males and females are similar, there are distinctive features in the management decisions that apply to female patients. At the start, we do not think of women as a special population, but the decisions that are different are, for convenience, discussed in this chapter.

### 12.2.1. Preoperative Evaluation

The history related to prior breast surgery is important for device positioning, including mastectomy, implants, or reconstruction. With prior surgery, operative reports should be solicited to aid in preoperative decision making. If there is a history of breast cancer, discussion with the patient and her oncologist should be undertaken to identify patients that may require magnetic resonance imaging (MRI) for surveillance. If a need for MRI is anticipated in the future, other options for treatment of OSA should be considered given the limitations of chest MRI with current UAS devices. (See Section 12.10.)

Preoperative physical examination should include a breast examination to identify prior incision sites and the presence of scar tissue that would influence surgical decision making. The same is true for men with prior chest or neck surgery, where prior surgery might change the approach to placement of the implant and its leads. In addition, one should recognize and identify whether/which implants were used in the reconstruction if the patient is unsure of the details of her prior surgery. At present there is no collection of group data to guide individual decision making.

## 12.2.2. Surgical Technique

Surgical incisions should be planned for not only the anatomic but also the functional considerations of the patient. If there are scars from previous chest or breast surgery, it is often possible to use them so as to minimize further scars. Additionally, the upper chest incision for the implantable pulse generator (IPG) should be positioned so the IPG will not be located under a bra strap; all else being equal, it should be slightly lower and more lateral than in men. This prevents the scar being visible if the patient wears clothing with a low neckline. The incision can also be positioned so that it overlies the upper third of the IPG. This places the incision lower on the chest without necessitating positioning of the IPG too low.

The lower chest incision should be placed so as not to lie in proximity to the location of an underwire. Discussion of this is necessary as fashions change. However, if improperly positioned, the patient may experience discomfort beyond that expected from the surgery. For both the upper neck (electrode placement) and lower chest (sensor) incisions, it is helpful to ask the patient directly about placement, in anticipation of marking out locations of the strap and underwire with a skin marker in the preoperative holding area so that incisions may be appropriately placed intraoperatively.

Intraoperatively, when encountering patients with larger breasts, the bulk of the breast tissue can be moved medially and superiorly and held with an adhesive drape to minimize the need for additional retraction during respiratory sensor placement. Larger breasts may permit the IPG to move more freely on the chest wall. This may result in causing the IPG to flip on its side postoperatively and over time can cause irritation for the patient and could chronically cause damage to the leads. Therefore, both the standard anchoring and accessory (medial) anchoring hole on the IPG should be used to secure the device to the pectoralis major (Figure 12.1). This will limit the mobility of the IPG.

## 12.2.3. Previous Breast Augmentation

Breast implants pose some challenge and a risk as there is the potential to injure the implant during tunneling of the respiratory sensor and due to possible difficulty encountered in positioning the IPG relative to the breast implant.

Current techniques for breast augmentation do not include placing the breast implant in a standard location. Options for positioning the implant include subfascial as well as both above and below the pectoralis major. It is recommended that when possible, old operative reports detailing the previous implant surgery be available so as to better

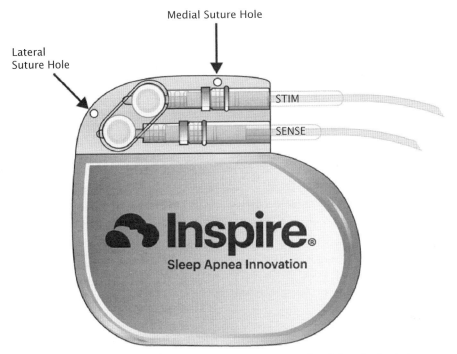

**FIGURE 12.1.** The Inspire IPG with standard (lateral) and accessory (medial) anchoring holes.

understand the position of the breast implant prior to UAS surgery. However, even implants that are placed deep to the pectoralis major will alter the anatomy of the muscle, making it possible to inadvertently pass through the muscle and injure the breast implant.

Techniques exist to minimize the potential for damage to a breast implant while tunneling. These include remaining immediately superficial to the pectoralis major fascia and dissecting under direct visualization as far as possible. In addition, ultrasound can be used intraoperatively to delineate the capsule of the implant so the surgeon can dissect around it. Finally, it is possible to consider dissecting inferior to the breast until beyond the medial extent of the implant and then directing dissection superiorly to the upper incision. In these cases, it may be helpful to make an additional sub-centimeter incision medial to the implant that would allow tunneling inferior to the breast and then dissecting superiorly (Figure 12.2). When such situations are anticipated, preoperative discussion should be undertaken with the patient as to the possible need for a fourth incision.

When considering placement of the IPG, the location of the breast implant dictates positioning. If the implant is below the pectoralis major, the IPG can be secured to the pectoralis major in a standard fashion. However, this is likely to make the IPG more visible to the patient. In patients whose breast implant is above the pectoralis major, it may be necessary to carefully dissect between the implant and the pectoralis major to create adequate space for the IPG on top of the pectoralis major.

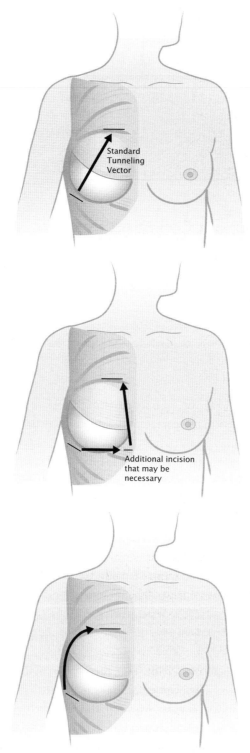

**FIGURE 12.2.** Depiction of tunneling in a standard fashion and an alternative method that can be used in a patient with a breast implant, inferior to the breast and possibly creating a fourth incision.

## 12.2.4. Breast Reconstruction

In patients who have undergone unilateral right mastectomy, it may be favorable to place the UAS device on the contralateral side (see Section 12.4). This will reduce the potential to damage any previous reconstruction and eliminate the need to operate in a scarred field. If the UAS device must be placed in the area of previous mastectomy, it is again helpful to obtain old operative reports. This will help to identify the extent of previous surgery (e.g., radical mastectomy in which the pectoralis major has been sacrificed), the type of reconstruction, and the presence of any implants. These factors will be crucial in identifying obstacles that may be encountered intraoperatively and in developing a surgical plan.

## 12.2.5. Post-Implant Considerations

Patients can be counseled that routine radiographic breast imaging is not contraindicated with a UAS system in place and should follow current guidelines. However, because of its location, the IPG may obscure some views of the breast with imaging such as mammography. This may necessitate special views as well as use of additional imaging modalities such as ultrasound for appropriate diagnosis.[1] The use of breast MRI for diagnosis and follow-up in the presence of the UAS implant should be done through radiology in consultation with the UAS company.

# 12.3. Down Syndrome

Due to the high prevalence of OSA in patients with Down syndrome, UAS has great potential as a therapeutic modality.

## 12.3.1. Features of Down Syndrome and Rationale for UAS

Down syndrome (trisomy 21) is the most common inherited chromosomal disorder, with an incidence of 1 in 700 births. It has many typical characteristic features, including a high prevalence of OSA. Some estimates place the prevalence in children at 50% to 100%, and this number may be near 100% in adults.[2] The high prevalence is a consequence of many risk factors, such as macroglossia, adenotonsillar hypertrophy, midface hypoplasia, obesity, and hypotonia.

Given the rates of OSA in the pediatric Down syndrome population and the incidence of adenotonsillar hypertrophy, tonsillectomy and adenoidectomy remains a mainstay of therapy. However, it has been established that these individuals remain at high risk for persistent OSA.[3] Continuous positive airway pressure (CPAP) is also an option that can be used for treatment, and adherence rates up to 65% have been described in adults with intellectual disabilities (this was not limited to individuals with Down syndrome).[4] However, this requires intensive training protocols that may not always be possible given caretaker limitations. Therefore, UAS has emerged as a potential treatment option for both adults and children with Down syndrome. The therapy has particular appeal because of the ease of use of the UAS device; caretakers can activate the device with limited need to have the patient participate in the process.

## 12.3.2. Evidence for UAS Therapy Use

Currently, while the literature is limited, there are publications supporting UAS in adults and children with Down syndrome. The first report of use in an adult was described in a case report in which the apnea–hypopnea index (AHI) was reduced from a baseline of 61.5 events per hour to 23.0 events per hour at 6 months.[5] This was followed by a case series of three adults who had reductions in the titrated AHI of 86% to 100%. It is important to note that adherence averaged 8.2 hours per night, which reflects excellent tolerance of therapy.[6]

UAS therapy has similarly been trialed in pediatric patients with Down syndrome. Twenty patients were implanted after failure of CPAP and after sleep endoscopy confirmed that they were appropriate candidates based on absence of complete concentric collapse at the palate. In this study, the baseline median AHI was reduced from 24.15 to a postoperative titrated AHI of 3.00. In addition, adherence was high, with a median nightly usage of 9.21 hours.[7]

Given the multiple factors that contribute to OSA in this population, UAS is not a treatment that can be expected to benefit all patients. However, given the studies to date and the established low morbidity, there is certainly great potential for use of this therapy in Down syndrome. Clearly, further study is warranted to establish any claims about short- and long-term efficacy.

# 12.4. Left-Sided Implants

By convention, the majority of UAS implants are performed on the right side. This is primarily so that implants will not be mistaken for cardiac implantable electronic devices (CIEDs) and so that the left side is preserved if patients should require a CIED in the future. However, there are clinical situations in which a left-sided implant may be desirable or necessary.

## 12.4.1. Clinical Indications for Left-Sided Implant

Indications for a left-sided implant may be due to patient preference such as occupational or recreational concerns. In addition, past medical treatments that have affected the right neck or chest may dictate the need for a left-sided approach (Box 12.1).

## 12.4.2. Technical Considerations

When preparing for a left-sided approach, incisions are planned in identical fashion as on the right and the patient is prepared as on the right (including placement of nerve

## BOX 12.1 Indications for Left-Sided Implants

Professional Activities or Personal Preference

    Athletes (right hand dominant)

    Hunters (concern putting gun stock on shoulder with existing implant)

    Law enforcement

Past medical care

    Previous surgery

        Radical mastectomy

        Unilateral breast reconstruction

        Thoracotomy with lobectomy or pneumonectomy

        Neck dissection

        Submandibular gland excision

        Previous UAS requiring revision

    Implanted device on right side

        Deep brain stimulation

        CIED

    Radiation therapy/scar on right

        Head and neck radiation

        Unilateral breast or chest radiation

integrity monitors in the left tongue). The operation proceeds in a similar fashion with some notable exceptions related to cuff placement and positioning of the respiratory sensor.

Placement of the cuff requires approaching the nerve from an inferior to superior direction. Many surgeons find this easier as the body of the mandible does not interfere with introduction of the cuff, which can be the case with the right-sided approach. Securing the anchor to the digastric tendon is identical to a right-sided operation.

The main difference in a left-sided approach is the placement and positioning of the respiratory sensor. Cardiac pulsations can interfere with normal respiratory sensor function. As a result, the sensor needs to be placed as far from the left ventricle as possible. While the sensor is still positioned between the external and internal intercostal muscles, the sensor needs to be positioned in a posterior direction to accommodate extra distance from the heart (Figure 12.3). It is important that the initial incision in the lower chest still be placed in a standard fashion anterior to the midaxillary line. This prevents inadvertent damage to the long thoracic nerve, which runs close to this anatomic landmark. As long as dissection is initiated anterior to the midaxillary line and maintained deep to the serratus anterior muscle in the plane between the external and internal intercostal

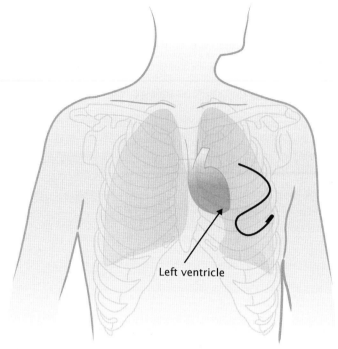

Left ventricle

**FIGURE 12.3.** Left-sided implant showing positioning of the respiratory sensor in a posterior direction and standard positioning of the tension-relieving loop.

muscles, the posterior positioning of the sensor tip should not put the long thoracic nerve at risk.

Given the current configuration of the respiratory sensor with two separate anchors to be secured, the surgeon also must account for the tension-relieving loop that is used. Two configurations of the loop can be employed. The first is with the loop positioned anteriorly and the second fixed anchor located in a more posterior location. This would position the proximal aspect of the lead in a more posterior location than normal as it approaches the IPG pocket. Alternatively, the second fixed anchor can be positioned in a more anterior location (Figure 12.4) with a more anterior position of the proximal lead as it approaches the IPG pocket.

Once the lead has been secured and coupled to the IPG, careful review of the respiratory waveform should be performed to ensure whether cardiac pulsations are being over-sensed. If significant cardiac artifact is identified, repositioning of the lead to a more inferior interspace may be considered.

## 12.4.3. Postoperative Considerations

Due to potential lack of awareness of UAS as a treatment for OSA, it is possible that a UAS device would be mistaken for a CIED. In addition, if patients require external cardioversion, there is greater risk with an indwelling left implant that it can be damaged

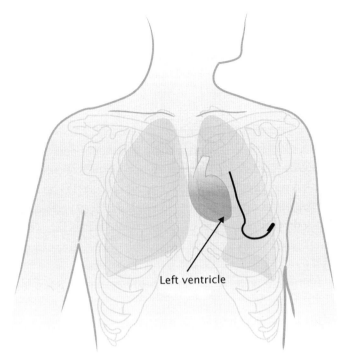

Left ventricle

**FIGURE 12.4.** Alternative configuration of tension-relieving loop.

by the electrical pulse. Patients should be counseled regarding these concerns and should inform any practitioners involved in their care (see Section 12.9 on cardioversion with implants).[8]

# 12.5. IPG Replacement

In the lifetime of the implanted patient, it is anticipated that there will arise a need to replace the IPG due to battery life or device dysfunction. This section will address the indications and technical aspects of IPG replacement.

## 12.5.1. Indications for IPG Replacement

Based on literature produced by the manufacturer, the IPG has a battery that is expected to last between 10 and 11 years (depending on the model implanted). In addition to battery depletion, other possible indications for replacing an IPG include damage to the device from iatrogenic injury and primary IPG failure.[8]

## 12.5.2. Replacing the IPG

When planning IPG replacement, patients should be counseled about the potential for complete device revision due to the possibility of damaging leads during the procedure. In addition, it is advised that an anteroposterior and lateral chest x-ray should be obtained preoperatively. This permits identification of the lead locations relative to the IPG to minimize the chance of injuring them when approaching the pocket. Patients should be prepared as in a primary case to include the neck and lower chest, and nerve integrity monitoring leads should be placed in the ipsilateral tongue.

The previous IPG incision should be used in the approach. However, it may be necessary to widen the incision slightly to facilitate device manipulation and to allow delivery of the device from the pocket. Monopolar cautery (see Section 12.8) should not be employed, and sharp dissection should proceed with caution. Palpation should be used frequently as the dissection proceeds more deeply and is used to potentially identify a superficial lead overlying the IPG. A dense capsule will be identified around the IPG, and this can be incised in the central portion of the wound. Once the capsule has been entered, dissecting with a hemostat and lifting the tissue can allow visualization into the pocket to minimize damage to the lead as the incision is fully extended. Typically the leads will also be encapsulated in a dense fibrous layer posterior to the IPG. This limits their mobility. As such, the IPG should not be delivered from the wound completely before removing the leads. Instead, it should be carefully mobilized superiorly without completely removing it from the pocket. This allows exposure of the lead–header interface and loosening of the set screws. After freeing the leads, the IPG can be safely removed without damaging them.

Based on CIED literature, there is a relatively high risk for device-related infection with IPG replacement.[9] This is thought to be due to the dense capsule surrounding the device, which is relatively avascular and prevents an adequate host immune response. Therefore, it is suggested that a 2 × 2-cm window be removed from the more superficial aspect of the capsule before introducing the new IPG into the pocket. This promotes granulation and the host response to the foreign body. Once complete, the pocket should be irrigated with bacitracin-infused saline.

At this point, the leads should be carefully dried and cleaned, a new IPG can be introduced into the field and the lead–header interface secured with the set screws. The IPG can be introduced into the pocket and secured to the chest wall in a standard fashion. Complete device interrogation should be performed, including stimulation, evaluation of respiratory sensing, and an impedance check. The device should be programmed to the patient's preoperative settings. Wound closure can be performed in a standard fashion.

Once the patient is awake in the recovery room, it is recommended that stimulation be carried out to ensure that the patient is tolerant of the device settings. It is not necessary to delay use of the UAS; patients can be instructed to begin using their device that evening. A sleep study should be performed within several months to confirm that there is still adequate control of OSA.

# 12.6. Revision Surgery

While it is a rare occurrence, revision surgery related to UAS implants has been reported. Revisions have included simple replacement of the IPG as well as lead replacement. Indications for revision are described in Box 12.2.

---

**BOX 12.2 Indications for Revision Surgery**

Primary device malfunction (leads or IPG)

Battery depletion

Dislodged leads (lead–header interface not adequately secured)

Mixed activation tongue motion due to inclusion of late hyoglossus nerve branches within the cuff

Unrecognized damage to leads with primary implant

Subsequent surgical procedures in the region of implant damaging leads or IPG

Iatrogenic injury from cardioversion/defibrillation

Patient injury from device manipulation within the pocket (pacemaker twiddler's syndrome)[10]

---

# 12.6.1. General Considerations for Revision Surgery

When device malfunction is recognized, it is important to engage the manufacturer's technical team to assist with diagnostic evaluation. Despite testing, it is not always possible preoperatively to identify which component of the system is dysfunctional. A preoperative chest x-ray may be helpful to identify the locations of the leads relative to the position of the IPG. In addition, a surprising amount of scar tissue develops after UAS surgery. This is not only a consequence of the degree of dissection of the primary surgery but also attributable to the foreign body reaction to the components of the system. As a result, revision surgery can be challenging, with distorted tissue planes. The surgeon should anticipate the potential for a much longer procedure than the initial implant. Finally, a general precaution for any revision surgery is the avoidance of monopolar cautery (see Section 12.8). See Section 12.5 for information about IPG replacement.

# 12.6.2. Replacement of Stimulation Lead

The replacement of a stimulation lead begins by opening the superior neck incision. This may require extending the incision to improve exposure. The lead will typically be located in the anterior or mid-portion of the incision and will be encountered relatively superficially, just deep to the platysma muscle. While it is possible to follow the lead down to its attachment to the digastric muscle and subsequently to the hypoglossal nerve, this is tedious and has the potential to injure the lead due to the degree of fibrotic tissue surrounding the lead. It is advantageous to try and identify the normal anatomic structures by dissecting deep to the submandibular gland in a standard fashion. If the ranine vein was not suture ligated during the initial procedure, its identification may serve as a useful landmark for nerve identification. However, it is helpful to suture ligate the vein during the revision surgery to limit bleeding around the nerve. If the revision is necessary due to poor tongue function secondary to late hyoglossus branches being included in the cuff, the anchor can be maintained on the digastric tendon, the cuff exposed and removed, and the nerve dissected to facilitate cuff repositioning. Nerve dissection can be technically demanding secondary to the fibrotic reaction. If the lead has been damaged, it needs to be removed from the nerve, the anchor released from the digastric tendon, and the lead–header interface disengaged. This requires opening the IPG pocket and removing the lead from its tunnel. Due to the tight capsule around the lead, it is best to cut either the cuff or the tip of the lead to allow it to slide through the tunnel. Once the new lead is placed, a new tunnel can be established from the neck incision to the IPG pocket and the lead can be resecured.

If extensive fibrosis prohibits safe dissection of the previously operated hypoglossal nerve, it is possible to place a new stimulation lead in the contralateral neck. This can be accomplished by approaching the unoperated neck in a standard fashion, placing the lead, and then tunneling the lead to the previously operated neck before tunneling down to the IPG pocket. This avoids tunneling the lead across the neck, in which it might overlie the laryngotracheal complex, and limits the potential to injure the anterior jugular veins. In this situation the old lead can be left in place. The major disadvantage to this technique is that the presence of the old lead negates the potential for patients to have MRI of any type in the future.

Once the stimulation lead cuff has been placed and the lead has been tunneled and attached to the lead–header interface, complete device interrogation should be performed and the device reprogrammed as warranted.

## 12.6.3. Sensor Lead Revision

Similar to stimulation lead revision, the procedure is initiated by incising through previous scar in the lower chest incision. As in any other device-related revision, monopolar cautery should be avoided. Once through the dermis, palpation should be carried out to identify the lead and ensure that it does not run superficially. Dissection is then carried carefully down to the level of the serratus anterior, where the lead will be encountered. The lead should be inspected to see whether it is rotated or is in a position that does not allow optimal sensing. If this is the case, it may be possible to slightly modify its position and resecure the lead without completely removing it from its pocket.

If it appears that the lead is damaged, it should be removed. This requires releasing the two anchors, extricating the sensor tip, and opening the IPG incision to allow the lead–header interface to be disengaged. The tight fibrotic capsule around the sensor tip makes it difficult to remove and often requires direct incision of the capsule. Given proximity to the pleura, dissection should proceed with caution to avoid creating a pneumothorax.

Once the lead has been removed, a new lead should be brought into the field, and it may be possible to replace the lead into the old location. However, if it is not possible to position it in its old pocket or interrogation of the respiratory wave yields an unacceptable waveform, a new location for the lead should be chosen. This can be accomplished by identifying another interspace either above or below the previous site. Alternatively, the lead can be positioned in the same interspace in a posterior direction (such as performed for a left-sided respiratory sensor). The advantage of this technique is that the tissues in this location have not been previously violated and less scar is present, which facilitates dissection. The anchors should be secured and tunneling should be performed to the upper chest incision.

At this point, the sensor lead should be resecured to the IPG and complete device interrogation should be carried out.

# 12.7. Surgical Procedures in Patients with an Existing UAS Device

If a patient with an existing UAS implant needs surgery, certain safeguards must be exercised to prevent injury to the patient and the device. It is important that patients discuss the need for elective surgery with their implanting surgeon so that it is possible to communicate among the care team (including surgeon and anesthesiologist with the implant surgeon) and discuss precautions.

## 12.7.1. General Precautions

During any surgical intervention, the patient's device should be turned off for the duration of the procedure. Ideally, bipolar cautery should be employed for hemostasis. If monopolar cautery is necessary, the minimum energy possible should be used and grounding of the patient should be performed such that no electrical energy would be transmitted through the UAS device. Electrical energy delivered through the UAS device not only risks damaging the implant but could also be transmitted through the stimulation lead and damage the hypoglossal nerve.

## 12.7.2. Procedures in the Region of the Implant

Due to the relatively recent introduction of UAS therapy, surgeons may have limited familiarity with the technology and its components. As a consequence, procedures performed in the vicinity of the implant have great potential to injure the device and necessitate revision of the implant. The care team, including the implant surgeon and the surgeon for upcoming procedure, should discuss routine precautions and site-specific concerns, including the location of the leads. It may be useful to obtain preoperative anteroposterior and lateral x-rays to help identify the location of the leads so as to minimize iatrogenic injury. If damage occurs during the procedure, the implant surgeon should be immediately notified to plan a revision.

## 12.7.3. Surgery Placing Another Electronic Implantable Device

The majority of implantable medical devices (IMDs) do not use bioelectric sensing and as such do not have the potential to interact with a UAS. In patients who need an electronic implantable device, it is important that representatives from the UAS device and the new electronic implant be present for the procedure to interrogate their respective devices and ensure that there is no interaction (see Section 12.8). Implants should be located as far from one another as technically possible, and settings should be used that minimize the potential for device interaction.

### 12.7.4. Postoperative Considerations

If an inpatient stay is required postoperatively following a procedure, the patient should bring the remote and plan to use it during any sleep periods. This minimizes the impact of OSA burden on postoperative care, especially immediately after anesthesia. The inpatient care team, including nurses, technicians, and physicians, must be informed of the presence of the UAS implant and educated on its use. The author has had a patient in whom nursing staff confiscated the remote control for the UAS device after the patient had activated the implant. When the patient attempted to contact nursing staff to have the remote returned, the staff became concerned due to slurred speech from stimulation and initiated a stroke protocol. This anecdote highlights the potential concerns that may occur for patients if the care team is not appropriately made aware regarding the patient's implant.

## 12.8. Implantable Medical Devices

The prevalence of IMDs is increasing. The majority of these devices are passive and do not employ bioelectric sensing. Therefore, they do not have potential to interact with UAS devices. However, given the comorbid conditions that are known to be correlated with untreated OSA, it is not uncommon to encounter patients who are already implanted with an *active* medical device or who may need to have an electronic medical device implanted. Some of the common active IMDs are listed in Box 12.3.

Active medical devices may interact with each other and alter the function of one another. For example, the stimulation produced by a UAS device might be sensed by an implantable cardiac-defibrillator and be identified as an arrhythmia, triggering an inappropriate intervention. Conversely, the shock delivered by the implantable cardiac-defibrillator could alter the function of the UAS or induce damage.[8] For this reason, it is imperative to obtain history in all patients related to the presence of an implanted device or if there is any history that might suggest future need for such a device. While the literature on use of UAS with other devices is not extensive, to date there have been no reports of device interaction.[11,12]

### 12.8.1. Implantation with CIEDs

Within the realm of IMDs, perhaps the most concerning situation in terms of potential interaction involves cardiac devices, where sensing of UAS stimulation could trigger an

---

## BOX 12.3 Commonly Encountered Implantable Medical Devices

Pacemakers

Internal cardiac defibrillators

Infusion pumps

Ventricular assist devices

Cochlear implants

Bone-anchored hearing aids

Neurostimulators

    Vagal nerve

    Spinal

    Phrenic nerve

    Sacral nerve

    Deep brain

---

inappropriate response from the cardiac implant. It is critical when implanting a UAS in a patient with a preexisting cardiac device that precautions be taken to minimize interaction. Therefore, some basic understanding of the function of these devices is helpful.

### 12.8.1.1. Stimulation Modes of UAS

With the Inspire hypoglossal nerve stimulator, different modes of stimulation can be used. As previously described, these can be altered to produce different effects on nerve stimulation and patient sensitivity to stimulation. The standard bipolar mode (+ - +) employs the central electrode within the stimulation cuff as the anode and the outer two electrodes within the stimulation cuff as the cathode. With this configuration, stimulation is confined in a narrow field within the cuff (Figure 12.5).

There is an alternative bipolar array (- + -) that reverses the configuration. Unipolar stimulation is also possible (off – off, - - -, - off -) and uses one or more of the cuff electrodes as the anode and the IPG as the cathode. Thus, the electrical field is not limited to the cuff and produces a wider field of stimulation (Figure 12.6).

### 12.8.1.2 Sensing of CIEDs

Cardiac devices have two basic modes of sensing arrhythmias related to the atria or ventricle: unipolar and bipolar. When bipolar sensing is being used, both the cathode and anode are on the same lead located near its tip. As a result, the sensing is confined to the chamber in which the implant resides, and there is less potential for over-sensing. With unipolar modes, the cathode is located on the lead and the anode is the pacemaker body.

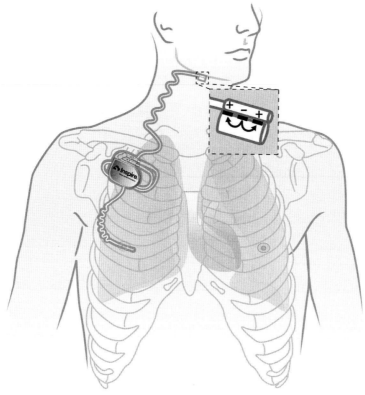

**FIGURE 12.5.** Bipolar configuration of UAS electrodes illustrating the narrow field of stimulation confined within the cuff.

Thus, sensing is not confined to the chamber of implant, and there is greater potential for myopotential over-sensing, given the wide field (Figure 12.7).

## 12.8.2. Basic Principles of Implantation

Prior to the planned operative intervention, evaluation by a cardiologist is warranted to ensure that the patient's cardiac status is optimized prior to general anesthesia. History should be obtained from the patient as to the type and manufacturer of the CIED. This should include information as to whether the patient is pacer dependent or independent. With knowledge of the make of the device, a representative from the manufacturer should be contacted so they can attend the UAS implant to interrogate and program the device.

Once in the operating room, if possible the CIED should be set to sense only-mode (this may not always be possible if the patient is pacer dependent). This is particularly relevant with an automatic implantable cardiac defibrillator (AICD) so as to prevent unintentional defibrillation during the procedure. To ensure patient safety, all AICD patients should have external defibrillator paddles placed in the event that the patient has an arrhythmia requiring intervention. UAS implantation should proceed in a standard fashion;

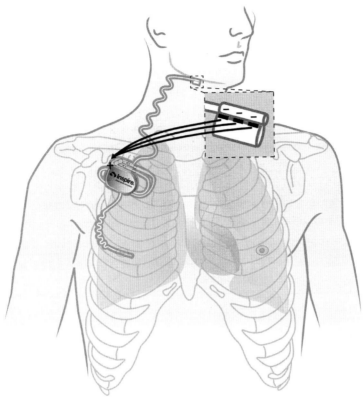

**FIGURE 12.6.** Unipolar configuration of UAS electrodes (- - -) showing the broad field of stimulation outside the cuff with the IPG serving as the anode.

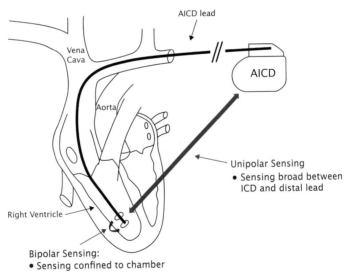

**FIGURE 12.7.** Cardiac electronic implantable device modes of sensing (not drawn to scale).

it is recommended that the UAS is placed as far from the CIED as possible (≥15 cm apart) and that bipolar cautery is used for hemostasis (to prevent damage to the CIED).

Once the UAS implant is in place, interrogation of both devices should be performed. The CIED should be set to maximum sensitivity so as to potentially capture any signals from the UAS. In addition, supra-therapeutic stimulation using unipolar settings and maximal stimulation (5 V) should be carried out to maximize potential for the cardiac sensing. Once complete, high-output pacing should be employed on the CIED to identify whether phrenic nerve capture causes UAS sensing.

## 12.8.3. Postoperative Considerations

Assuming that no interaction is identified during the procedure, it is recommended that, when possible, both devices be used in bipolar modes. This minimizes the potential for device interaction postoperatively. If the patient receives a defibrillation pulse, the UAS system should be interrogated to ensure that it functions normally and that the stimulation parameters set for the patient did not change.

## 12.8.4. Use of Other Electronic IMDs

To date, there is no literature regarding interaction of UAS with other non-cardiac implantable devices.[11,12] However, per the manufacturer's (Inspire Medical) literature, passive devices and those that do not use bioelectric sensing do not have the potential to interact with UAS therapy.

# 12.9. Cardioversion, Defibrillation, and Cardiac Procedures

There has been a well-established relationship between cardiac arrhythmias and OSA, particularly atrial fibrillation. In the Sleep Heart Study published in 2006, patients with sleep disordered breathing had an increased incidence of atrial fibrillation, nonsustained ventricular tachycardia, and complex ventricular ectopy. This was even after controlling for confounders. The cause is complex and likely multifactorial.[13,14] Given this relationship, it can be anticipated that there may be a need for intervention directed at cardiac arrhythmias in patients implanted with a UAS that may include cardiac ablations as well as external electrical cardioversion. To date there are no reported adverse interactions of cardiac ablation in patients with hypoglossal nerve stimulators. However, there are documented cases in which external electrical cardioversion or defibrillation has caused dysfunction of an implanted UAS.[8]

The electrical energy delivered from external cardioversion and defibrillation has the potential to damage the IPG as well as the leads associated with the UAS device. In addition, there is potential concern that the electrical energy could be transmitted via the stimulation lead and cause injury to the hypoglossal nerve. Fortunately, thus far in the history of UAS therapy, there have been no descriptions of any patient injury. In a publication by Vasconcellos et al., electrical cardioversion was responsible for causing dysfunction of UAS devices in several patients.[8] In each of these cases the IPG was damaged, necessitating replacement. It should be noted that all of the implants that incurred damage from cardioversion were of the Inspire II (2024) model. The newer Inspire IV (2028) model, which has been in production since 2017, is thought to be more resistant to damage from electrical energy.

## 12.9.1. Recommendations for Cardioversion/Defibrillation

Given the potential risk of damage to a UAS implant, precautions should be taken when performing electrical cardioversion. These include using the minimum energy possible when administering the shock, using biphasic waveforms, and paying careful attention to the positioning of the skin paddles so as to limit the energy transmitted through the UAS system. Skin paddles can be placed in different configurations, including anterolateral and anteroposterior. These allow conduction of the electrical shock through the heart to attempt to convert to sinus rhythm. Anteroposterior positioning of the paddles (Figure 12.8) is thought to be more protective of the device by virtue of not transmitting electrical energy through it. In contrast, anterolateral positioning poses a greater risk of implant damage as the energy cannot circumvent the implant.

## 12.9.2. Postoperative Considerations

Following cardioversion/defibrillation, patients may attempt to use their device as they normally would. However, if there is any question about dysfunction, the UAS implant should be interrogated to assess for normal function. Dysfunction can be limited to generator reset, which would simply require reprogramming. However, complete device malfunction can occur, which would require replacement of a component or all of the UAS system.

## 12.9.3. Protocol for Managing a Damaged Device

When dysfunction following cardioversion/defibrillation is noted, complete device interrogation should be performed that includes assessment of the respiratory sensor, stimulation with previously identified stimulation parameters, stimulation with alternative electrode configurations, and an impedance check. When damage to the IPG has occurred, it is the author's experience that the programmer will not be able to establish communication and neither identification of respiratory sensing nor stimulation will be possible. In such cases, revision surgery should be planned.

In most cases, revision surgery will only entail IPG replacement. However, the possibility of complete device revision, including replacement of the stimulation lead and respiratory sensor, should be anticipated, and the patient should be prepared and draped as per a standard implant procedure. This includes placement of nerve integrity

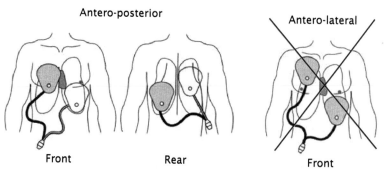

**FIGURE 12.8.** Positioning of paddles for cardioversion.

monitoring. Prior to the procedure it is helpful to obtain a lateral and anteroposterior chest x-ray to localize the leads relative to the IPG. This can help identify if leads have migrated and are in a position in which they could be transected when approaching the pocket of the IPG intraoperatively.

The operation should begin as one would perform with a replacement of IPG (see Section 12.5). Interrogation should be performed and all leads should be examined to ensure that there are no issues with the lead–header interface. At this point the leads should be disconnected from the IPG and a new IPG should be introduced into the field. Leads should be cleaned and dried and connected to the new IPG in standard fashion. The IPG should be placed back into the preexisting pocket, and interrogation of the device should proceed with a standard protocol as in placement of a new implant (see Chapter 7). If normal function is identified, the IPG should be secured to the chest wall in standard fashion, the pocket is closed, and the operation can be terminated. The device can be programmed with the patient's preoperative stimulation settings and the patient is instructed that immediate use of the device is acceptable. Plans should be made for a follow-up sleep study to ensure adequate control of the OSA.

If problems with either lead are noted, revision of the faulty lead should be performed (see Section 12.6.3).

# 12.10. MRI and Other Medical Devices

In patients who have a UAS implant, medical devices, therapeutic procedures, diagnostic procedures, and electromagnetic disturbances can potentially interact with the device and result in damage to the device or patient injury. As a consequence, it is important for implanting physicians to be aware of devices that might pose risk so they can counsel patients preoperatively and can manage potential issues after implantation.

## 12.10.1 MRI

The first commercially available generation of UAS (Inspire 3024) was MRI incompatible. However, the current generation (Inspire 3028) is considered MRI conditional and has

FDA approval for MRI of the head, extremities (excluding shoulder and hip), and cervical spine. Patients who have a medical condition that requires routine use or anticipated future need of MRI of the chest, abdomen, or neck should not be considered as appropriate candidates for UAS unless there are acceptable alternative imaging methods that yield similar diagnostic information as MRI and that would not be contraindicated with the implanted system.

General recommendations for MRI technique include a static magnetic field of 1.5T, a maximum scan time of 30 minutes out of any 90-minute period, and use of a cylindrical bore system. It is recommended that the imaging center contact the manufacturer to discuss more specific recommendations based on the type of scan being performed. Patients should be instructed to bring their device identification card and sleep remote to the imaging center. Prior to imaging, the implanted system should be confirmed to be MRI compatible and patients should be counseled regarding the possible interactions (e.g., vibration of the generator, electrode or generator heating, and stimulation of the tongue similar to therapy). Patients should be instructed to notify the scan operator if they identify any interaction, particularly if it becomes uncomfortable. Prior to the scan, confirmation of normal function of their system should be performed. This includes turning the system on with the sleep remote, confirming tongue protrusion, and ensuring the system is turned off with the remote.

During scanning, the sleep remote should not be brought into the magnet room. Patients should be monitored visually and audibly and scanning should be terminated if uncomfortable stimulation or heating occurs. On completion of the scan, patients should confirm normal function of their UAS system; if dysfunction is suspected, they should contact the implanting physician for interrogation of their device and reprogramming as necessary.

## 12.10.2. Medical Devices Contraindicated for Use with UAS Implants

Diathermy and transcranial magnetic stimulation are contraindicated for use with UAS due to the potential to damage the device or cause tissue injury at the electrode sites.

## 12.10.3. Medical Devices That Require Precautions

Each of the following devices can be used in patients with UAS implanted systems with precautions to avoid either implant damage or patient injury. Systems that have a return electrode should never be positioned to allow transmission of energy through any component of the UAS system.

Electrocautery used near the generator or leads can cause damage to the generator and potential damage to the hypoglossal nerve via transmission through the stimulation lead. If electrocautery is necessary, bipolar cautery should be used whenever possible.

Radiofrequency (or microwave) ablation should not be used in proximity to the implant. Current generated by the device can damage implant components or induce tissue damage.

Ultrasonic bone growth stimulators, transcutaneous electrical nerve stimulation, cryotherapy, and cryoablation can cause device damage or possible tissue injury and should be kept at least 6 inches from implanted components. Electromagnetic bone growth stimulators can result in unintended stimulation or generator reset and should be kept at least 18 inches from implant sites.

Radiation therapy can damage circuitry and should not be used directly over the generator. If this therapy is necessary, the device should be shielded.

Electroconvulsive therapy (ECT) can be used with the following recommendations: ECT electrodes should be placed as far from the UAS system as possible, ECT wires should be routed as far from the implant as possible, and therapy should be turned off during the ECT procedure.

## 12.10.4. Devices That Do Not Require Special Precautions

Diagnostic x-rays, computed tomography, fluoroscopy, and diagnostic ultrasound should not affect UAS systems and do not require special precautions. However, patients should inform the radiology technician that they have an implant and show them the location of implanted components.[15]

# 12.11. Infection in the Setting of UAS

While the exact incidence of UAS device-related infections is unknown, there is a known risk of infection with any implanted devices. In the literature on cardiac device infections, there is wide variability reported, with an incidence between 0.8% and 5.7%.[16–18]

## 12.11.1. Infection Prevention

Prevention of infection requires the use of meticulous sterile technique in conjunction with perioperative use of antibiotics. Approximately 30 minutes before the incision, a first-generation cephalosporin should be administered; administration can be repeated for extended cases based on the half-life of the antibiotic. In patients with known beta-lactam allergy, intravenous vancomycin can be given.[16,17] Additional measures that have been recommended for limiting infection include preparing the patient with an Ioban incise drape and adding bacitracin to the irrigation fluid that is employed intraoperatively.[19]

Routine administration of postoperative antibiotics is not recommended; this is in concordance with guidelines for other surgical implants.[20] However, special circumstances and surgeon judgment may dictate the use of postoperative antibiotics.

## 12.11.2. Management of Infections

Infections following placement of an implantable device may occur acutely in the immediate postoperative period but can also occur within 4 to 6 weeks after the implant.[21,22]

Most cases of infection will be apparent based on inflammatory changes such as erythema of the skin and swelling around incision sites. Differences in the normal healing pattern among patients may make recognition more challenging. More chronic infections may manifest as erosion of either the generator or associated leads through the skin. If an infection is suspected, patients should be seen urgently by the implanting surgeon for examination and initiation of treatment. The most common organisms seen in CIED infections include *Staphylococcus aureus* and coagulase-negative staphylococcus.[22,23]

Patients presenting with swelling that does not appear to be consistent with infection can be observed, and evacuation should be considered only if there is increased tension on the skin. If evacuation is necessary, it is recommended that the incision be reopened with a full surgical preparation. The contents are evacuated, cultures are obtained, any bleeding is meticulously controlled, and the pocket is flushed with bacitracin-infused saline. Reclosure is performed and a pressure dressing is applied.

Suspected superficial infections that do not involve the device may be diagnosed by erythema, swelling, discharge, and pain without evidence of a collection. Systemic symptoms are typically absent. These infections can be managed with topical application of mupirocin, with the choice of antimicrobial therapy based on the results of blood cultures or a wound culture (when possible). Empiric coverage against methicillin-resistant *S. aureus* (MRSA) and coagulase-negative staphylococcus should be considered immediately and should include intravenous vancomycin.

If infection involving the device is confirmed during exploration or by other means, successful treatment involves two steps: device explantation and antibiotic treatment.[24–26] During explantation, *all* components should be removed as bacterial contamination makes persistent infection likely if any remaining portions of the device are left in place. Cultures should be obtained of the infection site as well as the components of the device that are directly involved. Debridement of any nonviable tissue should be performed and all wounds irrigated with bacitracin-infused saline. Antibiotics should be administered for 10 to 14 days following explantation and are directed at the pathogens identified by culture.[23,26]

Reimplantation of a new system should not be performed until it is clear that there are no residual signs of infection. Ideally, the new device should be implanted on the contralateral side to avoid having to dissect through scar tissue and implant a fibrous nerve.

# 12.12. UAS Implants Outside of FDA Indications

Current indications for use of UAS to treat OSA in patients intolerant of CPAP include the following: moderate to severe OSA (AHI 15 to 65 events per hour) with <25% of central or mixed apnea, BMI ≤35, absence of complete concentric collapse on drug-induced sleep endoscopy, absence of neuromuscular disease, and no history of psychiatric disease. There are limited publications that assess the use of this therapy outside of these parameters.

## 12.12.1. BMI

Elevated BMI is known to have a significant impact on nearly all surgical treatments for OSA. Friedman et al. demonstrated that all patients with BMI ≥40 had failure of uvulopalatopharyngoplasty (UPPP).[27] While the negative impact of extreme BMI on outcomes with UAS is not disputed, moderately elevated BMI remains controversial. It has been previously established that as BMI increases, the likelihood of encountering the complete concentric pattern of palatal collapse also increases.[28] Thus, many patients with elevated BMI self-exclude from candidacy. However, in patients with elevated BMI but an appropriate pattern of airway collapse, there are conflicting data on outcomes.

In a publication by Huntley et al., a multi-institutional review that compared patients with BMI >32 to those <32 suggested there were no differences in outcomes.[29] However, in a subsequent publication analyzing the largest cohort of patients implanted, for every one-point increase in BMI there was a 9% reduced odds of success.[30] Thus, there is no definitive evidence for or against implanting patients with moderately elevated BMI. Current recommendations are that select patients with elevated BMI can be considered for implant by experienced surgeons.

## 12.12.2. Extreme AHI

The original feasibility trials for UAS had an upper AHI limit of 50. Within this cohort, there was no difference in outcomes as the AHI increased. As a result, the upper limit of AHI was raised to 65 in the Stimulation Therapy for Apnea Reduction (STAR) trial.[31] However, there are few published data that define outcomes in patients with AHI >65. In a recent publication by Patel et al., patients with an AHI >65 had similar surgical success defined by Sher criteria (AHI reduced by 50% with overall AHI <20). However, despite major reduction in disease burden, these patients had a higher rate of residual moderate OSA after treatment.[32] At this point there is insufficient information to make recommendations for this population. Thus, there is concern about the potential that patients with extreme AHI may be nonresponders to UAS therapy as well as concern that limiting this therapy to patients with AHI ≤65 may restrict a useful treatment modality that might be of benefit. Further research is warranted in this population.

## 12.12.3. Coexistent Psychiatric Disease

The prevalence of OSA with major psychiatric disorders is as high as 25.7%. These disorders include major depression, bipolar disorder, and schizophrenia.[32] In addition, the fifth edition of the American Psychiatric Association's *Diagnostic and Statistical Manual of Mental Disorders* recognizes that there exists a bidirectional relationship of OSA and psychiatric disorders.[33] The current literature suggests that treatment of OSA in these populations may have a positive impact on the psychiatric disease. This may be a consequence of decreasing inflammatory mediators as well as reducing sleep fragmentation and improving sleep continuity.[34] There are no published data regarding UAS for treatment of OSA in patients with coexistent psychiatric disorders, and the Stimulation Therapy for Apnea Reduction (STAR) trial excluded patients with known psychiatric illness.[35] Clearly, patients afflicted with psychiatric disease with comorbid insomnia are an at-risk population for whom this therapy may have benefit. Given the relatively low risks described with UAS, its use should be explored to determine potential benefit.

# 12.13. Conclusions

In the practice of UAS, clinicians may encounter special populations. Implanting physicians should familiarize themselves with some of these circumstances to anticipate patient needs and identify factors that may impact patient care.

# References

1. Heiser C, Thaler E, Soose R, et al. Technical tips during implantation of selective upper airway stimulation. *Laryngoscope*. 2018;128(3):756–762.
2. Simpson R, Oyekan A, Ehsan Z, et al. Obstructive sleep apnea in patients with Down syndrome: Current perspectives. *Nat Sci Sleep*. 2018;10:287–293.
3. Nehme J, LaBerge R, Pothos M, et al. Treatment and persistence/recurrence of sleep-disordered breathing in children with Down Syndrome. *Pediatr Pulmonol*. 2019;54:1291–1296.
4. Luijks K, Vandenbussche N, Pevernagie D, et al. Adherence to continuous positive airway pressure in adults with an intellectual disability. *Sleep Med*. 2017;34:234–239.
5. De Perck E, Beyers J, Dieltjens M, et al. Successful upper airway stimulation therapy in an adult Down syndrome patient with severe OSA. *Sleep Breath*. 2019;23:879–883.
6. Li C, Boon M, Ishman S, et al. Hypoglossal nerve stimulation in three adults with Down syndrome and severe obstructive sleep apnea. *Laryngoscope*. 2019;129(11):E402–E406.
7. Caloway C, Diercks G, Keamy D, et al. Update on hypoglossal nerve stimulation in children with Down syndrome and obstructive sleep apnea. *Laryngoscope*. 2020;130(4):E263–E267.
8. Vasconcellos A, Huntley C, Schell A, et al. Dysfunctional hypoglossal nerve stimulator after electrical cardioversion: A case series. *Laryngoscope*. 2019;129(8):1949–1953.
9. Johansen J, Jorgensen O, Moller M, et al. Infection after pacemaker implantation: Infection rates and risk factors associated with infection in a population-based cohort study of 46299 consecutive patients. *Eur Heart J*. 2011;32(8):991–998.
10. Salahuddin M, Cader F, Nasrin S, Chodhury M. The pacemaker-twiddler's syndrome: An infrequent cause of pacemaker failure. *BMC Res Notes*. 2016;9:32.
11. Ong A, O'Brien T, Nguyen S, Gillespie B. Implantation of a defibrillator in a patient with an upper airway stimulation device. *Laryngoscope*. 2016;126(2):E86–E89.
12. Parikh V, Thaler E, Kato M, et al. Early feasibility of hypoglossal nerve upper airway stimulator in patients with cardiac implantable electronic devices and continuous positive airway pressure-intolerant severe obstructive sleep apnea. *Heart Rhythm*. 2018;15(8):1165–1170.
13. Marulanda-Londono E, Chaturvedi S. The interplay between obstructive sleep apnea and atrial fibrillation. *Front Neurol*. 2017;8:668.
14. Mehra R, Benjamin E, Shahar E, et al. Association of nocturnal arrhythmias with sleep disordered breathing: The Sleep Heart Health Study. *Am J Respir Crit Care Med*. 2006;173(8):910–916.
15. Inspire technical guidance manual TG-00021 / Version 1.0, October 2018.

16. Eggimann P, Waldvogel F. Pacemaker and defibrillator infection. In Waldvogel FA, Bisno AL (eds), *Infections Associated with Indwelling Medical Devices*. Washington, DC: American Society for Microbiology Press, 2000:247.

17. Baddour L, Cha YM, Wilson W. Infections of cardiovascular implantable electronic devices. *N Engl J Med*. 2012;367:842–849.

18. Thaler E, Schwab R, Maurer J, et al. Results of the ADHERE upper airway stimulation registry and predictors of therapy efficacy. *Laryngoscope*. 2020;130(5):1333–1338.

19. Kramer A, Assadian O, Lademann J. Prevention of postoperative wound infections by covering the surgical field with iodine-impregnated incision drape (Ioban® 2). *GMS Krankenhhyg Interdiszip*. 2010;5(2):Doc08.

20. de Olivera JC, Martinelli M, Nishioka SA, et al. Efficacy of antibiotic prophylaxis before the implantation of pacemakers and cardioverter-defibrillators: Results of a large, prospective, randomized, double blinded, placebo-controlled trial. *Circ Arrhythm Electrophysiol*. 2009;2:29.

21. Klug D, Balde M, Pavin, D, et al. Risk factors related to infections of implanted pacemakers and cardioverter-defibrillators: Results of a large prospective study. *Circulation*. 2007;116:1349.

22. Sohail MR, Usian DZ, Khan AH, et al. Risk factor analysis of permanent pacemaker infection. *Clin Infect Dis*. 2007;45:166.

23. Sohail MR, Usian DZ, Khan AH, et al. Management and outcome of permanent pacemaker and implantable cardioverter-defibrillator infections. *J Am Coll Cardiol*. 2007;49:1851.

24. Karchmer AW, Longworth DL. Update on infections involving permanent pacemakers: Characterization and management. *Infect Dis Clin North Am*. 2002;16(2):477–505.

25. Chua JD, Wilkoff BL, Lee I, et al. Diagnosis and management of infections involving implantable elecrophysiologic cardiac devices. *Ann Intern Med*. 2000;133:604.

26. Baddour LM, Epstein AE, Erickson CC, et al. Update on cardiovascular implantable electronic device infections and their management: A scientific statement from the American Heart Association. *Circulation*. 2010;121:458.

27. Friedman M, Ibraham H, Joseph N. Staging of obstructive sleep apnea/hypopnea syndrome: A guide to appropriate treatment. *Laryngoscope*. 2004;114(3):454–459.

28. Vroegop AV, Vanderveken OM, Boudewyns AN, et al. Drug-induced sleep endoscopy in sleep disordered breathing: Report on 1,249 cases. *Laryngoscope*. 2014;124(3):797–802.

29. Huntley C, Steffen A, Doghramji K, et al. Upper airway stimulation in patients with obstructive sleep apnea and an elevated body mass index: A multi-institutional review. *Laryngoscope*. 2018;128(10):2425–2428.

30. Heiser C, Steffen A, Boon M, et al. Post-approval upper airway stimulation predictors of treatment effectiveness in the ADHERE registry. *Eur Resp J*. 2019;53(1):1801405.

31. Strollo PJ, Soose RJ, Maurer JT, et al. Upper airway stimulation for obstructive sleep apnea. *N Engl J Med*. 2014;370(2):139–149. doi:10.1056/nejmoa1308659

32. Patel J, Daniels K, Bogdan L, et al. Effect of gender, age, and profound disease on upper airway stimulation outcomes. *Ann Otol Rhinol Laryngol*. 2020;129(8):772–780.

33. Stubbs B, Vancampfort D, Veronese N, et al. The prevalence and predictors of obstructive sleep apnea in major depressive disorder, bipolar disorder and schizophrenia: A systematic review and meta-analysis. *J Affect Disord*. 2016;197:259–267.

34. Winokur A. The relationship between sleep disturbances and psychiatric disorders: Introduction and overview. *Psychiatr Clin North Am*. 2015;38(4):603–614.

35. Gupta MA, Simpson FC. Obstructive sleep apnea and psychiatric disorders: A systematic review. *J Clin Sleep Med*. 2015;11(2):165–175.

# Practical Aspects of Initiating and Maintaining a Multidisciplinary Program

Erica R. Thaler and Julianna Rodin

## 13.1. Critical Professional Elements

Two points of clarification need to be made at the outset about the contents of this chapter. First, while the initiation of an upper airway stimulation (UAS) program fundamentally involves the collaboration of a team of both a sleep medicine physician and a sleep surgeon, this chapter will be written from the perspective of an otorhinolaryngologist/head and neck surgeon. This is done because the sleep surgeon is critical in patient selection and education and, of course, in device implantation. Second, as currently there is only one commercially available UAS device that has been approved by the U.S. Food and Drug Administration (FDA) for patient use (Inspire [Inspire Medical Systems]), the chapter discussion will be tailored to this device. However, the concepts discussed for this particular device's program building are generalizable to any technological innovation in this arena.

The sleep surgeon will be familiar with more traditional ablative and reconstructive forms of sleep surgery and will have a method for patient selection of each of these kinds of surgeries. The integration of UAS surgery into a sleep surgeon's practice first requires some specialized education about the neuroanatomy involved. Most well-trained otorhinolaryngologist/head and neck surgeons do not have surgical experience with the complex anatomy of the distal branching of the hypoglossal nerve, nor the anterior anatomy of the Level 1 neck. It is imperative to understand this well for successful device implantation. Sanders and Mu have written a comprehensive article on tongue musculature that

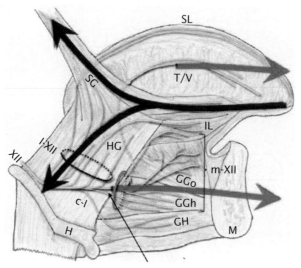

**FIGURE 13.1.** Tongue motion as determined by branches of the hypoglossal nerve. Anterior branching leads to forward motion (green arrows) through muscles T/V (transverse and vertical intrinsic muscles), GGo and GGh (Genioglossus), while posterior branching leads to retraction (red arrows) through muscles HG (Hyoglossus) and SG (Styloglossus). The black arrow marks the stimulation site SI (superior longitudinal) IL (inner longitudinal) H (Hyoid bone) G (geniohyoid). Dotted yellow line indicates the course of the nerve behind the muscle. The red circle indicates portions of the nerve responsible for retraction. Green circle indicates those responsible for protruding the tongue. Illustration courtesy of Inspire Medical Systems.

is worthy of study.[1] Further literature worthy of review includes O'Rahilly and Muller's article on the embryology and anatomy of the hypoglossal nerve.[2] Most relevant to UAS implantation is the understanding of which distal branching of the hypoglossal nerve is involved in tongue protrusion and tongue stiffening and which is involved in tongue retraction (Figure 13.1). It is also important to understand the muscular anatomy of the Level 1 neck with regard to location of the hypoglossal nerve (Figure 13.2). In particular, the relationships of the digastric muscle, mylohyoid muscle, and hyoglossus muscle with regard to the localization of and anterior branching of the hypoglossal nerve are of critical importance. Finally, it is important to be comfortable with the anatomy of the anterior chest wall. This may require some re-education on the part of the otorhinolaryngologist/ head and neck surgeon. As sensor lead placement requires dissection of the intercostal muscles, understanding the surgical approach and location of these muscles and of the intercostal neurovascular bundle is imperative (Figure 13.3).

Many adult sleep surgeons use drug-induced sleep endoscopy (DISE) in their practice as a method of guiding surgical decision making. There is dispute about the relevance and efficacy of DISE in improving patient outcomes.[3-5] Certainly, the diagnostic technique is evolving and there is much is to be explored about what information obtained during DISE is most useful in selecting surgical approaches. Currently, visual assessment of airway dimensions at multiple levels and some descriptive accounts of muscular prominence are the only aspects of DISE widely discussed in the literature. Some quantitative

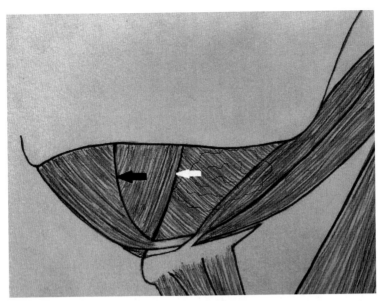

**FIGURE 13.2.** Tongue musculature of Level 1 neck. The black arrow points to the posterior edge of the digastric muscle. The white arrow points to the posterior edge of the mylohyoid muscle. The submandibular gland is illustrated just posterior to this. The anterior branches of the hypoglossal nerve lie deep to the mylohyoid, anterior to the submandibular gland. Reprinted with permission.

assessments have been proposed,[6,7] but to date they have not been shown to have any clear outcome benefit. Regardless, DISE studies were used in the preapproval investigation of the Inspire device, and certain findings appeared to be relevant for device efficacy or lack thereof. Therefore, DISE observations were incorporated into the selection criteria for Inspire implantation. As a result, the sleep surgeon establishing a UAS program must be comfortable with the use of DISE.

Comprehensive description of DISE and its interpretation is provided in Chapter 6. However, for the purposes of UAS patient selection, the ideal patient has some degree of anterior-to-posterior collapse at the base of tongue and anterior-to-posterior obstruction at the level of the soft palate (Figure 13.4). A circumferential pattern of obstruction at the palate is a contraindication to device implantation (Figure 13.5). Consensus opinion from experienced UAS surgeons is forming around the inadvisability of implanting patients with significant lateral musculature in the region of the soft palate (palatopharyngeus muscle) causing lateral-to-medial collapse. This is not, however, an absolute contraindication from the device manufacturer (Figure 13.6). The prospective UAS surgeon must gain familiarity with DISE and with proper identification of these anatomic and dynamic airway findings.

The next important facet of education and training is for the sleep surgeon and sleep medicine physician to go through the training course provided by Inspire Medical Systems. This guides the practitioners' education in all aspects of the UAS device: proper patient selection, how the device works, programming, troubleshooting, and, for the

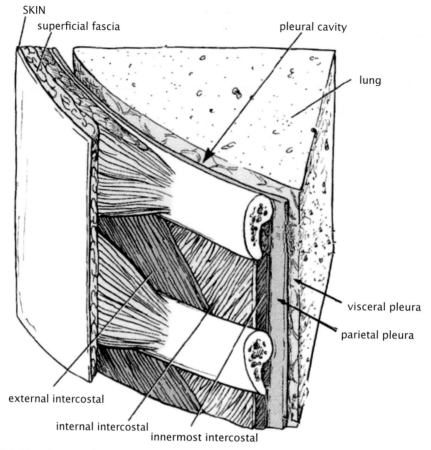

SKIN
superficial fascia
pleural cavity
lung
visceral pleura
parietal pleura
external intercostal
internal intercostal
innermost intercostal

**FIGURE 13.3.** Intercostal space. Reprinted with permission from Inspire Medical Systems.

surgeon, cadaver dissection and practice implantation. The sleep surgeon will then have a number of proctored cases once the program is initiated. These are, of course, critical to get past the surgical learning curve.

## 13.2. Multidisciplinary Professional Collaboration

There are many facets to the process of UAS program building that are somewhat different from the usual management of patients with obstructive sleep apnea (OSA) and require greater attention to multidisciplinary collaboration. Of course, as with any surgical sleep evaluation, it is important to have a comprehensive evaluation of the patient completed before the final surgical decision making occurs. This especially involves aspects of sleep disturbance other than OSA. For example, if there is a component of insomnia present, this is important to address as such a patient may have difficulty tolerating the nerve stimulation. Narcolepsy and restless leg syndrome are disorders that require medical

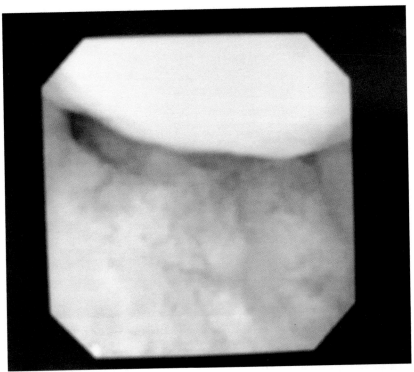

**FIGURE 13.4.** DISE photo showing anterior-to-posterior collapse of the retropalatal airway.

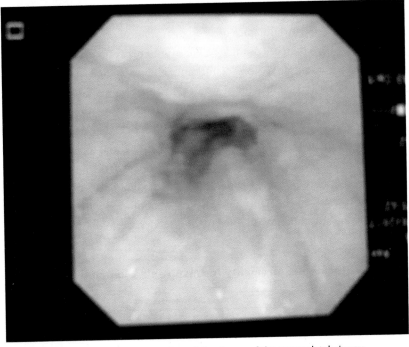

**FIGURE 13.5.** DISE photo showing circumferential collapse of the retropalatal airway.

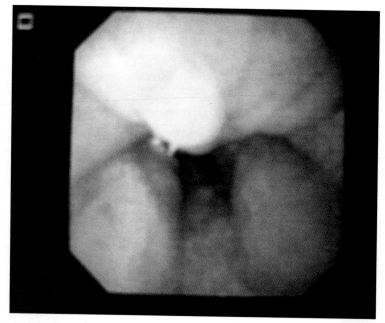

**FIGURE 13.6.** DISE photo showing prominent lateral musculature in the retropalatal airway.

management and should be treated prior to surgery if present. A significant proportion of central sleep apnea will detract from the success of implantation. Therefore, surgical decisions must be made taking into consideration these comorbid conditions. It is not sufficient to simply go by the device manufacturer's inclusion requirements (Table 13.1).

Beyond the multifactorial nature of sleep disturbance, other factors can play a role in the consideration of a patient's candidacy. For example, psychiatric disorders may need to be assessed prior to surgery. Sleep disturbance due to anxiety or depression should be considered. Cognitive impairment of whatever cause may make it difficult to handle even the relatively simple operational aspects of the device. A cardiologist's input is often necessary for a variety of reasons, including placement of the device if a pacemaker or defibrillator is already present (or consideration of any potential for device interference), anticoagulation management, and assessment of surgical risk of heart failure. Oral-maxillofacial evaluation is prudent if dentition or maxillary and mandibular anatomy may affect the outcome. In the neurologic realm, collaboration with a neurologist is important in assessing any patient with movement disorder, particularly involving the head

**TABLE 13.1. Inclusion Requirements for Inspire UAS Implantation**

|  | Acceptable Metrics |
| --- | --- |
| AHI range | 15–65 |
| BMI | <35 |
| DISE results | Anterior-to-posterior retropalatal collapse |

and neck. Patients with Down syndrome are being implanted successfully, particularly in the pediatric population; this is a situation that clearly requires collaboration with not only the managing physician but the caregiver as well, who may be responsible for the remote operation. Patients with prior procedures in the chest and neck, particularly oncologic, will require consultation with the treating physician. For example, patients with a history of breast cancer and reconstructive surgery may have specific anatomic considerations or imaging needs that need to be taken into account in any surgical planning.

A team of interested and committed physicians is important to build for a successful UAS program. When initiating such a program, the otorhinolaryngologist/head and neck surgeon is well equipped to serve as an educator for the many potentially involved disciplines. Lectures and demonstrations are important at the outset, as this is a technology most physicians will have not learned about in medical school or in their postgraduate training.

## 13.3. Integrated Approach

At our institution, we have found that patients do best if there is a clear pathway for them in the UAS implantation process. This involves collaboration with all members of the device implantation team and careful education of patients as they go through the implantation process. Inspire Medical Systems has developed useful patient education brochures and web-based educational portals that can be helpful with the latter. When a patient is first seen, they can be given a flow sheet to explain the process of surgical evaluation, implantation, activation, and usage (Box 13.1).

There are many important members of the team who make this process flow smoothly. The following team members are critical. On the sleep medicine side, a sleep medicine physician who has gone through the Inspire Medical Systems training and fully understands the relevant neuroanatomy and physiology that makes the device effective, the electrophysiology of the device, and appropriate selection criteria is critical. As sleep medicine physicians may be responsible for following the patients long term, it is important for them to be able to interrogate the device, alter settings where appropriate, and troubleshoot any device problems that arise over time. A sleep technician who is well trained in device titration and understands the technical aspects of the device is an important part of the team as well, particularly as the titration sleep study is so important to initial device success.

On the sleep surgical side, a larger team is necessary. The sleep surgeon's training and expertise is of paramount importance. A dedicated anesthesiologist who is well versed in care of the OSA patient as well as the DISE technique is very helpful. The anesthesia for DISE cases can be quite challenging to do correctly, and as this is an important piece of the preoperative assessment, it needs to be consistent. It is also helpful to have an operative team that is well versed in the procedural requirements, steps, and instrumentation. This

> ## BOX 13.1 Hypoglossal Nerve Stimulator Implantation (HGNS) Flow Sheet
>
> 1. Initial visit with a sleep surgeon, certified to perform HGNS implantation.
> 2. Drug-induced sleep endoscopy (DISE)—The surgeon will examine your airway with an endoscope while you are under light sedation in the operating room.
>
> If you are a candidate, the following office visits are required to insure you gain full benefit of your device.
>
> 1. Establish care with a sleep physician certified to assess patients with HGNS implants—This appointment is required because the sleep physician will make final adjustments and routine device checks after implantation.
> 2. Pre-operative appointment with the surgeon for HGNS implantation (sign consent and history & physical).
> 3. Implantation in operating room with the surgeon.
> 4. 1-week incision check with the surgeon.
> 5. 1-month activation with a nurse (remotes and instructions will be given at this appointment).
> 6. Follow-up titration in-lab sleep study 2 months after implantation (1 month after activation).
> 7. Follow-up with sleep physician to discuss sleep study results.
> 8. Yearly routine home sleep study.

includes the circulation and scrub nurses or technicians, the neuromonitoring personnel, and, of course, the Inspire Medical System representative who is present to interrogate the device after implantation but prior to wound closure to ensure proper placement. It is our experience that a good working relationship with the device representative makes the implantation procedure go smoothly and allows for optimization of device placement. The combination of all of these team members helps to minimize operative times.

Of further importance in the sleep surgery practice are office-based staff who are specially trained to help manage patients with the UAS device. It is useful to have a nurse practitioner, a registered nurse, and/or a medical assistant trained by Inspire Medical Systems who can interrogate the device, activate patients postoperatively, and do spot checks of the device and remote if any problems arise. This is of enormous benefit to patients, who inevitably will have device questions and considerations that arise regularly but may not require a physician's attention.

# 13.4. Administrative Approach

There are several facets on the administrative side of a successful UAS program that are worth attention. At the outset of the patient's interaction with the office, it is useful to have intake calls done by personnel who are fluent in the basic criteria for device implantation. It is possible to have patients screened by an administrative assistant who requests a sleep study of the patient to be available for review that has been done within the prior year. These studies are reviewed by the sleep surgeon prior to office appointments in order to ensure that the apnea–hypopnea index (AHI) and body mass index (BMI) criteria for Inspire implantation are met. This process is beneficial as many patients are self-referred and do not meet criteria for Inspire implantation, making the initial office visit disappointing—though it may still be possible to offer them alternative therapies for treatment of their OSA. Further, if the sleep study information is up to date, DISE scheduling and preoperative assessment may be done at the initial office visit, streamlining care.

For surgical scheduling and handling insurance approvals, it is useful to have an administrator who is conversant with the criteria that need to be met for implantation and who is familiar with the various insurance carriers' precertification requirements. Embedding these criteria in the patient's office notes is useful to facilitate the dialogue between the office staff and insurance carriers. The process of device implantation and the device itself are costly, and a careful review process and precertification done prior to implantation is prudent to avoid coverage problems once the process is under way. The surgery scheduler works with financial administrators to coordinate this process with the patient and to set expectations about what to anticipate with regard to timing.

While most currently practicing physicians have an electronic medical record that may be sufficient to follow each patient's course, it is beneficial to keep a privacy-protected, separate dataset regarding each patient's studies and outcomes. This dataset may include preoperative and postoperative polysomnograms, DISE videos and still photos, device settings, and any further testing or other interventions necessary to maximize outcome (such as awake endoscopy results for patients who have not achieved an acceptable result). While the motivation for this may be to facilitate research and outcome studies, it also proves useful for quick reference in the long-term management of patients and to facilitate comparison with similar clinical scenarios.

Finally, it is important to have good coordination between the sleep surgery and sleep medicine practices that are sharing UAS patients. Identifying administrative stakeholders to facilitate this coordination makes the process easier for patients. There is a lot of complex and unfamiliar testing to be done on the patient, particularly in the postoperative period in getting the device properly activated. When the surgical and medical offices work in concert, the patient can proceed through this process with better understanding of the parameters involved and with better confidence in the performance of the device.

Building a successful multidisciplinary UAS program requires some effort beyond the usual practice building that may be familiar to well-established physicians and surgeons. However, this sort of endeavor is emblematic of the direction that medicine is headed, with greater emphasis on team treatment of diagnoses, rather than isolated practitioners handing all aspects of care. Successful UAS implantation is a rewarding experience for the patient and physician alike and is certainly worth the effort required to initiate and maintain a program.

# 13.5. Economic Considerations

Inherent to the cost-effectiveness analysis for any OSA treatment are proof of success rates, therapy compliance, side effects, safety, diagnostic and management workflows, and long-term treatment outcomes. Historically, most OSA therapy outcomes and cost-effectiveness literature have focused on continuous positive airway pressure (CPAP) therapy improving quality of life, cardiovascular risks, days missed from work, motor vehicle accidents (MVAs), and mortality.[8–10] In a systematic review by Wickwire et al.,[8] seven of eight studies found that CPAP reduced healthcare use and costs when compared with no treatment. Wickwire et al.[8] also found that cost-effectiveness is strongly linked to the clinical effectiveness of OSA treatment. Thus, the economic benefit of positive airway pressure (PAP) therapy increased as patient adherence improved. It is timely to note that many past cost-effectiveness studies used traditional in-lab polysomnography (PSG) testing and face-to-face workflow models. In the current, evolving context of increased use of home sleep testing and telehealth workflows for uncomplicated OSA, further cost savings may be realized.[11–14]

In addition to CPAP cost-effectiveness studies, more recent non-CPAP outcome studies have emerged, including outcomes and comparative cost-effectiveness studies for oral appliances, upper airway surgeries, maxillomandibular advancement, and most recently UAS.[15–20] Comparing oral appliances (OA) and CPAP, Sadatsafavi et al.[15] and Sharples et al.[18] concluded that OA use was more costly but remained cost-effective for patients intolerant of CPAP or with lower CPAP adherence. Likewise, de Vries et al.[16] compared OA and CPAP cost-effectiveness and found better AHI reduction with CPAP but improved quality-adjusted life-years (QALYs) with OA. They concluded that OA was a good, cost-effective alternative for patients declining CPAP.[16] For middle-aged men with severe OSA, Tan et al.[21] compared the cost-effectiveness of no treatment, CPAP, and CPAP followed by surgery (palatopharyngeal and multilevel surgeries) and found these surgeries to be cost-effective for CPAP-intolerant patients.

Again, it is critical for cost-effectiveness models for an OSA therapy to show proof of AHI reduction, therapy compliance, low side effects, good safety, and improved long-term outcome measures. While it is a newer OSA treatment option, UAS has shown good AHI reduction, compliance, safety, and patient satisfaction with improvement of sleepiness, cardiovascular events, quality of life, and MVA metrics.[22–26] In a registry of 301 UAS patients, Boon et al.[22] found improved AHI and Epworth Sleepiness Scale (ESS) scores, good compliance, low complications, and high patient satisfaction. In a meta-analysis and review by Kompelli et al.,[26] UAS reduced mean AHI by 21.1 events per hour and oxygen desaturation index (ODI) by 15.0 by 12 months. In addition, improvement in quality of life and OSA clinical symptoms like sleepiness were seen with an increase in the Functional Outcomes of Sleep Questionnaire (FOSQ) score by 3.1 and reduction in the ESS score by 5.[26] Adverse events listed were few and relatively minor. Those mentioned were pain at 6.2%, tongue abrasion at 11%, internal device malfunction at 3%, external device malfunction at 5.8%, and other at 7% (which included paresthesias and lip weakness).[26] Furthermore, patients typically have long-term effects and good compliance with UAS. Woodson et al.[24] evaluated UAS outcomes at 5 years and found continued improvement in sleepiness, quality of life, and AHI response rate (defined as AHI <20 and >50% reduction). In a follow-up registry study that included 1,017 patients, device adherence averaged 5.6 hours per night, much higher than that of CPAP.[25]

As a newer OSA therapy, UAS has fewer studies detailing its long-term cost-effectiveness. In two studies by Pietzsch et al.,[27,28] the patient benefit and cost-effectiveness of UAS were compared to no therapy, given that most patients who undergo UAS are intolerant to CPAP. A Markov model was used to predict cardiovascular endpoints, MVAs, mortality, QALYs, and costs. Costs for UAS were obtained from Medicare reimbursement rates for 2013. Included in costs were all preprocedural and periprocedural costs (including PSG, DISE, and office visit), the cost of actual surgical implantation of the stimulator, annual follow-up costs, and the cost of eventual battery replacement in likely 10 years.[27] Total costs discounted over a lifetime were $286,497 for UAS compared to $243,543 for no treatment.[27] For the cohort, UAS led to a significantly reduced risk of cardiovascular events, MVAs, and mortality. This risk reduction in turn led to an increased mean survival and gain in life expectancy, resulting in a mean QALY gain of 1.70 over the patient's lifetime when compared to no treatment.[27] These authors also computed a 10-year and lifetime risk incremental cost-effectiveness ratio (ICER) in dollars per QALY under the assumption that all patients had the Stimulation Therapy for Apnea Reduction (STAR) trial reduction in AHI from 32.0 to 15.3.[27] ICER assesses the value of an intervention by taking the ratio of added costs to improvement in outcome, which in this study was defined as QALY. Pietzsch et al.[27] found the ICER to be 39,471 for lifetime, which is below the healthcare system's willingness-to-pay threshold ($50,000 to $100,000 per QALY in the United States). Thus, UAS appears to be a cost-effective OSA intervention compared with other well-accepted medical treatments. Interestingly, when assessed at 10 years, the ICER was 57,773, showing that upfront cost has more of an effect when future savings are not yet taken into account.[27] ICER also increased as UAS effectiveness was manipulated to be less effective at reducing MVA event rates and cardiovascular events and at improving quality of life.[27] Another study by Pietzsch et al.[29] also compared the cost-effectiveness of CPAP to no therapy. They reported an ICER of $15,915 per QALY, with discounted cost and QALY differences of $26,722 and 1.68 respectively.[29]

Thus, when comparing UAS and CPAP, UAS is less cost-effective, although it is still considered within the willingness-to-pay-threshold.

UAS is a successful OSA treatment option for improving subjective and objective outcomes. It also appears to be a cost-effective option, especially when evaluating its lifetime benefits. UAS improves AHI and ODI with a good safety profile while improving quality of life and other long-term outcomes. More recent studies also show lifetime cost-effectiveness despite the initial implantation costs.

# References

1. Sanders I, Mu L. A three-dimensional atlas of human tongue muscles. *Anat Rec.* 2013;296:1102–1114.
2. O'Rahilly R, Muller F. The early development of the hypoglossal nerve and occipital somites in staged human embryos. *Am J Anat.* 1984;1669:237–257.
3. DeVito A, Carrasco L, Ravesloot M, et al. European position paper on drug-induced sleep endoscopy: 2017 update. *Clin Otolaryngol.* 2018;43(6):1541–1552.
4. Kotecha B, DeVito A. Drug-induced sleep endoscopy: Its role in the evaluation of the upper airway obstruction and patient selection for surgical and non-surgical treatment. *J Thorac Dis.* 2018;10(Suppl):S40–S47.
5. De Vito A, Cammaroto G, Chong K, et al. Drug-induced sleep endoscopy: Clinical application and surgical outcomes. *Healthcare.* 2019;7(3):100.
6. Borek R, Thaler E, Kim C, et al. Quantitative airway analysis during drug-induced sleep endoscopy for evaluation of sleep apnea. *Laryngoscope.* 2012;122(11): 2592–2599.
7. Kezirian EJ, Hohenhorst W, De Vries N. Drug-induced sleep endoscopy: The VOTE classification. *Eur Arch Otorhinolaryngol.* 2011;268(8):1233–1236.
8. Wickwire EM, Albrecht JS, Towe MM, et al. The impact of treatments for OSA on monetized health economic outcomes: A systematic review. *Chest.* 2019;155(5):947–961. doi:10.1016/j.chest.2019.01.009
9. McDaid C, Griffin S, Weatherly H, et al. Continuous positive airway pressure devices for the treatment of obstructive sleep apnoea-hypopnoea syndrome: A systematic review and economic analysis. *Health Technol Assess.* 2009;13(4):iii–274. doi:10.3310/hta13040
10. Streatfeild J, Hillman D, Adams R, et al. Cost-effectiveness of continuous positive airway pressure therapy for obstructive sleep apnea: Health care system and societal perspectives. *Sleep.* 2019;42(12):zsz181. doi:10.1093/sleep/zsz181
11. Kim RD, Kapur VK, Redline-Bruch J, et al. An economic evaluation of home versus laboratory-based diagnosis of obstructive sleep apnea. *Sleep.* 2015;38(7):1027–1037. doi:10.5665/sleep.4804
12. Stewart SA, Penz E, Fenton M, Skomro R. Investigating cost implications of incorporating level III at-home testing into a polysomnography-based sleep medicine program using administrative data. *Can Respir J.* 2017;2017:8939461. doi:10.1155/2017/8939461
13. Lugo VM, Garmendia O, Suarez-Girón M, et al. Comprehensive management of obstructive sleep apnea by telemedicine: Clinical improvement and cost-effectiveness of a virtual sleep unit. A randomized controlled trial. *PLoS One.* 2019;14(10):e0224069. doi:10.1371/journal.pone.0224069
14. Isetta V, Negrín M, Monasterio C, et al. A Bayesian cost-effectiveness analysis of a telemedicine-based strategy for the management of sleep apnoea: A multicentre randomised controlled trial. *Thorax.* 2015;70(11):1054–1061.
15. Sadatsafavi M, Marra CA, Ayas NT, et al. Cost-effectiveness of oral appliances in the treatment of obstructive sleep apnoea-hypopnoea. *Sleep Breath.* 2009;13(3):241–252. doi:10.1007/s11325-009-0248-4
16. de Vries GE, Hoekema A, Vermeulen KM, et al. Clinical and cost-effectiveness of a mandibular advancement device versus continuous positive airway pressure in moderate obstructive sleep apnea. *J Clin Sleep Med.* 2019;15(10):1477–1485.

17. Tan MC, Ayas NT, Mulgrew A, et al. Cost-effectiveness of continuous positive airway pressure therapy in patients with obstructive sleep apnea-hypopnea in British Columbia. *Can Respir J.* 2008;15(3):159–165. doi:10.1155/2008/719231

18. Sharples L, Glover M, Clutterbuck-James A, et al. Clinical effectiveness and cost-effectiveness results from the randomised controlled Trial of Oral Mandibular Advancement Devices for Obstructive sleep apnoea-hypopnoea (TOMADO) and long-term economic analysis of oral devices and continuous positive airway pressure. *Health Technol Assess.* 2014;18(67):1–296. doi:10.3310/hta18670

19. Poullié AI, Cognet M, Gauthier A, et al. Cost-effectiveness of treatments for mild-to-moderate obstructive sleep apnea in France. *Int J Technol Assess Health Care.* 2016;32(1–2):37–45. doi:10.1017/S0266462316000088

20. Weatherly HL, Griffin SC, Mc Daid C, et al. An economic analysis of continuous positive airway pressure for the treatment of obstructive sleep apnea-hypopnea syndrome. *Int J Technol Assess Health Care.* 2009;25(1):26–34. doi:10.1017/S0266462309090047

21. Tan KB, Toh ST, Guilleminault C, Holty JE. A cost-effectiveness analysis of surgery for middle-aged men with severe obstructive sleep apnea intolerant of CPAP. *J Clin Sleep Med.* 2015;11(5):525–535. doi:10.5664/jcsm.4696

22. Boon M, Huntley C, Steffen A, et al. Upper airway stimulation for obstructive sleep apnea: Results from the ADHERE registry. *Otolaryngol Head Neck Surg.* 2018;159(2):379–385. doi:10.1177/0194599818764896

23. Strollo PJ Jr, Soose RJ, Maurer JT, et al. Upper-airway stimulation for obstructive sleep apnea. *N Engl J Med.* 2014;370(2):139–149. doi:10.1056/NEJMoa1308659

24. Woodson BT, Strohl KP, Soose RJ, et al. Upper airway stimulation for obstructive sleep apnea: 5-year outcomes. *Otolaryngol Head Neck Surg.* 2018;159(1):194–202. doi:10.1177/0194599818762383

25. Thaler E, Schwab R, Maurer J, et al. Results of the ADHERE upper airway stimulation registry and predictors of therapy efficacy. *Laryngoscope.* 2020;130(5):1333–1338. doi:10.1002/lary.28286

26. Kompelli AR, Ni JS, Nguyen SA, et al. The outcomes of hypoglossal nerve stimulation in the management of OSA: A systematic review and meta-analysis. *World J Otorhinolaryngol Head Neck Surg.* 2018;5(1):41–48. doi:10.1016/j.wjorl.2018.04.006

27. Pietzsch JB, Liu S, Garner AM, et al. Long-term cost-effectiveness of upper airway stimulation for the treatment of obstructive sleep apnea: A model-based projection based on the STAR trial. *Sleep.* 2015;38(5):735–744. doi:10.5665/sleep.4666

28. Pietzsch JB, Richter AK, Randerath W, et al. Clinical and economic benefits of upper airway stimulation for obstructive sleep apnea in a European setting. *Respiration.* 2019;98(1):38–47. doi:10.1159/000497101

29. Pietzsch JB, Garner A, Cipriano LE, Linehan JH. An integrated health-economic analysis of diagnostic and therapeutic strategies in the treatment of moderate-to-severe obstructive sleep apnea. *Sleep.* 2011;34(6):695–709. doi:10.5665/SLEEP.1030

# The Future in Upper Airway Stimulation Therapy

David T. Kent

## 14.1. The History of Hypoglossal Nerve Stimulation

Understanding present gaps in upper airway stimulation (UAS) research requires a careful assessment of its history and development, which began shortly after the invention of continuous positive airway pressure (CPAP) in 1981. In 1987 Miki et al. published a short report in *The Tohoku Journal of Experimental Medicine* describing how they transorally stimulated the genioglossus muscle in six anesthetized dogs and found that activation of the muscle, using voltages between 10 and 20 V at 0.2 ms duration, progressively decreased resistance up to 50 Hz,[1] at which point the curve flattened (Figure 14.1). In this preclinical model, the effect occurred at several intraluminal pressures and was the proof-of-concept that muscle stimulation could reduce airflow resistance. In 1989, the same group followed up with a short report of submental "genioglossus" muscle activation in patients with obstructive sleep apnea (OSA), reporting improvements in the apnea–hypopnea index (AHI) and time in deep sleep This observation caught the attention of international researchers.[2]

A series of subsequent animal and human experiments progressed through the 1990s.[3-8] Several groups demonstrated promising improvements in upper airway resistance in animal models.[5,7,9,10] Eisele et al. demonstrated that proximal or distal activation of the feline hypoglossal nerve was comparable as long as stimulation captured the medial branches of the hypoglossal nerve projecting to the genioglossus muscle.[5] Isolated activation of distal lateral branches to the extrinsic retrusor muscles of the tongue appeared less effective. The safety and feasibility of chronic electrode implantation and UAS

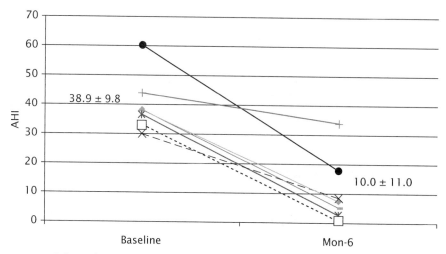

**FIGURE 14.1** Relationship between geniglossus muscle stimulation frequency and opened upper airway (Raw) of a dog. From Miki H, Hida W, Shindoh C, et al. Effect of electrical stimulation of genioglossus muscle on upper airway resistance in anesthetized dogs. *Tohoku J Exp Med.* 1987;153(4):397–398. doi:10.1620/tjem.153.397

were demonstrated by Goding et al., who implanted six dogs with a hypoglossal cuff electrode.[11] The implant was activated after 1 month. After 2 months of stimulation, no injury to the chronically stimulated hypoglossal nerve was identified, suggesting that this approach was relatively safe.

Experiments with human UAS began in the United States in parallel with ongoing animal studies. Initial physiology experiments in humans avoided the invasiveness of hypoglossal cuff electrode placement by substituting submental electrodes and/or transoral fine-wire genioglossus muscle electrodes.[3,6,8,12] Results were more variable due to patient discomfort with temporary electrode stimulation, with some investigators reporting that any improvements in ventilation were likely attributable to neurologic arousal instead of reduced pharyngeal collapse.[8]

In 1997, Eisele et al. implanted 15 volunteers undergoing other open surgical procedures of the neck with a tripolar cuff electrode around the hypoglossal nerve.[4] Seven subjects received a proximally placed cuff electrode just distal to the ansa hypoglossi, while eight underwent more distal placement of the cuff electrode on the branches to just the genioglossus muscle. In five patients with OSA, overnight stimulation during polysomnography (PSG) was successful, with significant improvements in ventilation (184.5 ± 61.7 ml/s) observed below stimulation thresholds leading to arousal from sedated sleep. Greater improvements in ventilation were observed with the more distal cuff placement, but statistical significance was lacking. Again, this suggested some degree of efficacy, and safety in implantation

Based on the human and animal experimental data, several efforts toward commercially implantable products began in the late 1990s. Device stimulation parameters were informed by prior experiments. Schwartz et al. and other groups observed tetanic contraction of the genioglossus muscle increasing up through 50 Hz.[2,7] Stimulation voltages during initial submental or transoral electrode experiments were high, generally requiring values >10 V for adequate muscle recruitment.[2,3,8] Evidence from implanted cuff experiments suggested that with close contact of the stimulation electrode to the hypoglossal nerve, significantly lower stimulation voltages could be used, decreasing the need for higher stimulation levels and the likelihood of patient arousal.[4] Substantial muscle tension occurred at a frequency of 0.2 ms, consistent with values observed for tension in other skeletal muscle experiments.[13]

# 14.2. First- and Second-Generation UAS Trials

Results of the first formal feasibility phase I trial for a chronically implanted device were published in 2001.[14] Eight patients were implanted with the Inspire I system (Medtronic Inc., Minneapolis, MN). The device consisted of an implantable pulse generator (IPG) connected to a half-cuff tripolar stimulation cuff electrode and a respiratory pressure sensor placed through a hole drilled in the manubrium. The main selection criteria were AHI >10; three of the eight patients were also selected based on overnight manometric pressure studies suggesting primarily hypopharyngeal obstruction. Stimulation was initiated 1 month after surgery, and serial PSGs were completed at 1, 3, and 6 months postoperatively. Mean (standard deviation) AHI decreased from 52.0 (20.4) to 22.6 (12.1) events per hour in non–rapid-eye-movement (NREM) sleep and from 48.2 (30.5) to 16.6 (17.1) events per hour in rapid-eye-movement (REM) sleep. No changes in tongue anatomy (hypertrophy, fasciculations, or atrophy) were observed. Importantly, pharyngeal critical closing pressure ($P_{crit}$) improved by $3.98 \pm 2.31$ cm $H_2O$, with increases in maximum inspiratory flow at a given upstream pressure from $75.8 \pm 98.4$ ml/s to $261.4 \pm 123.8$ ml/s. Of note, the greatest improvement in flow was observed in the three patients identified for implant candidacy through manometric studies of pressure drop across the nasopharynx to the hypopharynx. While initial results were promising, five of the eight devices had hardware failures within the first 6 months of use.

Initial implant data and general enthusiasm for UAS as a viable treatment modality led to second-generation device trials. The Stimulation Therapy for Apnea Reduction (STAR) phase II trial was the first to open in 2010 with a feasibility study to ascertain what factors were best associated with Inspire II (Inspire Medical Systems, Inc., Minneapolis, MN) device response.[15] The second-generation device incorporated a similar stimulation cuff and IPG design to the first, but exchanged the manubrial respiratory pressure sensor for one placed between the intercostal muscles in the fourth or fifth intercostal space. The feasibility study was conducted in two phases, in which the first few patients informed the selection criteria of the last few patients. In the first phase, criteria for implant was a body mass index (BMI) <35 kg/m$^2$ and any value of AHI $\geq$25. Twenty-two patients underwent implantation, and PSG evaluation of 20 patients at 6 months yielded 6 responders, as defined by the Sher criteria (50% reduction in AHI and AHI <20).[16] Analysis of baseline characteristics determined that the combined criteria of AHI ≤50 and BMI <32 kg/m$^2$ were associated with therapy success ($p = .01$). The presence of complete circumferential palatal collapse was observed in all nonresponders of a subset of 7 patients (3 responders, 4 nonresponders) who underwent drug-induced sleep endoscopy (DISE) prior to implant. These findings in terms of BMI, AHI, and DISE led toward criteria that informed subsequent studies of the device.

In the second phase of this safety and feasibility trial, 9 additional patients were prospectively selected using the criteria of BMI ≤32 kg/m$^2$ and AHI 20 to 50, without complete concentric palatal collapse during DISE (only 1 patient had a baseline AHI of 60). Seven of the 8 patients completing 6-month post-implant PSG were responders by the Sher criteria, with overall AHI reduced from 38.9 ± 9.8 to 10.0 ± 11.0 ($p < .01$); in 4 patients the AHI was <10 (Figure 14.2). These findings determined enrollment criteria for the STAR trial, published in 2014.[17]

The STAR trial, a U.S. Food and Drug Administration (FDA) phase III trial, enrolled 126 patients with moderate to severe OSA intolerant of positive airway pressure (PAP) treatment. Based on feasibility study data, patients were excluded from enrollment for BMI >32 kg/m$^2$ or complete concentric collapse of the palate during DISE, as well as a history of hypoglossal nerve palsy or other neuromuscular disease, a history of severe cardiopulmonary disease, significant upper airway anatomic abnormalities, or active psychiatric or comorbid sleep disorders confounding functional assessment. Therapy was activated 1 month after implantation. Importantly, subjects underwent a repeat diagnostic PSG immediately prior to activation. Due to natural night-to-night variation in OSA disease burden, some subjects displayed sleep disordered breathing as severe as 65 events per hour during the repeat diagnostic study. Device titration PSGs were completed at 2 and 6 months postoperatively, followed by an efficacy PSG without device adjustment

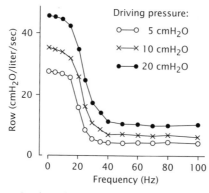

FIGURE 14.2 Summary of part 2 subjects' AHI at baseline and 6 months after implantation. From Van De Heyning PH, Badr MS, Baskin JZ, et al. Implanted upper airway stimulation device for obstructive sleep apnea. *Laryngoscope*. 2012;122(7):1626–1633. doi:10.1002/lary.23301

at 12 months. Notable in the study supplemental material is that there were a number of PSG titrations to optimize therapy, but these had to stop 1 month before the 12-month follow-up.

Mean AHI decreased in the STAR trial from 32.0 ± to 15.3 ± 16.1 events per hour. The mean ODI decreased from 28.9 ± 12.0 to 13.9 ± 15.7. Metrics of subjective symptoms, including the Functional Outcomes of Sleep Questionnaire (FOSQ) and the Epworth Sleepiness Scale (ESS), were also measured at 12 months. The FOSQ score increase was clinically meaningful, from 14.3 ± 3.2 to 17.3 ± 2.9. The average ESS score at 12 months normalized (11.6 ± 5.0 to 7.0 ± 4.2). Oxygen saturation <90% during sleep decreased from 5.4% to 0.9%. A consecutive cohort of 46 responders (by Sher criteria) were randomized to therapy withdrawal for 1 week after the 12-month visit. Significant increases in AHI (25.8 vs. 7.6 events per hour, $p < .001$) and ODI (23.0 vs. 6.0, $p < .001$) were observed in the therapy-withdrawal group. Average AHI increased in the therapy-withdrawal group by 18.2 versus 1.7 in the therapy-maintenance group (difference in mean score changes: 16.4 ± 12.0; $p < .001$). Based on this phase II trial of 12 months, in April 2014, the FDA approved the therapy for use and listed criteria for eligibility roughly based on the phase II trial.

Meanwhile, other companies had developed and were testing neurostimulation approaches. Results from a 12-month trial of the aura6000 system (ImThera Medical Inc., San Diego, CA) were published earlier in 2013.[18] The aura6000 differs from the Inspire device in several ways. The stimulation cuff is placed on the proximal hypoglossal nerve prior to the division of the medial (protrusor) and lateral (retrusor) branches. It contains six independent electrodes arranged in a radial fashion around the nerve and is designed to take advantage of the concept of the tongue as a muscular hydrostat, where optimal coactivation of innervated muscles maintains tongue shape through protrusion.[19] The IPG is rechargeable and works on a closed-loop duty cycle as opposed to coordination with any biological signal input, such as respiratory effort.

Trial eligibility criteria for the aura6000 were similar to those of the STAR trial. Eligible patients were required to demonstrate PAP intolerance, with AHI ≥20, BMI 25 to 40 kg/m², age 25 to 70 years, modified Mallampati score from I to III, and palatine tonsils assessed as grade 0, 1, or 2. A DISE was not required. Patients were excluded for pregnancy, central sleep apnea, syndromic craniofacial abnormality, enlarged tonsils (grade 3 or 4), diagnosis of restless leg syndrome or insomnia, obstructive nasal polyps, active substance abuse, and other medical factors. Thirteen of 14 patients were successfully implanted with the device; hardware failure occurred in one implant procedure. Therapy was activated 3 to 4 weeks after surgery and was titrated upward to determine sensory and activation thresholds for each electrode. Endoscopic pharyngoscopic examination determined which electrodes yielded the greatest improvements in awake pharyngeal patency. Patients then underwent an initial device titration PSG. Twelve months later, therapy was again adjusted under fiberoptic pharyngoscopy with the use of 2 mg midazolam to mimic the natural sleep state prior to overnight titration PSG.

All 13 subjects completed evaluation at 12 months. Ten of the 13 were reported as therapy responders. Overall, AHI decreased from $45.2 \pm 17.8$ to $21.0 \pm 16.5$ ($p < .001$). ESS score decreased from $11 \pm 7$ to $8 \pm 4$ ($p = .09$). Of the 3 nonresponders, 1 was observed to have a significantly hypertrophied uvula, 1 displayed predominant central sleep apnea, and the third was the largest (BMI = 39 kg/m²) subject with the most severe OSA (AHI = 80).

A second single-arm, open label study of the aura6000 was opened in 2013 with similar eligibility criteria (Targeted Hypoglossal Neurostimulation 2 trial; ClinicalTrials. gov ID: NCT01796925). A third trial (Targeted Hypoglossal Neurostimulation 3 trial; ClinicalTrials.gov ID: NCT02263859) was opened in 2014 and designed as a parallel-arm, 4-month study with the experimental group having therapy activated 1 month after implantation and the control group having therapy activated only after the month 4 visit and PSG assessment. As of this writing, 57 patients have been enrolled in THN2 and 138 patients in THN3, but no results have yet been published. ImThera Medical, Inc. was acquired in 2018 by LivaNova, PLC.

A third implanted stimulation system, the Hypoglossal Nerve Stimulation (HGNS) system (Apnex Medical, Inc., St. Paul, MN), was implanted into 31 patients as part of a multicenter, single-arm, open-label trial undertaken at Austrian and U.S. clinical sites.[20] Requirements for participants were failed PAP therapy; moderate to severe OSA; BMI ≤37 kg/m² (in the United States); AHI 20 to 100; non-REM AHI ≥15; and hypopneas making up at least 80% of obstructive events. Patients with a history of prior upper airway surgery, significant upper airway anatomic abnormalities, >5% central or mixed apneic events, untreated comorbid sleep disorders, and other major medical issues were excluded.

Kezirian et al. published 12-month outcomes in 2014. At 12 months, implanted subjects were observed to use the HGNS device on $86 \pm 16\%$ of nights for $5.4 \pm 1.4$ hours per night. Seventeen (55%) subjects achieved surgical success as defined using the Sher criteria (AHI decrease of ≥50% and <20 residual events per hour). Overall, AHI improved significantly from baseline ($45.4 \pm 17.5$ to $25.3 \pm 20.6$; $p < .001$) and was stable compared to 6-month post-implant values. Subjective improvements were realized as well, with FOSQ scores improving from $14.2 \pm 2.0$ to $17.0 \pm 2.4$. Two patients experienced stimulation lead cuff displacements requiring revision surgery and one patient experienced an infection requiring device explant. This HGNS device was withdrawn before FDA assessment of mid-phase III studies and is not commercially available for clinical use.

Bilateral stimulation of the hypoglossal nerve is also under active development. The Bilateral Hypoglossal Nerve Stimulation for Treatment of Obstructive Sleep Apnoea (BLAST OSA) trial was an open-label, single-arm trial in the United Kingdom, France, and Australia investigating the effect of the Genio system (Nyxoah SA, Mont-Saint-Guibert, Belgium) in 27 patients, with 6-month outcome data published in 2020.[21] The Genio system is a bilateral nerve stimulator implanted through a submental incision.

A paddle electrode is placed across each genioglossus nerve, and the device is powered transdermally by an activation unit and disposable adhesive patch. It operates on a duty cycle instead of synchronizing with any biophysiologic signals. Similar to other trials, eligible patients were CPAP intolerant with age 21 to 75 years; BMI ≤32 kg/m$^2$; AHI 20 to 60; and absence of complete concentric collapse of the soft palate during DISE. At 6 months, 22 patients had completed the protocol. AHI decreased from 23.7 ± 12.2 to 12.9 ± 10.1 ($p < .001$). ESS score decreased from 11.0 ± 5.3 to 8.0 ± 5.4 ($p = .01$) and FOSQ score increased from 15.3 ± 3.3 to 17.2 ± 3.0. Larger trials (ClinicalTrials.gov ID: NCT03868618 and NCT04031040) are planned for further evaluation of device safety and efficacy.

# 14.3. UAS Knowledge Gaps and Current Research Efforts

The preceding review of UAS physiology research and device development highlights gaps in understanding critical to future successful patient treatment that can be classified into four broad categories: (1) UAS device design, (2) patient selection criteria, (3) long-term therapy outcomes, and (4) combination therapy. Such tactical concepts of future improvements in therapy are now feasible given that all therapies to date use a common management pathway to some degree or another. How general management will evolve will depend on device design and digital footprints for diagnosis and therapy adjustments.

## 14.3.1. UAS Device Design

The difference between existing UAS devices is due to not only technical design decisions but also differences in underlying philosophies regarding maintenance of pharyngeal patency. Current variations in existing designs include proximal or distal hypoglossal nerve placement (excluding the retrusor branches to the hyoglossus and styloglossus muscles), phasic or tonic stimulation patterns, and unilateral or bilateral nerve stimulation.

The aura6000 functions differently from other unilateral UAS devices. It is placed on the proximal hypoglossal nerve and uses a tonic stimulation strategy, as opposed to other UAS devices, which depend primarily on unopposed phasic genioglossus muscle activation for dilation of the pharyngeal airway. Prior animal and human experiments confirmed the importance of the genioglossus muscle for improvements in ventilation and pharyngeal collapsibility.[3–7,9–11] Importantly, Eisele demonstrated that activation of the medial branches of the hypoglossal nerve (with subsequent downstream contraction of the genioglossus muscle) yielded greater improvements in ventilation and collapsibility than isolated activation of other extrinsic tongue musculature via the lateral branches of the hypoglossal nerve.[5] These findings informed the development of multiple UAS devices, including Inspire, which excludes retrusor branches of the hypoglossal nerve via selective placement on only the medial division.

A competing model acknowledges the role of the genioglossus muscle but highlights the incompressibility of the tongue at physiologic pressures as a musculature hydrostat.[19] Under this model, co-activation of various muscle groups reshapes the tongue as it remains isovolumic, leading to protrusion, elongation, flattening, and internal stiffening that can have varying effects on pharyngeal patency and stiffness due to either increased drag on lateral pharyngeal walls during protrusion or direct stiffening of tongue retrusor muscles (hyoglossus and styloglossus) that make up a portion of the pharyngeal wall. The muscular hydrostat model emphasizes the role of tongue musculature beyond the genioglossus and is employed by the ImThera device, which uses six monopolar electrodes arranged in a helical formation inside the stimulation cuff. The electrodes are then sequentially tested to identify optimal combinations for improving pharyngeal patency during stimulation of the proximal hypoglossal nerve. Instead of operating on a duty cycle or timing respiration, the electrode combinations are cycled to maintain a shifting but overall tonic pattern of tongue contraction. Tonic stimulation and proximal nerve placement decrease the number of device components and may simplify implantation. Limited reports suggest that varying the pattern of nerve activation can affect pharyngeal patency (as measured via ultrasound),[22] but available outcome data do not currently suggest therapeutic superiority to other stimulation strategies.

Other UAS devices are implanted more distally on the medial branch of the hypoglossal nerve innervating the genioglossus muscle, the geniohyoid muscle (a branch of the first cervical spinal nerve traveling with the extracranial hypoglossal nerve), and intrinsic tongue musculature. Various phasic stimulation strategies are used to avoid potential neuromuscular fatigue. The Genio system from Nyxoah operates on a constant duty cycle, whereas the Inspire system (and the prior HGNS system from Apnex) paces respiration through measurement of chest wall respiratory cycles. The current Inspire system now uses a piezoelectric sensor placed in the intercostal space conceptually to detect deformation of the chest wall, triggering stimulation close to end-expiration. Apnex used impendence measures of chest wall excursion. The extent to which these efforts to refine the timing of stimulation in relation to respiration effects on outcome is not known.

Currently, the differences in device philosophy and design have not yielded dramatic differences in outcomes.[17,18,20,21] It would seem trivial to assume that the bilateral hypoglossal nerve stimulation design of the Genio device would more effectively dilate that pharynx than unilateral stimulation devices. An investigation of tongue protrusion in 20 patients implanted with the Inspire device reported that patients with a greater degree of bilateral tongue protrusion during unilateral hypoglossal nerve stimulation yielded more significant dilation of the retropalatal pharynx than did patients with a more pronounced ipsilateral protrusion pattern.[23] The authors hypothesized that improved retropalatal dilation effects may be partially mediated by a greater degree of anterior mechanical traction on the soft palate through the bilateral palatoglossus muscles, which would suggest that bilateral hypoglossal nerve stimulation would provide superior retropalatal space dilation and improved ventilation. Nevertheless, a prior physiology experiment in rabbits did not show significant differences between the two stimulation modalities in terms of inspiratory peak flow, intrathoracic pressure changes, or tidal volume.[24] Physiology experiments evaluating unilateral versus bilateral stimulation effects have not been conducted in humans outside of the ongoing Genio device trials. Pacing strategy also does not seem to dramatically affect therapy outcomes. While airway cross-sectional area is generally smallest at end-expiration,[25-28] UAS devices paced to time stimulation to end-expiration have not demonstrated markedly superior performance to those using tonic stimulation or duty-cycle strategies.[17,18,20,21]

The lack of differences in outcomes may speak more to the similarities between treated populations than it does differences in UAS device design. Clinically meaningful differences in inspiratory flow and other respiratory metrics may be difficult to demonstrate due to a "ceiling" effect: The dramatic improvements in ventilation with even just unilateral stimulation in good anatomic candidates often eliminate flow limitation and restore ventilation to physiologic or near-physiologic levels.[29] Goding et al. demonstrated that unilateral stimulation restored an average of 77% of maximal possible flow in a canine model.[11] Prior feasibility study data yielded poor results in a loosely selected cohort of patients, but a highly selected cohorts of patients clinically treated with unilateral UAS achieved surgical cure (defined as AHI <5) in 70% of recipients.[15,30] Such high success rates in similar populations make it difficult to prove the superiority of alternative stimulation modalities without much larger cohorts.

## 14.3.2. UAS Patient Selection Criteria

Patient selection criteria for current-generation UAS devices are similar for important reasons. Feasibility study data for the STAR phase III trial suggested that UAS therapy responders meet anatomic criteria including BMI $\leq$32 kg/m², with an AHI <50 and lack of complete circumferential collapse at the palate during DISE.[15] These findings were derived from a post hoc analysis of 22 implanted patients, and only 7 of them underwent DISE prior to implantation. Despite the small study population size, these implant criteria have underpinned implant candidacy criteria for thousands of UAS patients since publication. Most available data come from Inspire device recipients as it is the only FDA-approved UAS device at the time of this writing.

Much effort has been focused at the request of the FDA on approval of the Inspire device in April 2014 on retrospective and concurrent analyses after approval of UAS recipients to better understand responder criteria. In a review of 584 patients implanted with the Inspire device across multiple research and clinical cohorts, Kent et al. reported that greater improvement in the postoperative AHI was associated with a higher preoperative AHI (−0.74 events per hour; 95% confidence interval [CI]: −0.82, −0.67), older patient age (−0.10 events per hour; 95% CI: −0.20, −0.00), and lower BMI (0.52; 95% CI: 0.22, 0.83).[31] The Adherence and Outcome of Upper Airway Stimulation for OSA International Registry (ADHERE registry) is a multicenter post–FDA approval database that monitors the outcomes of Inspire patients implanted as part of regular clinical care.

Heiser et al. reported post hoc associations of demographic factors with treatment success, as defined by the Sher criteria.[16,32] For each 1-year increase in age, there was a 4% increase in odds of success, and for each 1-unit increase in BMI, there was a 9% reduction in odds of success. Age was the only statistically significant predictor of treatment success in a multivariate regression analysis.

Reasons for age-related associations were therapy success are unclear. Age-associated changes decreases in hyoepiglottic ligament elasticity have been hypothesized to augment the effect of UAS in older individuals.[32,33] Phenotypic analysis of 10 young and 10 elderly patients with OSA using the PALM scale ($P_{crit}$, arousal threshold, loop gain, and muscle responsiveness) determined that older patients had a more collapsible airway (ventilation at 0 cm $H_2O$ = 3.4 ± 0.9 vs. 1.5 ± 0.7 L/min; $p$ = .05), a decreased minute ventilation on CPAP (8.2 ± 0.5 vs. 6.1 ± 0.4 L/min; $p$ < .01), and lower loop gain (5.0 ± 0.7 vs. 2.9 ± 0.5; $p$ < .05).[34] The observed increase in pharyngeal collapsibility correlates with other reports of increased pharyngeal collapsibility in the elderly.[35,36] Decreased minute ventilation suggests that end-expiratory lung volume in the elderly may be decreased (although this was not explicitly measured). Decreased end-expiratory lung volume has been associated with pharyngeal collapsibility in multiple studies due to a decline in tracheal traction effects on the pharynx.[37–41] The exact anatomic factors predisposing to collapsibility may also vary with age. Vincini et al. reported that older patients were less likely to display lateral pharyngeal wall collapse, and Green et al. reported separately that patients with lateral wall collapse were less likely to achieve successful reductions in AHI with a variety of surgical interventions.[42,43] The greater role of anatomic collapsibility in elderly patients (as opposed to nonanatomic factors, such as loop gain) may be one factor associated with greater benefit from anatomy-modifying therapies such as UAS.

Anatomic collapsibility as a greater proportion of the driving mechanism for OSA in the elderly should not be confused with a significantly greater amount of anatomic collapsibility in this age group. The available evidence still suggests that UAS as a monotherapy ultimately has a limited ability to modify pharyngeal collapsibility, which may explain the decreased efficacy observed in feasibility trials and post hoc analyses of clinical data.[15,31,32] Early animal studies confirmed that at least part of the therapeutic mechanism to UAS is a reduction in pharyngeal collapsibility.[7] However, increasing weight is associated with increasing pharyngeal collapsibility, and, by extension, a higher probability of complete concentric collapse of the palate.[44] This may be mediated by decreased airway caliber and increasing tissue pressure from peripharyngeal fat deposition, as well as reduced longitudinal traction on the pharynx due to abdominal visceral fat deposition and decreased end-expiratory lung volumes.[37,38,40,41,45] Conversely, weight loss is associated with decreased pharyngeal collapsibility.[46]

Circumferential palatal collapse likely represents increased lateral wall compliance and/or peripharyngeal tissue pressure diffusely ascending from the oropharynx to the velopharynx. The effect of UAS tongue protrusion is translated to the soft tissues of the oropharynx and velopharynx via direct mechanical traction on the soft tissues and decreased lateral tissue pressure. Increasing laxity of the lateral walls may decrease the impact and distance over which mechanical traction translates, especially as one moves farther away from the oropharyngeal tongue to the velopharynx. Nevertheless, pharyngeal fat deposition and resulting increases in peripharyngeal tissue pressure can differ between individuals with comparable BMI,[47] which may partially explain why some individuals with BMI >32 kg/m$^2$ can be successfully treated with UAS if carefully selected.[48] More severe and diffuse airway collapse has been positively associated with AHI and BMI.[44]

Ultimately, a variety of patient factors likely influence UAS candidacy and deserve further study. Research into nonanatomic physiologic mechanisms underpinning OSA continues.[49] For most patients with OSA, the BMI and lack of complete concentric collapse criteria will limit access to therapy. However, as we have shown in the preceding discussion, the anatomic properties underlying these criteria are poorly understood. The exclusion of patients with complete concentric palatal collapse across several device trials is based primarily on feasibility study DISE examination of only 7 patients.[15] AHI, BMI, and circumferential palatal collapse are all likely proxy markers for anatomic factors that respond variably to UAS, including tongue and palatal collapse severity, the degree of coupling between the palate and the tongue during protrusion, lateral wall compliance, and peripharyngeal tissue pressure. More research is needed to ascertain what criteria predict therapy success in patients with complete circumferential palatal collapse, more severe OSA, and BMI >35 kg/m$^2$.

## 14.3.3. Long-Term UAS Outcomes and Combination Therapy

Five-year outcomes of the STAR trial were published in 2018.[50] Of the original 126 patients, 97 completed the protocol and 71 completed PSG. AHI decreased from 32.0 ± 11.8 to 12.4 ± 16.3. ESS score decreased from 11.6 ± 5.0 to 7.0 ± 5.0, and FOSQ score increased from 14.3 ± 3.2 to 18.0 ± 2.2. Of the 71 patients completing PSG assessment, 75% were treatment responders, with an overall responder rate of 63% at 5 years.

Long-term PSG and subjective symptom outcomes have not been reported for other devices. Data exploring the impacts of UAS (and other surgical treatments) on diseases associated with OSA, including hypertension, myocardial infarction, and stroke, are also needed. The Cardiovascular Endpoints for Obstructive Sleep Apnea with Twelfth Nerve Stimulation (CARDIOSA-12) Trial (ClinicalTrials.gov ID: NCT03359096) is an ongoing randomized, double-blinded crossover study with an enrollment goal of 80 designed to evaluate the impact of UAS on 24-hour ambulatory and nocturnal blood pressures along with several other secondary endpoints.[51] Enrolled patients are implanted with the Inspire UAS device as part of routine clinical care. After a washout period of 1 week, patients are randomized to subtherapeutic UAS settings or therapeutic settings for 28 days followed by sympathetic and vascular testing. After a second washout week, patients are switched to the other intervention arm for another 28 days prior to final testing. Results are expected to provide insight into proxy markers of downstream cardiovascular disease risk.

There is also a growing appreciation in sleep medicine for the potential of combined medical and surgical interventions to comprehensively manage OSA in patients with only partial responses to monotherapy. Initial efforts have been made to assess the impact of prior upper airway surgery on UAS outcomes.[52–54] Nevertheless, the potential for combination with other medical treatments exists, including positional therapy, mandibular advancement devices, weight loss, and even PAP. Use of UAS with PAP or mandibular advancement devices may permit de-escalation of medical therapy intensity for patients, improving tolerance and compliance. Further work is needed to explore what therapy combinations are most tolerable and effective.

## 14.4. Beyond UAS

Modest additions to the candidate pool for UAS may be discovered in the coming years through refined phenotyping techniques, but a large population of patients with OSA (primarily those with class II and III obesity) are unlikely to benefit significantly from hypoglossal nerve monotherapy. The commonly used term "upper airway stimulation" is somewhat misleading, as the hypoglossal nerve is only one of many neuromuscular mechanisms that work to support the structure of the upper airway, coordinating tonic and phasic contraction with respiratory effort through a finely balanced network of opposing muscles forces and tension.[55–62] Future progress will likely move beyond isolated hypoglossal nerve stimulation to other support mechanisms of the upper airway.

Device-related adverse effects from UAS in currently implanted patients include tongue-related discomfort with stimulation, tongue abrasion on the teeth, and xerostomia. Forty percent of participants in the STAR trial reported discomfort with tongue stimulation alone.[17] Advancements in biophysiologic signal detection have the potential to reduce device-related discomfort in the future. Newer generations of equipment may be able to detect sleep and wake states by monitoring respiratory, heart rate, and accelerometry data, and may even be able to detect impending respiratory events by monitoring these or other data channels. Such advances would permit new devices to activate automatically on detection of the sleep state and would also permit de-escalation of stimulation intensity in scenarios such as non-supine sleep and unobstructed breathing.

Advances beyond current device modifications are under way. Medical trials are currently under way evaluating the ability of neuromodulating agents to amplify input to respiratory motor neuron groups.[63] Efferent motor nerves of the upper airway may also be controlled by modifying afferent input to respiratory and upper airway motor control centers of the central nervous system. Recent research suggests that electrical or tactile auricular stimulation or nasal insufflation has the potential to modify central respiratory control centers.[64–66] In the pharynx, stimulation of the internal branch of the superior laryngeal nerve in a canine model evoked ipsilateral genioglossus electromyographic activity, demonstrating promise for control of pharyngeal afferents.[67]

## 14.5. Conclusions

A review of the development of UAS reveals gaps in our current knowledge base regarding the physiologic mechanisms at work and patients' response to therapy. While multiple stimulation modalities have been proposed, only one is currently approved by the FDA for clinical use. Future research needs include a better understanding of the benefits and limitations to variations in device designs, including pacing strategy and the need for unilateral versus bilateral stimulation. Although not yet available for clinical use, there are new device designs currently undergoing clinical trials. Patient selection criteria continue to be refined, and research efforts are under way to better understand the long-term impacts of UAS therapy and how different therapy modalities can be combined for more effective treatment. Neuromodulating agents and neurostimulation of afferent feedback pathways from the upper airway provide promising new avenues for augmenting the effect of UAS.

## References

1. Miki H, Hida W, Shindoh C, et al. Effect of electrical stimulation of genioglossus muscle on upper airway resistance in anesthetized dogs. *Tohoku J Exp Med.* 1987;153(4):397–398. doi:10.1620/tjem.153.397

2. Miki H, Hida W, Chonan T, et al. Effects of submental electrical stimulation during sleep on upper airway patency in patients with obstructive sleep apnea. *Am Rev Respir Dis.* 1989;140(5):1285–1289. doi:10.1164/ajrccm/140.5.1285

3. Decker MJ, Haaga J, Arnold JL, et al. Functional electrical stimulation and respiration during sleep. *J Appl Physiol.* 1993;75(3):1053–1061. doi:10.1152/jappl.1993.75.3.1053

4. Eisele DW, Smith PL, Alam DS, Schwartz AR. Direct hypoglossal nerve stimulation in obstructive sleep apnea. *Arch Otolaryngol Head Neck Surg.* 1997;123(1):57–61. doi:10.1001/archotol.1997.01900010067009

5. Eisele DW, Schwartz AR, Hari A, et al. The effects of selective nerve stimulation on upper airway airflow mechanics. *Arch Otolaryngol Head Neck Surg.* 1995;121(12):1361–1364. doi:10.1001/archotol.1995.01890120021004

6. Schwartz AR, Eisele DW, Hari A, et al. Electrical stimulation of the lingual musculature in obstructive sleep apnea. *J Appl Physiol.* 1996;81(2):643–652. doi:10.1152/jappl.1996.81.2.643

7. Schwartz AR, Thut DC, Russ B, et al. Effect of electrical stimulation of the hypoglossal nerve on airflow mechanics in the isolated upper airway. *Am Rev Respir Dis.* 1993;147(5):1144–1150. doi:10.1164/ajrccm/147.5.1144

8. Guilleminault C, Powell N, Bowman B, Stoohs R. The effect of electrical stimulation on obstructive sleep apnea syndrome. *Chest.* 1995;107(1):67–73. doi:10.1378/chest.107.1.67

9. Oliven A, Odeh M, Schnall RP. Improved upper airway patency elicited by electrical stimulation of the hypoglossus nerves. *Respir Int Rev Thorac Dis.* 1996;63(4):213–216. doi:10.1159/000196547

10. Bishara H, Odeh M, Schnall RP, et al. Electrically-activated dilator muscles reduce pharyngeal resistance in anaesthetized dogs with upper airway obstruction. *Eur Respir J.* 1995:1537–1542. doi:10.1183/09031936.95.08091537

11. Goding Jr GS, Eisele DW, Testerman R, et al. Relief of upper airway obstruction with hypoglossal nerve stimulation in the canine. *Laryngoscope.* 1998;108(2):162–169. doi:10.1097/00005537-199802000-00003

12. Edmonds LC, Daniels BK, Stanson AW, et al. The effects of transcutaneous electrical stimulation during wakefulness and sleep in patients with obstructive sleep apnea. *Am Rev Respir Dis.* 1992;146(4):1030–1036. doi:10.1164/ajrccm/146.4.1030

13. Hultman E, Sjöholm H, Jäderholm-Ek I, Krynicki J. Evaluation of methods for electrical stimulation of human skeletal muscle in situ. *Pflugers Arch*. 1983;398(2):139–141. doi:10.1007/bf00581062

14. Schwartz AR, Bennett ML, Smith PL, et al. Therapeutic electrical stimulation of the hypoglossal nerve in obstructive sleep apnea. *Arch Otolaryngol Head Neck Surg*. 2001;127(10):1216–1223. doi:10.1001/archotol.127.10.1216

15. Van De Heyning PH, Badr MS, Baskin JZ, et al. Implanted upper airway stimulation device for obstructive sleep apnea. *Laryngoscope*. 2012;122(7):1626–1633. doi:10.1002/lary.23301

16. Sher AE, Schechtman KB, Piccirillo JF. The efficacy of surgical modifications of the upper airway in adults with obstructive sleep apnea syndrome. *Sleep*. 1996;19(2):156–177. doi:10.1093/sleep/19.2.156

17. Strollo PJ, Soose RJ, Maurer JT, et al. Upper-airway stimulation for obstructive sleep apnea. *N Engl J Med*. 2014;370(2):139–149. doi:10.1056/NEJMoa1308659

18. Mwenge GB, Rombaux P, Dury M, et al. Targeted hypoglossal neurostimulation for obstructive sleep apnoea: A 1-year pilot study. *Eur Respir J*. 2013;41(2):360–367. doi:10.1183/09031936.00042412

19. Zaidi FN, Meadows P, Jacobowitz O, Davidson TM. Tongue anatomy and physiology, the scientific basis for a novel targeted neurostimulation system designed for the treatment of obstructive sleep apnea. *Neuromodulation*. 2013;16(4):376–386. doi:10.1111/j.1525-1403.2012.00514.x

20. Kezirian EJ, Goding GS, Malhotra A, et al. Hypoglossal nerve stimulation improves obstructive sleep apnea: 12-month outcomes. *J Sleep Res*. 2014;23(1):77–83. doi:10.1111/jsr.12079

21. Eastwood PR, Barnes M, MacKay SG, et al. Bilateral hypoglossal nerve stimulation for treatment of adult obstructive sleep apnoea. *Eur Respir J*. 2020;55(1). doi:10.1183/13993003.01320-2019

22. Fleury Curado T, Otvos T, Klopfer T, et al. Synergistic co-activation of lingual protrusors and retractors is required to stabilize the upper airway during sleep. In *Predictors of Sleep Disordered Breathing and Response to Treatment*. American Thoracic Society International Conference Abstracts, 2018. doi:10.1164/ajrccm-conference.2018.197.1_MeetingAbstracts.A7777

23. Heiser C, Edenharter G, Bas M, et al. Palatoglossus coupling in selective upper airway stimulation. *Laryngoscope*. 2017;127(10):E378–E383. doi:10.1002/lary.26487

24. Bellemare F, Pecchiari M, Bandini M, et al. Reversibility of airflow obstruction by hypoglossus nerve stimulation in anesthetized rabbits. *Am J Respir Crit Care Med*. 2005;172(5):606–612. doi:10.1164/rccm.200502-190OC

25. Morrell MJ, Badr MS. Effects of NREM sleep on dynamic within-breath changes in upper airway patency in humans. *J Appl Physiol*. 1998;84(1):190–199. doi:10.1152/jappl.1998.84.1.190

26. Morrell MJ, Arabi Y, Zahn B, Badr MS. Progressive retropalatal narrowing preceding obstructive apnea. *Am J Respir Crit Care Med*. 1998;158(6):1974–1981. doi:10.1164/ajrccm.158.6.9712107

27. Schwab R, Gefter W, Hoffman E, et al. Dynamic upper airway imaging during awake respiration in normal subjects and patients with sleep disordered breathing. *Am Rev Respir Dis*. 1993;148(5):1385–1400. doi:10.1164/ajrccm/148.5.1385

28. Walsh JH, Leigh MS, Paduch A, et al. Evaluation of pharyngeal shape and size using anatomical optical coherence tomography in individuals with and without obstructive sleep apnoea. *J Sleep Res*. 2008;17(2):230–238. doi:10.1111/j.1365-2869.2008.00647.x

29. Schwartz AR, Barnes M, Hillman D, et al. Acute upper airway responses to hypoglossal nerve stimulation during sleep in obstructive sleep apnea. *Am J Respir Crit Care Med*. 2012;185(4):420–426. doi:10.1164/rccm.201109-1614OC

30. Kent DT, Lee JJ, Strollo PJ, Soose RJ. Upper airway stimulation for OSA: Early adherence and outcome results of one center. *Otolaryngol -Head Neck Surg*. 2016;155(1):188–193. doi:10.1177/0194599816636619

31. Kent DT, Carden KA, Wang L, et al. Evaluation of hypoglossal nerve stimulation treatment in obstructive sleep apnea. *JAMA Otolaryngol Head Neck Surg*. 2019;145(11):1044–1052. doi:10.1001/jamaoto.2019.2723

32. Heiser C, Steffen A, Boon M, et al. Post-approval upper airway stimulation predictors of treatment effectiveness in the ADHERE registry. *Eur Respir J*. 2019;53(1):1801405. doi:10.1183/13993003.01405-2018

33. Irvine LE, Yang Z, Kezirian EJ, et al. Hyoepiglottic ligament collagen and elastin fiber composition and changes associated with aging. *Laryngoscope*. 2018;128(5):1245–1248. doi:10.1002/lary.27094

34. Edwards BA, Wellman A, Sands SA, et al. Obstructive sleep apnea in older adults is a distinctly different physiological phenotype. *Sleep.* 2014;37(7):1227–1236. doi:10.5665/sleep.3844

35. Kirkness JP, Schwartz AR, Schneider H, et al. Contribution of male sex, age, and obesity to mechanical instability of the upper airway during sleep. *J Appl Physiol.* 2008;104(6):1618–1624. doi:10.1152/japplphysiol.00045.2008

36. Eikermann M, Jordan AS, Chamberlin NL, et al. The influence of aging on pharyngeal collapsibility during sleep. *Chest.* 2007;131(6):1702–1709. doi:10.1378/chest.06-2653

37. Heinzer RC, Stanchina ML, Malhotra A, et al. Lung volume and continuous positive airway pressure requirements in obstructive sleep apnea. *Am J Respir Crit Care Med.* 2005;172(1):114–117. doi:10.1164/rccm.200404-552OC

38. Hoffstein V, Zamel N, Phillipson EA. Lung volume dependence of pharyngeal cross-sectional area in patients with obstructive sleep apnea. *Am Rev Respir Dis.* 2018;130(2):175–178. doi:10.1164/arrd.1984.130.2.175

39. Joosten SA, Sands SA, Edwards BA, et al. Evaluation of the role of lung volume and airway size and shape in supine-predominant obstructive sleep apnoea patients. *Respirology.* 2015;20(5):819–827. doi:10.1111/resp.12549

40. Squier SB, Patil SP, Schneider H, et al. Effect of end-expiratory lung volume on upper airway collapsibility in sleeping men and women. *J Appl Physiol.* 2010;109(4):977–985. doi:10.1152/japplphysiol.00080.2010

41. Stadler DL, McEvoy RD, Bradley J, et al. Changes in lung volume and diaphragm muscle activity at sleep onset in obese obstructive sleep apnea patients vs. healthy-weight controls. *J Appl Physiol.* 2010;109(4):1027–1036. doi:10.1152/japplphysiol.01397.2009

42. Vicini C, De Vito A, Iannella G, et al. The aging effect on upper airways collapse of patients with obstructive sleep apnea syndrome. *Eur Arch Otorhinolaryngol.* 2018;275(12):2983–2990. doi:10.1007/s00405-018-5163-5

43. Green KK, Kent DT, D'Agostino MA, et al. Drug-induced sleep endoscopy and surgical outcomes: A multicenter cohort study. *Laryngoscope.* 2019;129(3):761–770. doi:10.1002/lary.27655

44. Vroegop AV, Vanderveken OM, Boudewyns AN, et al. Drug-induced sleep endoscopy in sleep-disordered breathing: Report on 1,249 cases. *Laryngoscope.* 2014;124(3):797–802. doi:10.1002/lary.24479

45. Catcheside PG, Ryan MK, Sprecher KE, et al. Abdominal compression increases upper airway collapsibility during sleep in obese male obstructive sleep apnea patients. *Sleep.* 2017;32(12):1579–1587. doi:10.1093/sleep/32.12.1579

46. Schwartz AR, Gold AR, Schubert N, et al. Effect of weight loss on upper airway collapsibility in obstructive sleep apnea. *Am Rev Respir Dis.* 1991;144(3 Pt 1):494–498. doi:10.1164/ajrccm/144.3_Pt_1.494

47. Kim AM, Keenan BT, Jackson N, et al. Tongue fat and its relationship to obstructive sleep apnea. *Sleep.* 2014;37(10):1639–1648. doi:10.5665/sleep.4072

48. Huntley C, Steffen A, Doghramji K, et al. Upper airway stimulation in patients with obstructive sleep apnea and an elevated body mass index: A multi-institutional review: Impact of BMI on upper airway stimulation. *Laryngoscope.* 2018;128(10):2425–2428. doi:10.1002/lary.27426

49. Eckert DJ, White DP, Jordan AS, et al. Defining phenotypic causes of obstructive sleep apnea: Identification of novel therapeutic targets. *Am J Respir Crit Care Med.* 2013;188(8):996–1004. doi:10.1164/rccm.201303-0448OC

50. Woodson BT, Strohl KP, Soose RJ, et al. Upper airway stimulation for obstructive sleep apnea: 5-year outcomes. *Otolaryngol Head Neck Surg.* 2018;159(1):194–202. doi:10.1177/0194599818762383

51. Dedhia RC, Quyyumi AA, Park J, et al. Cardiovascular endpoints for obstructive sleep apnea with twelfth cranial nerve stimulation (CARDIOSA-12): Rationale and methods. *Laryngoscope.* 2018;128(11):2635–2643. doi:10.1002/lary.27284

52. Huntley C, Vasconcellos A, Doghramji K, et al. Upper airway stimulation in patients who have undergone unsuccessful prior palate surgery: An initial evaluation. *Otolaryngol -Head Neck Surg.* 2018;159(5):938–940. doi:10.1177/0194599818792191

53. Mahmoud AF, Thaler ER. Upper airway stimulation therapy and prior airway surgery for obstructive sleep apnea. *Laryngoscope.* 2018;128(6):1486–1489. doi:10.1002/lary.26956

54. Kezirian EJ, Heiser C, Steffen A, et al. Previous surgery and hypoglossal nerve stimulation for obstructive sleep apnea. *Otolaryngol Head Neck Surg.* 2019;161(5):897–903. doi:10.1177/0194599819856339

55. Mortimore IL, Douglas NJ. Palatopharyngeus has respiratory activity and responds to negative pressure in sleep apnoeics. *Eur Respir J.* 1996;9(4):773–778. doi:10.1183/09031936.96.09040773

56. Guilleminault C, Hill MW, Simmons FB, Dement WC. Obstructive sleep apnea: Electromyographic and fiberoptic studies. *Exp Neurol.* 1978;62(1):48–67. doi:10.1016/0014-4886(78)90040-7

57. Mortimore IL, Douglas NJ. Palatal muscle EMG response to negative pressure in awake sleep apneic and control subjects. *Am J Respir Crit Care Med.* 1997;156(3 I):867–873.

58. Mathur R, Mortimore IL, Jan MA, Douglas NJ. Effect of breathing, pressure and posture on palatoglossal and genioglossal tone. *Clin Sci.* 2015;89(4):441–445. doi:10.1042/cs0890441

59. Mortimore IL, Mathur R, Douglas NJ. Effect of posture, route of respiration, and negative pressure on palatal muscle activity in humans. *J Appl Physiol.* 2017;79(2):448–454. doi:10.1152/jappl.1995.79.2.448

60. Kuna ST. Respiratory-related activation and mechanical effects of the pharyngeal constrictor muscles. *Respir Physiol.* 2000;19:155–161. doi:10.1016/S0034-5687(99)00110-3

61. Roberts JL, Reed WR, Thach BT. Pharyngeal airway-stabilizing function of sternohyoid and sternothyroid muscles in the rabbit. *J Appl Physiol.* 1984;57(6):1790–1795. doi:10.1152/jappl.1984.57.6.1790

62. Tachikawa S, Nakayama K, Nakamura S, et al. Coordinated respiratory motor activity in nerves innervating the upper airway muscles in rats. *PLoS One.* 2016;11(11):e0166436. doi:10.1371/journal.pone.0166436

63. Taranto-Montemurro L, Messineo L, Sands SA, et al. The combination of atomoxetine and oxybutynin greatly reduces obstructive sleep apnea severity: A randomized, placebo-controlled, double-blind crossover trial. *Am J Respir Crit Care Med.* 2019;199(10):1267–1276. doi:10.1164/rccm.201808-1493OC

64. Donic V, Tomori Z, Gresova S, et al. Treatment of sleep apnea syndrome by electrical auricle stimulation using miniaturized system of second generation. *Sleep Med.* 2017;40:e80–e81.

65. Sowho MO, Woods MJ, Biselli P, et al. Nasal insufflation treatment adherence in obstructive sleep apnea. *Sleep Breath.* 2015;19(1):351–357.

66. Hernández AI, Pérez D, Feuerstein D, et al. Kinesthetic stimulation for obstructive sleep apnea syndrome: An "on-off" proof of concept trial. *Sci Rep.* 2018;8(1):1–7. doi:10.1038/s41598-018-21430-w

67. Maurer JT, Perkins J. Innovative neuromodulation concepts for the treatment of obstructive sleep apnea. *Laryngorhinootologie.* 2019;98(S 02):S189–S190. doi:10.1055/s-0039-1686800

# Index

*For the benefit of digital users, indexed terms that span two pages (e.g., 52–53) may, on occasion, appear on only one of those pages.*

Tables, figures and boxes are indicated by *t, f* and *b* following the page number